PRACTICAL
PHYSIOLOGY

Other important CBS books in physiology

PRACTICAL PHYSIOLOGY

RAJ KAPOOR MD

Professor
Department of Physiology
Vardhman Mahavir Medical College and
Safdarjung Hospital
New Delhi, India

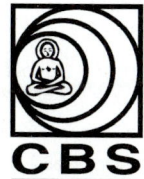

CBS

CBS Publishers & Distributors Pvt Ltd

New Delhi • Bengaluru • Pune • Kochi • Chennai

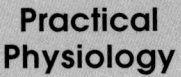 **Practical Physiology**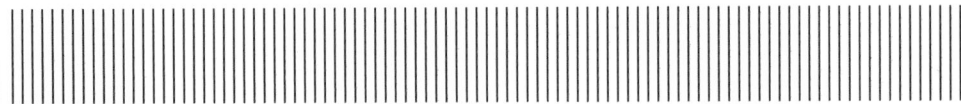

ISBN: 978-81-239-1861-7

First Edition: 2010
Reprint: 2011, 2015

Published by Satish Kumar Jain and produced by Vinod K. Jain for
CBS Publishers & Distributors Pvt Ltd
4819/XI Prahlad Street, 24 Ansari Road, Daryaganj,
New Delhi 110 002, India.
Ph: 23289259, 23266861/67   Fax: 011-23243014

Website: www.cbspd.com
e-mail: delhi@cbspd.com
cbspubs@vsnl.com
cbspubs@airtelmail.in

Branches

• Bengaluru: Seema House 2975, 17th Cross, K.R. Road,
  Banasankari 2nd Stage, Bengaluru 560 070, Karnataka
  Ph: 26771678/79   Fax: 080-26771680   e-mail: bangalore@cbspd.com

• Pune: Shaan Brahmha Complex, 631/632 Basement, Appa Balwant Chowk,
  Budhwar Peth, next to Ratan Talkies, Pune 411 002, Maharashtra
  Ph: 020-24464057/58   Fax: 020-24464059   e-mail: pune@cbspd.com

• Kochi: 36/14 Kalluvilakam, Lissie Hospital Road, Kochi 682 018, Kerala
  Ph: 0484-4059061-65   Fax: 0484-4059065   e-mail: cochin@cbspd.com

• Chennai: 20, West Park Road, Shenoy Nagar, Chennai 600 030, TN
  Ph: 044-26260666, 26208620   Fax: 044-45530020   email: chennai@cbspd.com

Printed at: Paras Offset Pvt. Ltd., C-176, Naraina Industrial Area Phase-I, New Delhi

to

---

my parents
Late Shri Yad Ram and Smt Lachho Devi

my wife
Mrs Rajni Bala

and

my respected teachers

Preface

The main objectives which were kept in mind at the time of writing this practical book are as follows.

- It is prepared as per the new curriculum of MCI for First Prof MBBS students.
- To give more importance to non-invasive human experiments.
- To give the quantity and quality of practical knowledge which really an undergraduate student requires.
- To provide them ideal graphs so that they can analyse them and can apply their theoretical knowledge to understand them.
- To give them almost all the typical records of animal experiments so that unnecessary killing of animals can be avoided.
- To use the advanced scientific equipment in conducting various experiments and clinical tests, however, photographs of the various equipment which were used previously have also been incorporated in the book.
- Photographs showing eliciting of the various tests in clinical examination have been incorporated in this book.
- Experiments for postgraduate students have also been incorporated.

The duration of the first professional MBBS has been decreased from one and a half to one year for the last few years. There is increase in the syllabus because as more research is taking place in the basic sciences and clinical field. Day-by-day advance investigations are coming in the medical field to study the functions of various organs and systems required in making the diagnosis. Because of both the reasons there is a lot of stress of study on the medical students. Can we decrease some amount of workload on the students without affecting their knowledge of basic aspects of clinical studies? In this book I have tried my best to keep the balance between the practical workload on the medical student and knowledge required by them. More attention has been given to the clinical physiology as compared to animal experiments. Various photographs have been incorporated showing eliciting of the various tendon jerks and other clinical tests so that students can easily learn the clinical examination of the patient. These photographs will be helpful in improving the clinical skill of medical students.

We should have kind attitude towards the experimental animals rather than sacrificing the animals unnecessarily. We should use the good and typical previous experimental records for study purposes. Here in the manual I have given the copies of typical graphs recorded by myself in my postgraduation training at PGIMS, Rohtak, and during my senior residency at Lady Hardinge Medical College, New Delhi. The graphs which are not available in original have been drawn by me keeping in view of the scientific accuracy. At the end of the UG experiments, PG practicals are given. The graphs given in the PG practicals can also be used to teach the UG students to understand the physiological bases of body functions. I have also gone through the practical manuals of different medical colleges before writing this book. The various practical books consulted before writing this book for clarification of various doubts are Wintrobe's Clinical Haematology, de Gruchy's Haematology, Practical Physiology by VG Ranade, Practical Physiology by CL Ghai, Hutchinson's Clinical Methods, Experimental Physiology by BL Andrews, Experimental Physiology by DT Harris, and Fundamental of Experimental Pharmacology by MN Ghosh.

Some important *viva voce* questions have been given at the end of each experiment. No answer is given with them so that student will try to use his theoretical knowledge to find out the answers. However, the answers of certain questions which are supposed to be difficult or not easily available have been given along with the questions.

I am thankful to my respected teachers Dr (Mrs) KK Mahajan, who has been the Professor and Head Department of Physiology, PGMS, Rohtak, and at Himalayan Institute of Medical Sciences, Dehradoon; Dr RK Marya, Professor, Department of Physiology (currently teaching in Malaysia), Dr (Mrs) Sushma Sood, Professor and Head, Department of Physiology, PGMS, Rohtak; Dr (Mrs) Indu Khurana, Professor, Department of Physiology, and all other teachers who were working there at the time of my postgraduation at Medical College, Rohtak. The training given to me in Medical College really brought me at the stage of writing this practical book with so much confidence.

I am sincerely thankful to Dr (Mrs) Asha Gandhi, Professor and Head, Department of Physiology, Lady Hardinge Medical College, New Delhi, for her constant encouragement to me to write the practical book. She appreciated my practical skills which was a real encouraging force behind me to write this book.

I am grateful to Dr (Mrs) Shobha Dass, Director-Professor and Head, Department of Physiology, Vardhman Mahavir Medical College, New Delhi, for her valuable suggestions and encouragement to write this practical book.

I am highly thankful to Mr GK Meena, medical student, who offered himself as a volunteer to be the subject to elicit various tendon reflexes. This is his greatness that he came forward for this purpose.

I am thankful to Late Shri BR Sharma and the team of CBS Publishers & Distributors for their effort to make this practical physiology book for undergraduate students. I am also thankful to Mr Chand S Naagar and Nishi Verma of Limited Colors for their effort to improve the quality of diagrams, graphs, and page layout.

My thanks are also due to my daughter Miss Chandni, a physiotherapist, for drawing the diagrams of blood cells (colour plate) under my supervision and for her help at various stages of writing this book.

I am also thankful to my wife Mrs Rajni Bala for her help in writing the book, because of her cooperation I was able to spare the time for writing this book.

In spite of the great care taken by me and the editorial team of publishers, some errors may have escaped our notice. I shall appreciate if these errors are brought to my notice and I will definitely try to rectify them. The suggestions and comments of the readers in improving the book are always welcome!

Raj Kapoor

Contents

Section 3: HUMAN EXPERIMENTS

Section 4: MAMMALIAN EXPERIMENTS

(For Postgraduate Students)

General Instructions to Students

I. General Guidelines

1. Read the instructions carefully regarding the objectives of the experiment and means available to carry it out.
2. Acquaint yourself thoroughly with the apparatus and if not satisfied take the help of your table teacher.
3. Never undertake anything without understanding why you are doing it. If there is any doubt, take the help of your tutor.
4. When you have obtained and analyzed your results, you are in a position to discuss them. If your result differs from the others, do not accept the conclusion that your result is wrong. Review what you have done carefully and if you cannot find technical error, submit your result for discussion to your tutor.
5. Summarize your result as briefly and concisely as possible in your practical file/manual.

II. Guidelines for Laboratory Procedures

1. Check the laboratory schedule at least one day in advance. Read the assigned experiment and bring the certain instruments required in the experiment, e.g. disposable injection needle 24 gauge, pen torch, stethoscope, tuning fork, and dissection box containing pithing needle, scalpel, scissors, and forceps.
2. Student must wear white overall in the laboratory.
3. Student must bring the practical manual for the practical class in the lab.
4. Some experiments are supposed to be performed by the students while others are demonstrated by the teacher only.
5. Equipment required for each day's experiment may be checked out at the distribution table. At the completion of experiment or termination of laboratory period, all the equipment must be returned in the same condition as when they were received.
6. During laboratory period confine your conversation to the subject of the experiment and while talking use a moderate tone. A quiet laboratory is conducive to good results.
7. Maintain neatness all the time during the experiment. All cotton, gauze, or paper, whether dry or wet, must be put in the wastebin.
8. Before leaving the laboratory get your observations checked by your table teacher. All the equipment must be left in the proper order and all the switches should be turned off. The table top should be cleaned.

9. The student should take his/her own record; if the student is not able to take the record because of some unavoidable reason, he/she should draw the expected record in the manual and analyze it.

III. Guidelines to Write the Records

1. Every student has to maintain a record of the experiment performed and the demonstration attended.
2. Record should be maintained as follows:
    (i) Neat and clean well-labelled diagram, if any, or to paste the record or graph in the manual.
    (ii) Observations and calculations.
    (iii) Result and discussion.
    (iv) Write the answers of the questions given at the end of each experiment.
3. The practical records should be checked by the allotted teacher at regular time intervals.

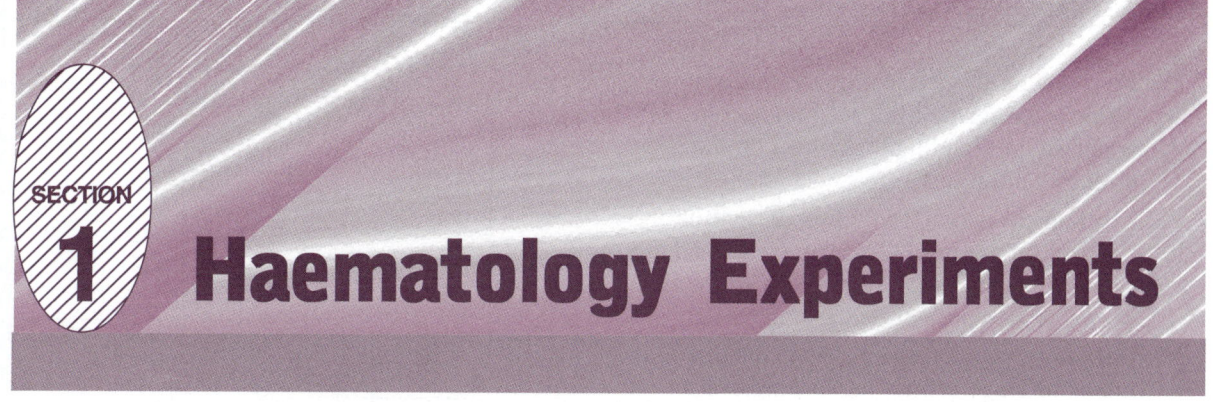

Haematology Experiments

To study the compound microscope and observe common interfering objects under low power and high power

APPARATUS

A compound microscope, glass slide, cover slip, sand, milk, wool thread, cotton fibres, hair and starch granules (crushed potato).

Compound Microscope

Microscope was invented by Antoni van Leeuwenhoek. Various parts of the microscope (Fig. 1.1.1) are as follows:

1. **Base:** Horseshoe-shaped base which provides stability to the microscope.
2. **Limb:** It joins the base to the optical part of the microscope by hinge joint.
3. **Handle:** It is a curved part which joins body tube to the stage of microscope.
4. **Body tubes:** Outer vehicle tube is attached with the handle. It can be moved up and down by coarse and fine adjustment screws, present on the upper part of the handle. Upper end of the inner tube has eyepiece of ten times (10×) magnification lens. Lower end of outer tube has revolving nose piece which contains three objective lenses with low power (10×), high power (40 or 45×) and oil immersion lens (100×).

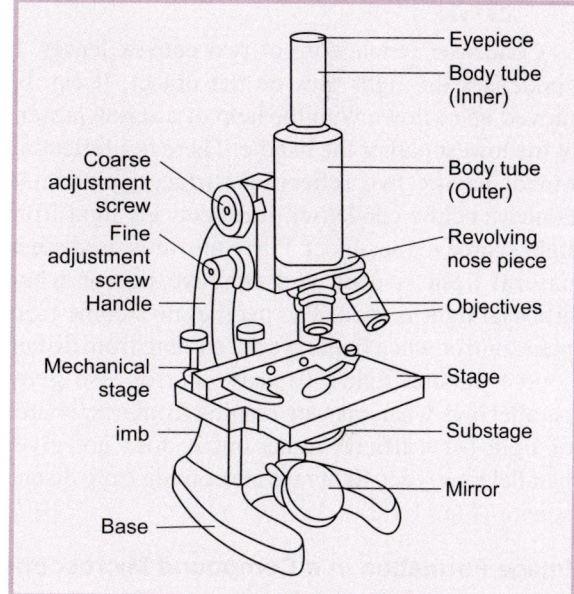

Fig. 1.1.1: Compound microscope.

Identification of objectives: Each objective marked with its magnifying power that is 10×, 40×, 45× and oil.

Magnification by using various objectives:

Total magnification = Magnification by eyepiece × magnification by objective

(i) Low power (10×): $10 \times 10 = 100$ times
(ii) High power (45×): $10 \times 45 = 450$ times
(iii) Oil immersion lens (100×): $10 \times 100 = 1000$ times

1

5. **Fixed stage:** It is a fixed square platform with a hole in the centre. Slide or counting chamber is placed on it and light rays fall on the slide through central hole.

6. **Mechanical stage:** Two clips present on the fixed stage, are used to shift the slide side to side and backward and forward with the help of two screws present on the stage.

7. **Substage:** Under the fixed stage there is movable stage which has a diagram and a condenser. Aperture size of the diaphragm can be adjusted with the help of a knob present on its side.

Condenser is made up of two convex lenses. It condenses the light rays on the object. It can be moved up or down with the help of a screw present at the lowest part of the handle. There is a reflecting mirror having two reflecting surfaces, plane and concave below condenser. It reflects the light from light source to the object. Plane mirror is used when natural light is used and concave mirror when artificial light is used. The parallel rays come from plane mirror when light rays are coming from distant source (natural light). Concave mirror also gives parallel rays when rays are coming from near source of light (or artificial light) but it does not gives parallel rays when light rays are coming from distant source (Fig. 1.1.2).

Image Formation in a Compound Microscope

(i) Objective forms real, inverted and enlarged image.

(ii) Eyepiece forms virtual, erect and enlarged image (Fig.1.1.3).

Adjustment of Intensity of Illumination

General Principle

When we use low power (10×) objective, a large area of field is visualized, a so we need less illumination. When oil immersion lens (100×) is used, very small area of the field is visualized, requiring highest illumination so that sufficient light reaches up to the eyepiece (Fig. 1.1.4).

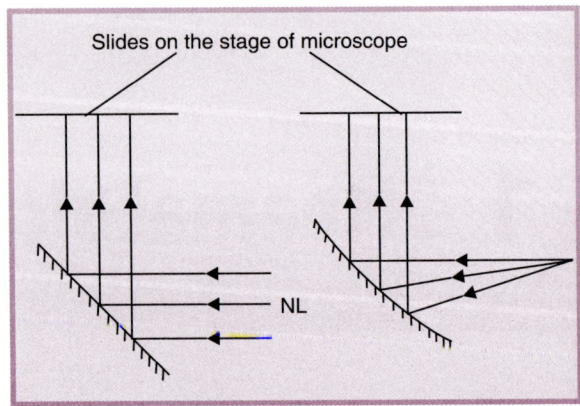

Slides on the stage of microscope

NL

Fig. 1.1.2: Reflection of light rays from plane mirror and concave mirror of a compound microscope when the source of light is natural (NL) or artificial (AL).

Means to increase the intensity of illumination:

1. Aperture size of diaphragm

   Small size—less illumination

   Big size—more illumination

2. Position of condenser

   Lowest position—minimum illumination

   Highest position—maximum illumination

3. Type of reflecting mirror

   Plane mirror—less illumination

   Concave mirror—more illumination

Use of Cedar Wood Oil or Liquid Paraffin in Oil Immersion Objective

Refractory index of cedar wood oil or liquid paraffin is equal to that of glass, it prevents the divergence (spreadingout) of light rays and the image formed will be more clear when we use it with oil immersion lens (Fig. 1.1.5).

Binocular compound microscope (Fig. 1.1.6).

• Two eyepieces are there in the microscope.

• No reflecting mirror

• Inbuilt light source

• *At the time of focusing stage move up or down not the body tube holding eyepiece.*

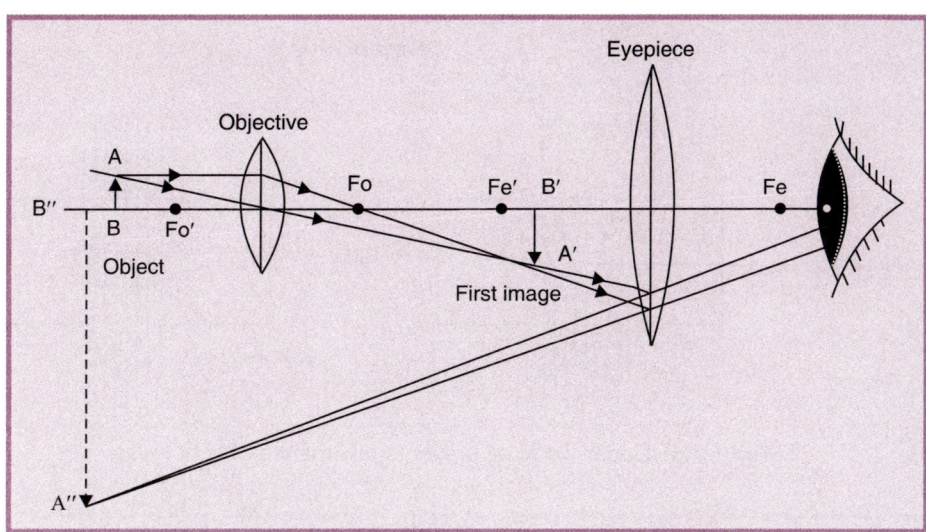

Fig. 1.1.3: Image formation in a compound microscope.

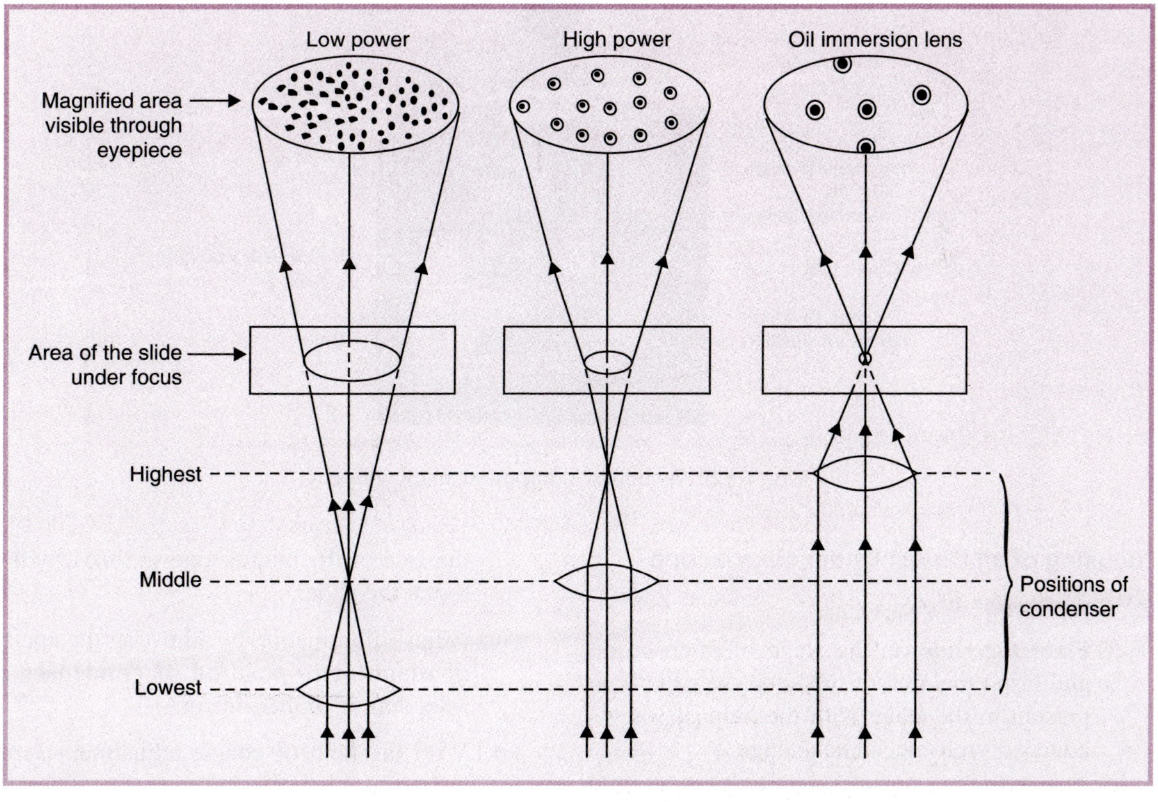

Fig. 1.1.4: Position of condensers in relation to examination of slide under various objectives of a compound microscope.

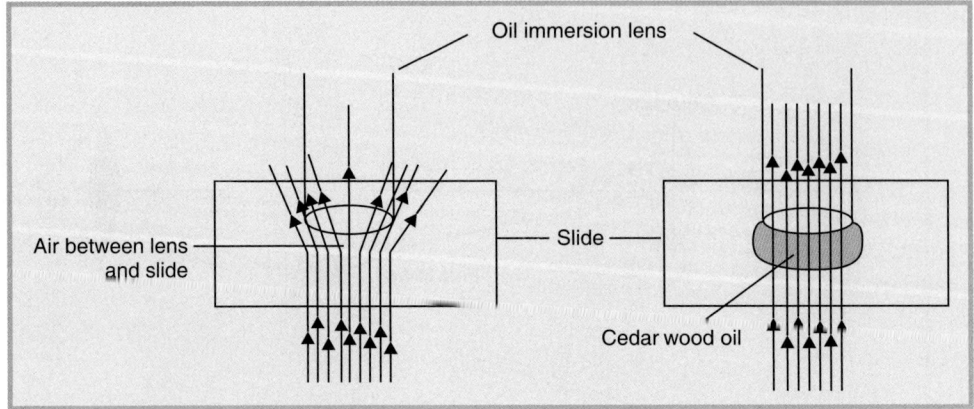

Fig. 1.1.5: Cedar wood oil prevents divergence of light rays.

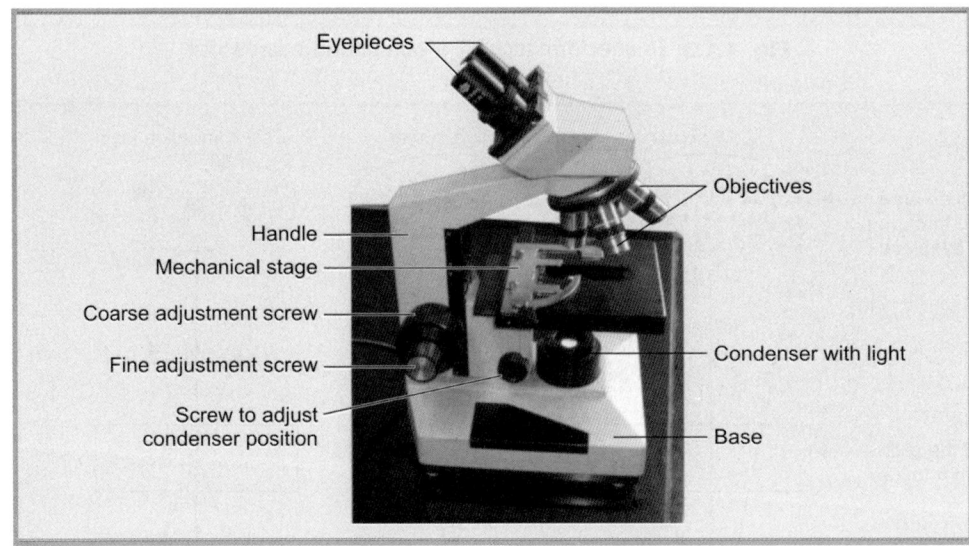

Fig. 1.1.6: Binocular compound microscope.

Focusing of an Object Under Microscope

(a) Low Power

(i) Place the slide on the stage of microscope and bring the area of the slide over the hole present in the stage with the help of screws attached with mechanical stage.

(ii) Then bring low power objective over the slide and adjust its position a few mm above the slide. During this process constantly look from the side of the microscope so that it will not touch the slide.

(iii) Adjust illumination by adjusting the aperture of diaphragm, position of condenser and selection of proper mirror.

(iv) With the help of coarse adjustment screws move the objective up and simultaneously look into the microscope till the object is visualized.

(v) Now with the help of fine adjustment screw further focus the object till it becomes clearly visible.

(b) High Power

(i) First focus the object under low power.

(ii) Turn the nose piece and bring high power objective over the slide.

(iii) Adjust the fine adjustment screw till view becomes clear.

(iv) Adjust the illumination so that object becomes very clear.

(c) Oil Immersion Lens

(i) Put a drop of cedar wood oil after placing the slide on the stage just over the area which has to be focused.

(ii) Dip the oil immersion lens very carefully with the help of coarse adjustment screw by constantly looking from the side of microscope so that it will just dip in the oil without touching the slide.

(iii) Do fine focusing with the help of fine adjustment screw by raising the objective till its view becomes very clear.

(iv) Illumination is adjusted to the maximum by all the ways discussed (fully open diaphragm and highest position of condenser).

Precautions

1. Eyepiece and objective of the microscope must be clean.

2. Do not use dry cotton to clean the lens. Xylene with soft cloth should be used for this purpose.

3. Do not use spirit to clean lenses since it may dissolve the fixing material of the lens.

4. Do not lower the objective grossly without looking from the side of the microscope.

5. Always keep the microscope vertical at the time of shifting it from one place to the other.

Focusing

Focus all the objects first in low power and then under high power as follows.

1. Sand (Dust) Particles

Place a little quantity of sand mixed in water on the slide and put a coverslip on it and examine. Translucent and opaque particles of different shapes and sizes are seen.

2. Air Bubble

Put a drop of distilled water on the slide and place a coverslip over it, in such a way that it will have air bubbles.

Air bubbles are clear spaces with dark boundaries because of refraction from the boundaries of air bubble (Fig. 1.1.7).

3. Fat Globule

Take a drop of milk on the slide and put a coverslip. Fat globules are seen as circular objects having fine clear boundary.

4. Wool Fibres

Place wool fibres on a drop of water on the slide and put a coverslip over it and examine under microscope.

These fibres are translucent having no twists.

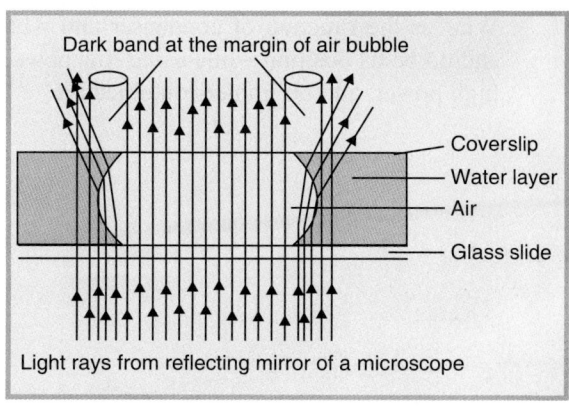

Fig. 1.1.7: Appearance of boundaries of air bubble under oil immersion lens.

5. Cotton Fibres

Put some cotton fibres in a water drop on glass slide, cover it with coverslip and examine under microscope.

These are translucent fibres having twists (oblique marking) at various sites.

6. Human Hair

Place some hair on a slide, cover it with coverslip and examine.

These are dark coloured objects some time lighter in the centre and darker in periphery (cortex and medulla).

7. Starch Particles

(i) **Unstained:** Take a drop of mixture of crushed potato in water on a slide and put a coverslip on it. Examine under microscope.

Starch particles are pear-shaped objects with concentric rings and pointed hilus on one side.

(ii) **Stained:** Add a drop of iodine solution to starch particles and examine under microscope.

Particles appear blue in colour having concentric rings and pointed hilus on one side.

Objectives of the Experiment

At the end of the class students should be able to

1. Identity different parts of microscope with their functions.
2. Tell total magnification under low power, high power, and oil immersion objectives.
3. Focus the objects under low power, high power, and oil immersion objectives.
4. To identity the various common interfering objects in the slide.

QUESTIONS AND ANSWERS

1. How will you identity the various objectives?
2. What is the role of cedar wood oil/liquid paraffin in oil immersion lens?

Ans. Cedar wood oil has the same refractory index as that of glass so it prevents the divergence of light rays coming from the slide and makes the view more clear.

3. What is the function of condenser and what should be its position while using low power, high power, and oil immersion objective?

4. What are various types of surfaces of the mirror present in the microscope and in which situation they are used?
5. What type of image do you observe in the microscope?
6. Why is the boundary of air bubble darker?

Ans. Light rays coming from the boundaries of air bubble divert their path and because of deficiency of light in this region they look dark.

EXPERIMENT 1.2

To study haemocytometer and to collect blood sample

A. HAEMOCYTOMETER

Haemocytometer is an apparatus used to do count of various blood cells (RBC, WBC, eosinophil, and platelets). It consists of RBC, and WBC pipette and a thick slide (Neubauer's chamber).

1. RBC Pipette

(i) This consists of a glass stem having capillary tube in it which opens in a bulb containing red bead and opposite to the bulb again there is a small stem. This small stem is connected to the red coloured mouth piece with the help of a rubber tube (Fig. 1.2.1).

(ii) The stem has three markings, 0.5, 1.0 and 101. From the tip of the pipette to the marking 1.0 there are 10 equal divisions. These are simple divisions not any specific unit like: mm, ml, and cu.mm.

(iii) The stem has the capacity of one part and bulb has 100 parts.

(iv) Bead of the pipette serves two purposes one mixing of the blood with diluting fluid and

other act as an identification mark of RBC pipette.

2. WBC Pipette

This pipette is similar in shape except size of bulb is smaller, markings are 0.5, 1.0 and 11, and bulb contains white bead and colour of the mouthpiece is white (Fig. 1.2.2).

3. Neubauer's Chamber (Counting Chamber)

(i) This is a thick glass slide having central platform divided into two positions with the help of H-shape groove or trench (Fig.1.2.3).

(ii) On both the sides of lateral groove there are raised ridges of a height of 0.1 mm (1/10 mm) from the central platform. When a coverslip is placed on the ridges, a space of 0.1 mm height is created below the coverslip on the central platform.

(iii) Counting chamber (Grid) is made up of ruled area of 3 mm × 3 mm size on each central platform (Fig.1.2.4). Each central area is further divided by triple lines into 9 squares of equal size (1 square mm each).

(iv) Four corner squares are further divided into 16 squares of equal size. These four corner squares are used to do total leucocytic count (TLC).

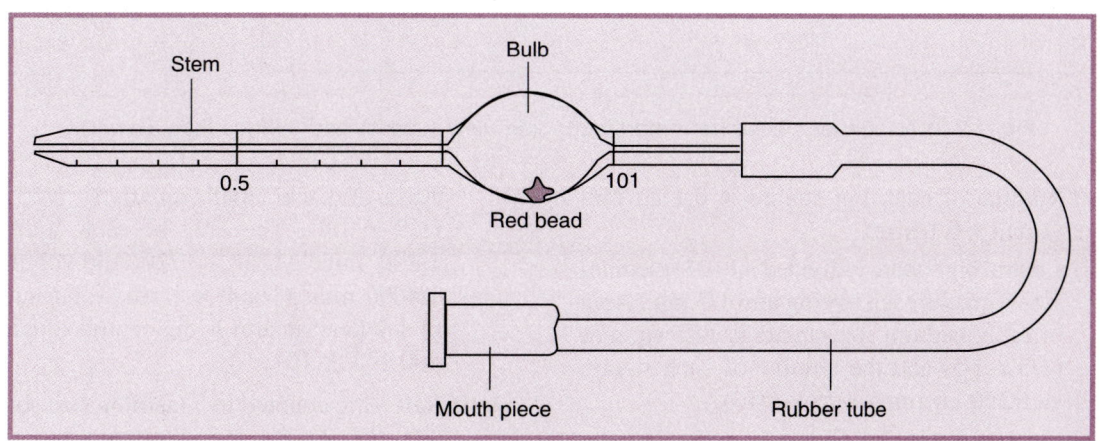

Fig. 1.2.1: RBC pipette.

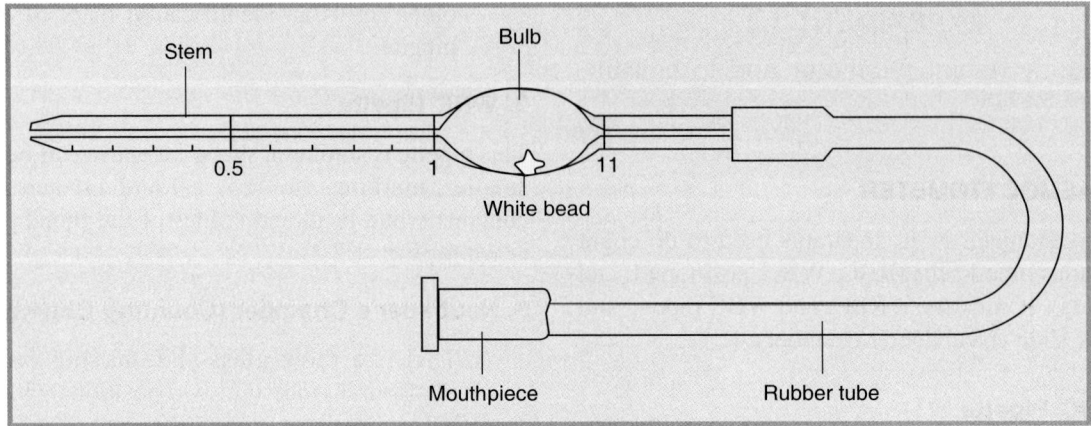

Fig. 1.2.2: WBC pipette.

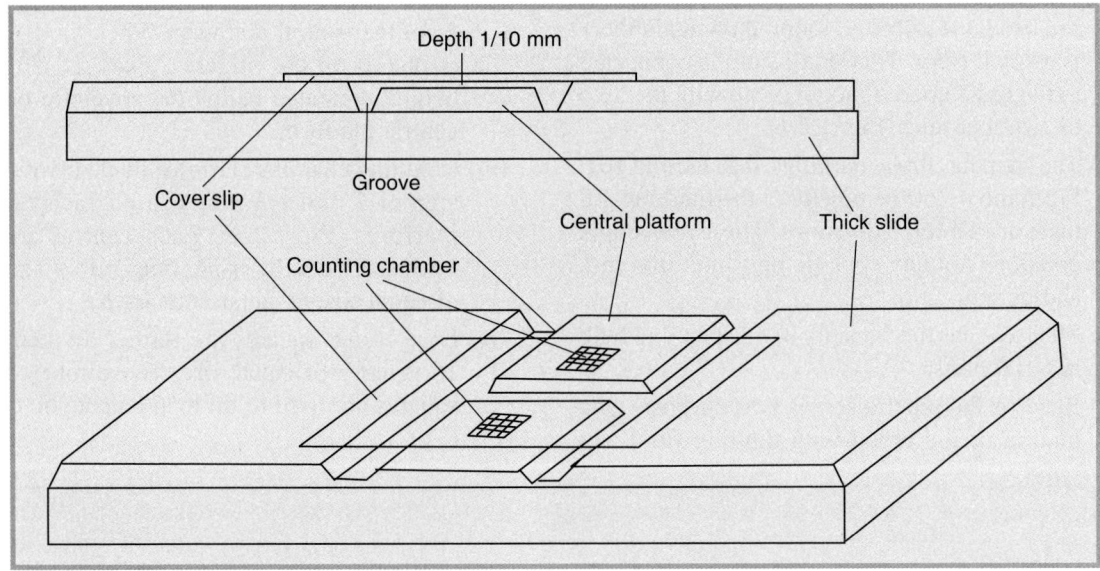

Fig. 1.2.3: Neubauer's chamber (improved), side view (upper) and surface view (lower).

(v) Volume of each big square is 0.1 cu mm (1 mm × 0.1 mm).

(vi) Central big square is divided into 25 (medium size) squares each having arm 1/5 mm. Area of each medium size square is 1/25 sq. mm (1/5 × 1/5) and the volume of each square is 1/250 cu mm (1/25 × 1/10).

(vii) Further these medium size squares are divided into 16 small squares of equal size.

Area of each small square is 1/20 mm (1/5 × 1/4). The area of each square is 1/400 mm² (1/20 × 1/20) an volume is 1/4000 mm³ (1/400 × 1/10). Total number of smallest squares is big central square are 400 (25 × 16).

(viii) RBCs are counted in 5 medium size squares (R1, R2, R3, R4, R5), four corners and one central.

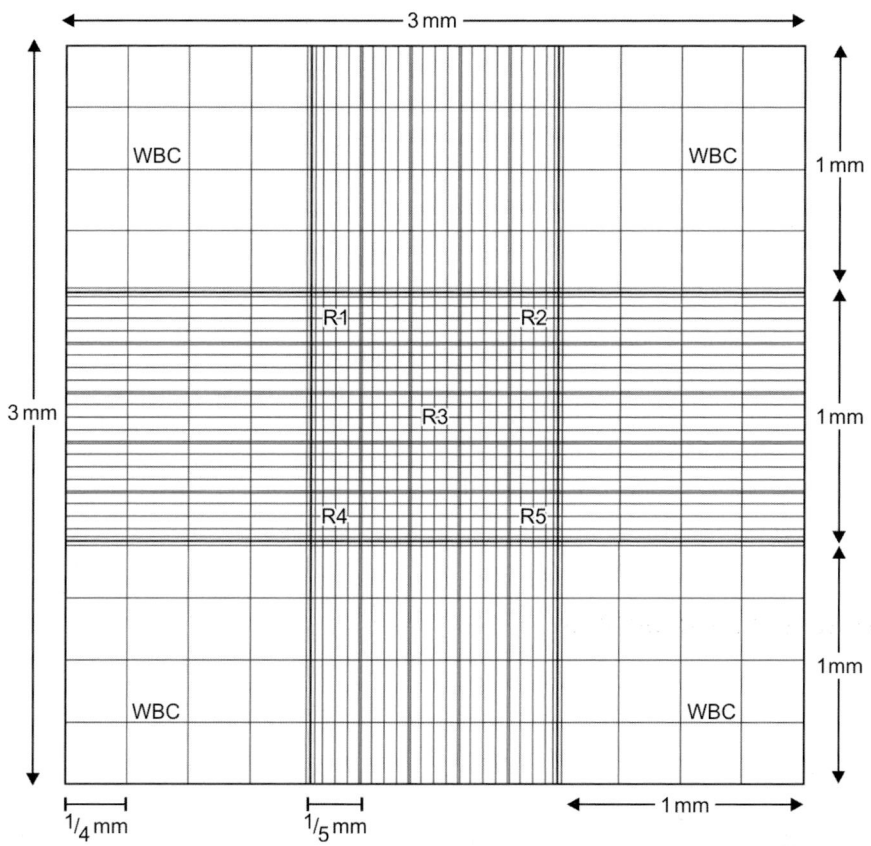

Fig. 1.2.4: Counting chamber (Neubauer's chamber) under low power of a compound microscope.

Use of Counting Chamber

RBC chamber

RBC, Platelet and reticulocyte count.

WBC chamber

WBC and Eosinophils count.

Procedure

  (i) Clean the Neubauer's chamber in soap solution and let it dry.

 (ii) Place it on the stage of microscope and focus counting chamber in low power and study all the squares carefully.

(iii) Turn the nose piece of microscope and focus the chamber under high power. Study all the squares carefully.

Charging of Chamber

This involves introducing diluted blood in Neubauer's chamber below coverslip.

Remove the chamber from the stage of the microscope and place a coverslip over the chamber. Now take coloured solution (eosin in water) in the RBC pipette and touch the tip of pipette near the edge of the coverslip on central platform at an angle of about 45 degrees. As the fluid enters below the coverslip because of capillary action, immediately remove the pipette.

Precautions

  1. Chamber should be clean, dry, and grease free.

  2. There should not be overcharging (flow of

fluid in side trenches) or under charging (incomplete filling of the chamber).

3. Do not hold the coverslip from its flat side (it will leave fingerprints), hold it from the edges.

4. If over changing is there wash the chamber and recharge.

Objectives

At the end of the class student should be able to:

1. identity RBC and WBC pipette;

2. identity the various squares of Neubauer's chamber;

3. tell the size and volume of big, medium, and small squares;

4. charge the Neubauer's chamber.

B. COLLECTION OF BLOOD SAMPLE

Blood is collected for various haematological investigations.

Capillary Blood

(i) It can be collected from fingertip and ear lobule in adult and heal in case of newborn or infant.

(ii) Take 20–24 gauge sterilised disposable hypodermic needle for this purpose.

(iii) Clean ring finger of left hand (preferably ring finger) with spirit swab and left it dry. Sterilisation is effective when spirit dries up and spirit causes haemolysis when it comes in contact with blood.

(iv) Give 2–3 mm deep prick at centre of the tip of ring finger so that free flow of blood will be there.

(v) After collection of blood sample put a spirit swab at pricking site and hold it there for 2–3 minutes (till bleeding stops).

(vi) Do not squeeze the finger for collection of blood, it will cause dilution of blood because tissue fluid mixes with blood.

Venous Blood

(i) Take 5 ml disposable syringe with 19–20 gauge needle.

(ii) Support the arm of the subject on the edge of the table and locate the vein in antecubital fossa (area).

(iii) Clean the area with spirit swab and let it dry. Do not touch the area again with finger once it is cleaned.

(iv) Apply rubber or cloth tourniquet firmly around the arm to occlude venous return. Ask the subject to close and open the fist repeatedly so as vein gets engorged with blood.

(v) Place the thumb of your left hand on the skin about 4–5 cm distal to the vein to be pricked so that vein will not slip.

(vi) Introduce the needle into the skin and push the needle on the side of vein, when needle enters the vein resistance felt to cease.

(vii) Draw the blood in syringe slowly to the required quantity (slowly means not faster than the filling of vein).

(viii) Release the tourniquet and withdraw the needle after putting the fresh spirit swab at the site of the puncture of skin.

(ix) Ask the subject to press the swab at the site of puncture for 2–3 minutes (till bleeding stops).

(x) Eject the blood from the syringe after removing needle in the vial having anti-coagulant. For serum no anticoagulant is required in the vial.

Anticoagulant Used

1. Ethylenediamine tetra-acetic acid (EDTA):
   - Calcium chelating agent
   - No effect on blood cells
   - 2.4 mg dry powder in a vial for 2 ml of blood. (1.2 mg/ml of blood)
   - Used for ESR and PCV measurement.

2. Sodium citrate:
   - Calcium chelating agent
   - 0.4 ml of 3.8% solution for 1.6 ml of blood
   - Used for ESR and collection of blood from donors
3. Double oxalate mixture:
   - Potassium oxalate and ammonium oxalate in the ratio of 2:3.
   - Single oxalate is not used mainly to measure PCV. Because potassium oxalate causes shrinkage of cells and ammonium oxalate causes increase in volume of the cells.
4. Heparin:
   - Solution or powder may be used according to need.
   - Does not affect cell volume.

Precautions

1. Must not interchange the pricking needle.
2. Preferably use a needle for pricking once.
3. If necessary to reuse the needle in the same subject, sterilise it on spirit lamp (as spirit does not kill hepatitis virus).
4. Do not use single oxalate anticoagulant for measuring PCV.
5. Destroy the needle before disposing it off.

Objectives

At the end of the class students should be able to:
 (i) Collect blood sample.
 (ii) Tell the names of common anticoagulants used and their mechanism of action.

QUESTIONS AND ANSWERS

1. Why ring finger of left hand is preferred for pricking?
Ans. Because palmar fascia from the palm does not extends up to ring finger. So there are no chances of spread of infection if occurs during pricking. Other reason is the ring finger of left hand comes in contact least as compared to the other fingers of same hand or of the opposite during working, so chances of pain and infections are less.
2. How will you sterilise a pricking needle?
3. Why should we not squeeze the finger for taking the blood?
4. How will you differentiate between RBC and WBC pipette.
5. What is mechanisms of action of different anticoagulant?
6. What measures will you take to prevent the haemolysis at the time of collection of blood?
Ans. Haemolysis can be prevented by:
 (i) Using the clean vial to collect the sample.
 (ii) Taking the sample by wide-gauze needle (No. 24 or less).
 (iii) Withdrawing the blood slowly from the vein.
 (iv) Delivering the blood gently after removing the needle from the syringe in the vial.

EXPERIMENT 1.3

Determination of red blood cell (RBC) count

APPARATUS

Neubauer's chamber (thick slide), RBC pipette, diluting fluid, microscope, coverslip, pricking needle, and spirit swab.

RBC Diluting Fluid (Hayem's Fluid)

1. *Sodium chloride* (NaCl): 0.5 gm, to maintain isotonicity of fluid
2. *Sodium sulphate* (Na_2SO_4): 2.5 gm, which prevent rouleaux formation.
3. *Mercuric chloride* ($HgCl_2$): 0.25 gm, act as preservative (antibacterial and antifungal)
4. *Distilled water* (H_2O): 100 ml.

PRINCIPLE

Red blood cells are counted in diluted blood and actual count is calculated by multiplying by dilution factors.

PROCEDURE

1. Take about 3–5 ml Hayem's fluid in a watch glass.
2. Prick the ring finger after cleaning it with spirit swab.
3. Wipe off the first drop of blood. Suck the next drop in RBC pipette exactly up to 0.5 mark, taking care that there should be no air bubble. If excess blood has been drawn, remove it by touching the pipette on the cotton swab very carefully.
4. Wipe off the blood sticking around the tip of the pipette with cotton swab.
5. Now suck the Hayem's fluid in the pipette up to mark 101.
6. The pipette is then kept horizontally between palms and rolled gently for a minute to mix the blood with diluting fluid.

7. Focus Neubauer's chamber under low power (10×) objective of microscope.
8. Remove the chamber from microscope and place a coverslip on it.
9. Discard first 2–3 drops of fluid from the pipette which is unmixed fluid present in the stem of the pipette.
10. Charge the Neubauer's chamber:
    (i) Small drop of fluid is allowed to form at the tip of the pipette.
    (ii) Bring the tip of the pipette near the edge of the coverslip on central platform in such a way that it will make an angle of about 45° with central platform.
    (iii) Fluid will be drawn in capillary space below the coverslip. Once the fluid enter below coverslip immediately remove the pipette from central platform.
11. Wait for 3–5 minutes to settle the cells and put the charged Neubauer's chamber under low of microscope. With the help of fine focusing see that there should be the uniform distribution of RBCs, if it is not recharge the chamber again.
12. Focus the Neubauer's chamber under (40×) high power and count the cells in five medium size square shown in Fig. 1.3.1 (R1, R2, R3, R4, and R5). There are 16 small squares in each medium size square so the total small squares are 80.

Rules for Counting the Cells

(i) Any cell which is touching the line is counted in the same square.
(ii) Counting is started from left and upper border of square.
(iii) Among the tripple line central line should be considered as a main line for counting of cells.
(iv) Cells of lower and right border should also counted at the end of each row.

For example: In medium size square R1 (Fig. 1.3.2) the number of cells are as follows:

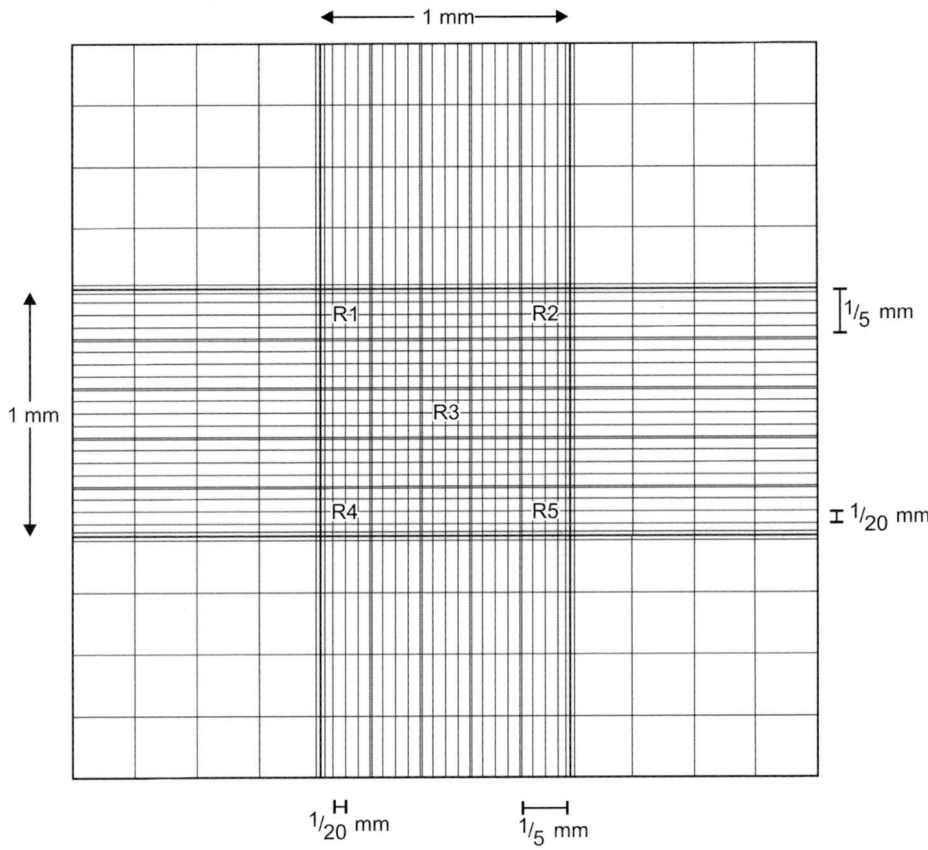

Fig. 1.3.1: Counting chamber (Neubauer's chamber) under low power of a compound microscope.

Square 1–2 cells

Square 2–1 cell

Square 3–3 cells

Square 9–2 cells

Square 11–2 cells

Square 12–1 cell

Total cells in R1 square = 10.

During counting enters the number of cells present in different small squares in the square drawn on a paper in a similar way as in Neubauer's chamber (Fig. 1.3.2).

CALCULATIONS

Dilution factor: 0.5 part of blood mixes in total 100 parts of mixture (99.5 parts diluting fluid). Fluid present in the stem (1.0 part) does not take part in mixing. This is why 2–3 drops of fluid (present in stem) is discarded before charging the chamber.

$$\text{Dilution factor} = \frac{\text{Total volume of bulb}}{\text{Volume of blood taken}}$$
$$= \frac{100}{0.5} = 200$$

Area of medium size square (R)

$$= 1/5 \times 1/5 = 1/25 \text{ mm}^2$$

Depth of chamber = 1/10 mm

Volume of each medium size square (R)

$$= 1/25 \times 1/10 = 1/250 \text{ cu mm}$$

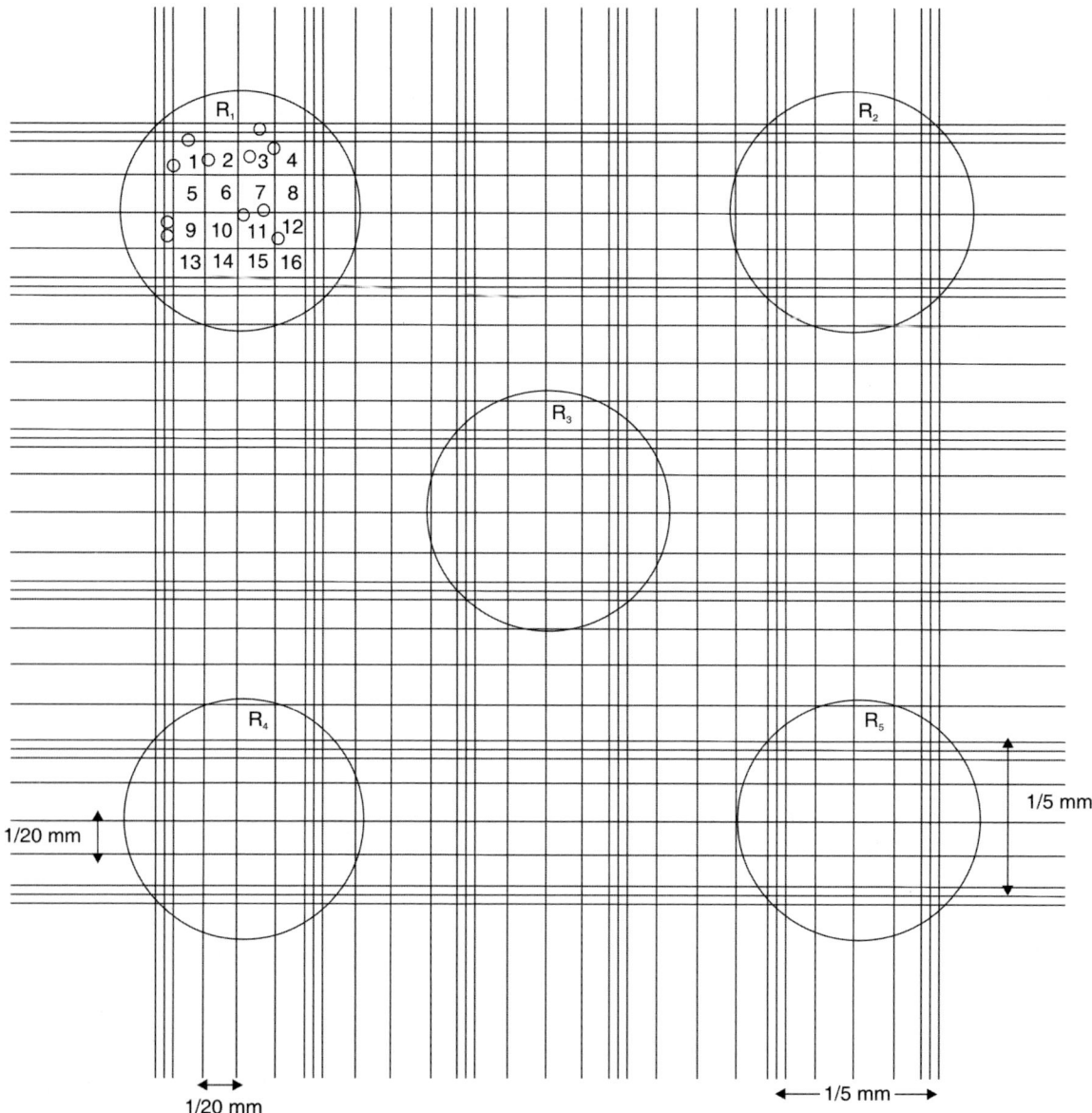

Fig. 1.3.2: Each circle denotes the field which is visualised at one time under high power of a compound microscope.

Total volume of 5 square $(R_1 + R_2 + R_3 + R_4 + R_5)$

$\quad = 1/250 \times 5 = 1/50$ cu mm

Suppose total number cell counted in five

$\quad (R_1 + R_2 + R_3 + R_4 + R_5)$ squares = N

Number of cells counted in $1/50$ mm^3 in diluted blood

$\quad = N$

Number of cells counted in 1 mm^3 diluted blood

$\quad = N \times 50$

Number of cell in 1 mm^3 undiluted blood

$$= N \times 50 \times 200$$

RBC count $\qquad = N \times 10000/mm^3$

Normal RBC Count

In adult male – 5.5 million/cu.mm (5–6 million)

In adult female – 4.8 million cu.mm (4.5–5.5 million)

Result and Comments

Write down the result and comment accordingly

Precautions

1. RBC pipette, Neubauer's chamber and cover-slip should be clean and dry.
2. Hold the coverslip from its edges not from its flat surfaces.
3. Don't take more time in filling the pipette with blood (blood will clot in the pipette).
4. There should not be under charging or over charging.

Physiological Variations

1. Age: In newborn baby it is more.
2. Sex: More in male.
3. High attitude: Increase RBC count at high attitude.

Pathological Variations

1. Hypoxia.
2. Polycythemia vera.

Objectives

At the end of the class students should be able to:

(i) do RBC count of his own blood.

(ii) tell normal value of RBC count.

(iii) enumerate physiological and some patholo-gical conditions which effect erythrocyte count.

QUESTIONS AND ANSWERS

1. What is the normal value of RBC count in adult male and female?
2. How will you differentiate RBC and WBC pipette?
3. What are the functions of bead in the pipette?
4. What are the units of markings on the pipette?
5. How much is the dilution in RBC pipette and why?
6. Why there is a need to dilute the blood for RBC count?

Ans. Because the RBC count is very high and in undiluted blood it is very difficult to count the cells under microscope.

7. What are the other uses of RBC pipette?

Ans. RBC pipette can used for platelets count and sperm count.

8. Why is it important to discard 2–3 drops of fluid before charging the chamber?
9. How is the RBC count affected, when the chamber is under or over charged?
10. How will you clean the pipette blocked by a blood clot?

Ans. It should be cleaned with N/10 HCl or hydrogen peroxide.

11. What is the importance of rules of counting of RBC?

Ans. If we follow this rule during counting of RBCs we will not miss any cell and will not count any cell twice.

12. Will you count the WBCs during RBC count and how will it affect RBC count?

Ans. WBCs should be avoided during counting of RBCs but smaller white cells are difficult to exclude during counting. Even if these cells are included during counting it will not affect the RBC count because WBC count is very less as compared to RBC count.

13. What is the approximate error in RBC count by this method?

Ans. It is about ± 20%.

14. Is there any other accurate method for determination of RBC count?

Ans. Yes, it is done by electronic cell counter which is accurate and more reliable method. By this method error is about 2%.

15. What are the physiological factors responsible for polycythemia?

16. What is the composition of Hayem's fluid and what is the role of various ingredients in fluid?

EXPERIMENT 1.4

Determination of total leukocyte count (TLC)

APPARATUS

Neubauer's chamber, WBC pipette, diluting fluid, microscope, coverslip, prickling needle and spirit swab.

WBC diluting fluid (Turk's fluid):
1. Gentian violet: 1% 1ml, stains nuclei of WBCs.
2. Glacial acetic acid: 3 ml to destroy RBCs and platelets (destroy cell membrane).
3. Distilled water: To make 100 ml.

PRINCIPLE

White blood cells are counted in diluted blood and actual count is calculated by multiplying it by dilution factor.

PROCEDURE

1. Take 3–5 ml Turk's fluid in a watch glass.
2. Prick the ring finger of left hand after cleaning it with spirit swab.
3. Wipe off first drop of blood. Suck next drop of blood in WBC pipette exactly up to 0.5 mark, taking care that there should be no air bubble. If excess blood has been drawn, remove it by touching the pipette on cotton swab very carefully.
4. Wipe off the blood sticking around the tip of the pipette with cotton swab.
5. Now suck the Turk's fluid in the pipette up to mark 11.
6. Hold the pipette in between palms and mix the blood with diluting fluid by rolling it gently.
7. Focus the Neubauer's chamber under low power and charge the chamber after discarding 2–3 drops of fluid from the pipette in this same way as in RBC count.
8. Let the cells settle for 3–5 min, and keep the Neubauer's chamber again under low power

of microscope and count WBC in outer four corner squares.
9. During counting WBC enter, the number of cells counted in different squares in the squares drawn on a paper (Fig. 1.4.1).

CALCULATIONS

Dilution factor: 0.5 part of blood mixes in total 10 part of mixture in bulb (9.5 parts diluting fluid). Fluid present in the stem (1.0 part) does not take part in mixing. This is why 2–3 drops of fluid is discarded before charging.

$$\text{Dilution factor} = \frac{\text{Total volume of bulb (10 parts)}}{\text{Volume of blood taken (0.5 part)}}$$

$$= 20$$

Area of a big square $= 1 \times 1 = 1 \text{ mm}^2/\text{mm}^2$

Depth of chamber $= 1/10 \text{ mm}$

Volume of a big square $= 1 \times 1/10$

$$= 0.1 \text{ mm}^3/\text{mm}^3$$

Volume of four squares $= 0.4 \text{ mm}^3$

Total number of cells counted in four corner squares

$$= N$$

Number of cells in 0.4 mm^3 of diluted blood $= N$

Number of cells in 1 mm^3 of diluted blood

$$= N / 0.4$$

Number of cells in 1 mm^3 of undiluted blood

$$= N/ 0.4 \times 20 = N \times 50$$

Normal WBC count : 4000–11000 / cu mm.

Precautions

All the precautions are similar as in RBC count.

Variations in WBC Count

Leucocytosis

Physiological: Severe muscular exercise, pregnancy and food intake.

Pathological: Acute pyogenic infection, e.g. abscess, pneumonitis, appendicitis.

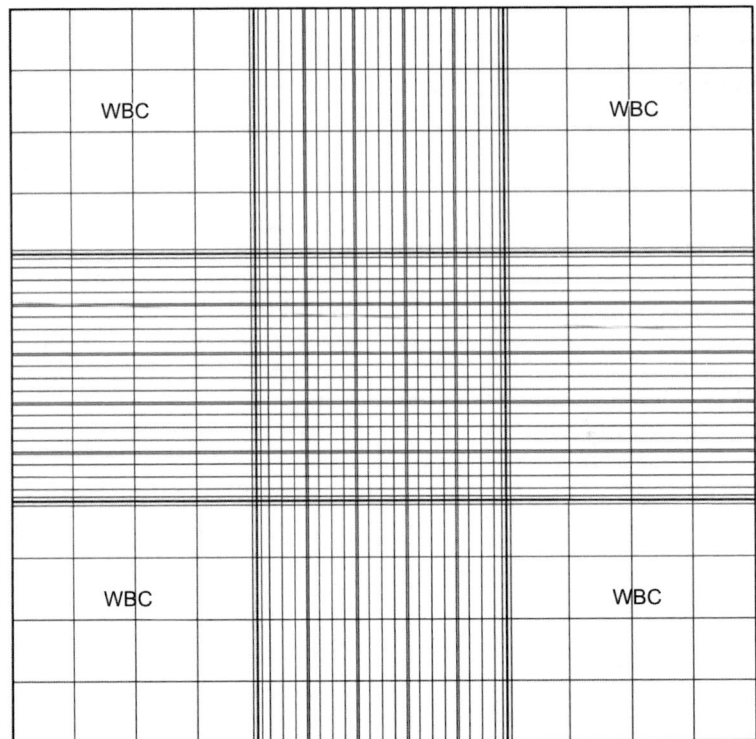

Fig. 1.4.1: Counting chamber (Neubauer's chamber) under low power of a microscope.

Leucopenia

Pathological: Bone marrow depression, e.g.chlor-amphenicol, aplastic anaemia.

Result and Comments

Write down the result and give your comments accordingly.

OBJECTIVES OF THE EXPERIMENT

At the end of the class students should be able to

  (i) determine WBC count of his own blood,

  (ii) tell normal value of WBC count,

  (iii) enumerate certain conditions in which WBC count increases and decreases.

QUESTIONS AND ANSWER

1. What is the normal value of WBC count?
2. How much is the dilution in WBC pipette?
3. What are the constituents of Turk's fluid and what are the functions of each ingredient?
4. What is the leucocytosis and leucopenia?
5. How will you differentiate between leuco-cytosis and leukaemia?

Ans. In lecocytosis WBC count is less than 50000 per cu mm and in leukaemia it is more. In leukaemia immature white cells are seen in the blood film.

6. What are the causes of leucopenia?

EXPERIMENT 1.5

Estimation of Haemoglobin by Sahli's method

APPARATUS

Haemoglobinometer, pricking needle and spirit swab.

Haemoglobinometer

It is a box which contains:

1. Comparator: It consisted of a box having one slot for Sahli's (haemoglobin) tube and two non fading standard brown tinted glass pieces for matching the colour of diluted blood. A translucent white glass is fitted at the back to provide uniform illumination for matching the colour (Fig. 1.5.1).

2. Sahli's tube (Haemoglobin tube): It is a graduated tube having markings on two sides. On one side in gm% (gm per 100 ml) from 0 to 24 and other side 0–170%. Gram % means Hb in gm per 100 ml of blood. Simple per cent means percentage of haemoglobin in relation to normal value of Hb which is considered as 100 %.

3. Haemoglobin pipette: It is a simple pipette having capillary tube in it. This is connected to the teat (mouthpiece) through a rubber tube. There is a marking on the pipette indicating 20 cu mm (0.02 ml) volume.

4. Stirrer: Simple glass rode used to mix the blood with acid or distilled water.

5. Simple rubber dropper: To add acid or water drop by drop.

PRINCIPLE

Known quantity of blood (Hb) is mixed with N/10 HCl leading to formation of acid haematin which gives brown colour. Now mixture containing acid haematin is diluted with distilled water till its colour matches standard colour in the glass fitted in the comparator. Value of Hb is noted down from the Sahli's tube.

PROCEDURE

1. With the help of a dropper, take N/10 HCl in Sahli's tube up to mark 20%.

2. Under all aseptic conditions give a bold prick on the tip of ring finger with the help of pricking needle.

3. Wipe off the first drop of blood and suck the blood from the second drop in Hb pipette up to mark 20 cu mm.

4. Wipe the tip of the pipette with the help of cotton to remove sticked blood around the tip.

5. Blow out the blood from the pipette in to acid in Sahli's tube and rinse the pipette with the same.

6. Mix the blood in acid with stirrer and wait for 10 minutes.

7. Dilute the mixture by adding distilled water drop by drop till the colour of mixture matches with standard colour in comparator.

8. Each time you have mix it with help of stirrer after adding the distilled water.

9. Once the colour is matched lift the stirrer up and note down the reading in Sahli's tube by taking the lower miniscus in consideration.

10. Usually in coloured solution upper meniscus is considered for taking the reading but it is a transparent coloured solution and lower meniscus can be recorded.

11. Now add one more drop of distilled water and mix it properly. If colour is still matching note down the reading, if it is lighter it shows reading taken before dilution was correct. If not add a drop of distilled water again and match the colour. If it is lighter it shows that reading taken just before last dilution is correct.

12. Reading is expressed in Hb gm/100 ml of blood.

Normal Value of Haemoglobin

Male adult – 15.5 gm/100 ml (14–18 gm%)

Female adult – 14 gm/100 ml (12–15.5 gm%)

Newborn – 16.5/100 ml

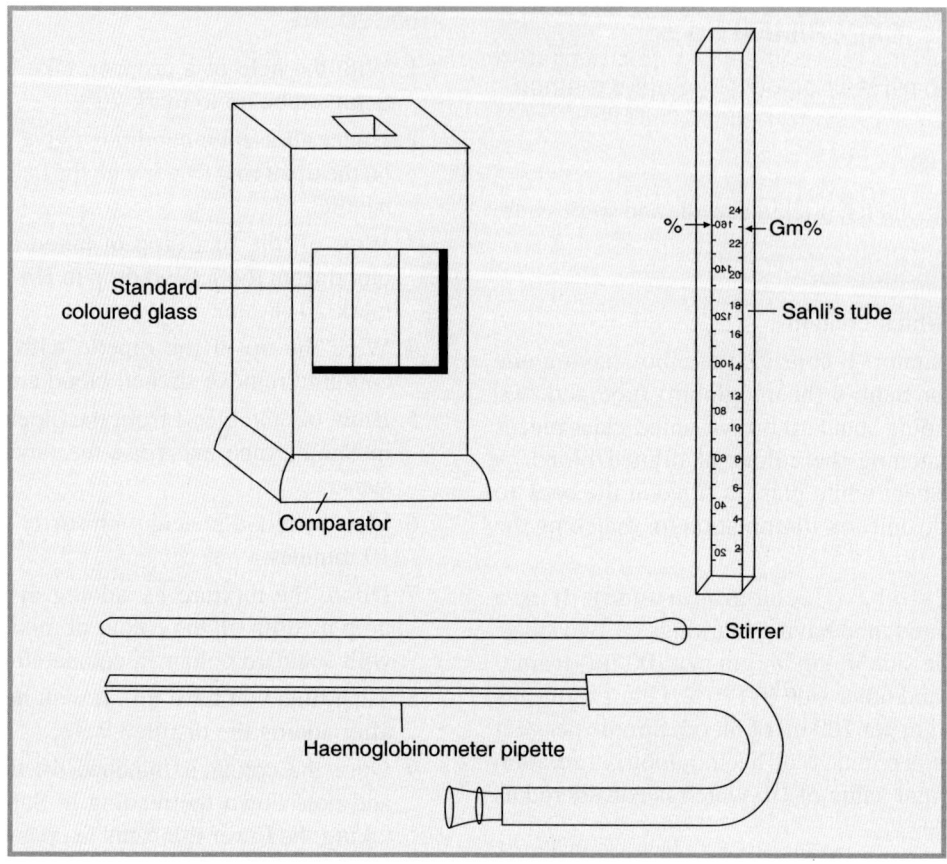

Fig. 1.5.1: Sahli's haemoglobinometer.

PRECAUTIONS

1. Haemoglobin pipette and Sahli's tube should be clean and dry before use.

2. Suck the blood exactly up to the mark of 20 cu mm.

3. There should not be any air bubble in the pipette with blood.

4. Wait for 8–10 minutes after adding the blood in acid.

5. Add distilled water drop by drop to avoid over dilution.

6. The matching of colour should be done against natural source of light or electrical tube light (white light).

Other Methods Used for Hb Estimation

1. Cyanmethaemoglobin Method

In this method blood is first treated with potassium cyanide and potassium ferricyanide, which forms methaemoglobin. Light absorbed by this is compared with standard solution in photo-electric calorimeter.

2. Alkali Haematin Method

Alkali is used to form alkali haematin and colour is matched with standard.

3. Iron Estimation Method

It is based on the principle that 100 gm Hb contains 347 mg of iron. Value of iron is estimated in blood which gives value of Hb.

4. Vanslyke's Method

The amount of oxygen combine with Hb is measured. One gm of Hb can carry 1.34 ml of oxygen. So quantity of oxygen is measured in 100 ml of blood.

5. Tallquist Scale Method

In this method a drop of blood is absorbed on a absorbent paper and colour of this paper is matched with standard.

6. Copper Sulphate Method

It is a rapid method for estimation of approximate level of Hb and it is used in large surveys.

OBJECTIVES

Student should be able to:

  (i) tell the principle used in determination of Hb by Sahli's method,
 (ii) estimate Hb of his own blood,
(iii) tell the normal value of Hb,
(iv) enumerate other methods of Hb estimation.

QUESTIONS AND ANSWERS

1. What is the principle of estimation of Hb by Sahli's method?

2. What is N/10 HCl and how will you prepare it?

Ans. One normal solution of HCl is having 36.5 gm (H:1 + Cl:35.5) HCl in one litre of solution. N/10 HCl is prepared by dissolving 3.65 gm of HCl in one litre of distilled water.

3. What is the normal value of Hb in adult?

4. Which meniscus of acid haematin is considered for taking the reading and why?

5. Why do we wait after adding the blood to HCl for 10 minutes?

Ans. This is the time required to convert the Hb of the blood in acid haematin.

6. Why do we take HCl up to mark 20% in Sahli's tube?

Ans. This is the minimum quantity of HCl which is required to convert total Hb present in the tube. If the quantity of HCl is less it will be insufficient to convert the whole of the Hb in to acid haematin. If the quantity of HCl is more than 20% it will not affect the result in healthy subjects but it will be the wastage of HCl. In case of patients of severe anaemia it may affect the result. For example in a patient there is 4.0 gm of Hb and HCl taken in the tube is up to 50% mark it will be already diluted than the standard colour in the haemoglobinometer.

7. Why do not we keep the stirrer outside once we have started to mix the blood and distilled water?

Ans. It may lose the (drop of) mixture present with the stirrer.

8. What are the experimental errors which effect Hb level?

Ans. Experimental error may be because of:

   (i) Quantity of the blood taken in the pipette may be less or more.
  (ii) Air bubble in the blood column in the pipette.
 (iii) Fading of the colour of standard glass rods of comparator.

9. How will you calculate the oxygen carrying capacity of blood?

Ans. It can be calculated after estimating the haemoglobin of the subject. One gram of Hb combines with 3.36 ml of oxygen, with this we can calculate the total oxygen carried by the Hb present in 100 ml of blood.

10. Enumerate some other methods of Hb estimation.

11. What is anaemia?

12. What is the grading of anaemia?

Ans. Grading of severity of anaemia is as follows:

    (i) Mild anaemia: Hb 8–12 gm%

    (ii) Moderate anaemia: Hb 5–8 gm%

    (iii) Severe anaemia: Hb less than 5 gm%

13. What are the physiological and pathological causes of increase and decrease Hb in blood?

Ans. A. Physiological causes:

    (i) Sex: Higher in male.

    (ii) Age: Hb decreases with age. In newborn it is about 16.5 gm per 100 ml.

    (iii) Pregnancy: Hb decreases in pregnancy.

    (iv) High altitude: At high altitude there is increase in Hb.

B. Pathological causes:

    (i) Hb decreases in anaemia.

    (ii) It increases in polycythaemia.

EXPERIMENT 1.6

Preparation of blood smear (film) and identification of various cells

APPARATUS

4–5 glass slides, compound microscope, pricking needle, spirit swab, cedar wood oil/liquid paraffin, Leishman's stain, wash bottle, buffered water and staining tray.

Leishman's Stain

1.5 gm powder of Leishman's stain is dissolved in one litre of acetone free methyl alcohol. Leishman's stain contains two dyes, eosin and methylene blue. Eosin is an acidic dye that stains basic structures like RBC and granules of eosinophil. It is pink or red in colour. Methylene blue is a basic dye that stains acidic structures like nucleus or granules of basophils. It is blue in colour. Acetone free methyl alcohol is a fixative for smear.

   (i) Fixation of smear is because of precipitation of proteins by alcohol which prevent washing off of the film.

   (ii) It preserves the cells in whatever chemical and metabolic state they are at the time of staining.

   (iii) Acetone if present will cause shrinkage or even lysis of the cells.

PRINCIPLE

Blood smear is prepared, stained with Leishman's stain and cells are identified under oil immersion lens.

PROCEDURE

(A) Preparation of Blood Smear

1. Selection of a spreader: Take one slide a spreader which has smooth edge. It should be done by careful look on the narrow edge of the slide or by moving a thumb smoothly on its edge. But, the slide should be washed with soap and water after touching its edge, to remove grease particles from its edges.

2. Take 3–4 clean and dry glass slides and keep them on filter paper or any clean white paper placed on the table.

3. Prick the ring finger of left hand with the help of pricking needle under all aseptic conditions.

   Put a small size of blood drop on each glass slide about half centimeter from it's narrow edge on the right side. Place the blood drop on the same way on other slides also.

4. Now put the spreader on left side of blood drop at the angle 45° as shown in Fig. 1.6.1.

5. Give left to right movement to the spreader so that blood comes along the edge of the spreader. Further give side to side movement so that blood comes along the whole edge of spreader.

6. Now spread the blood by giving smooth, uniform and rapid movement to the spreader up to the left edge of the slide. Repeat the same procedure with rest of the slides.

7. Dry the smear by waving the slides in the air for some time.

8. Now observe the all smears whether they are satisfactory or not (Fig. 1.6.2). A good smear has following characteristics:

   (i) It is tongue shaped, having head, body, and tail. Head is the area where blood drop is placed. Body is the area between head and tail. Tail is the last part of the smear.

   (ii) It should cover two-thirds of the slide.

   (iii) It should not be thick.

   (iv) There should not be marks or blank spaces in the smear.

9. After selecting a good smear with naked eyes focus it under low power of the microscope. The smear should be thin enough to have single layer of cells. There should not be rouleaux formation or clumping of cells.

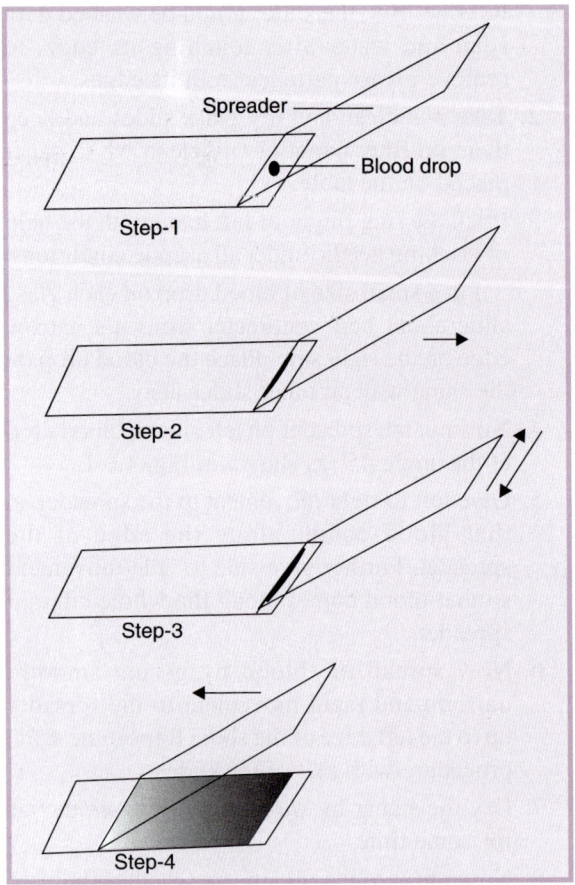

Fig. 1.6.1: To make blood smear.

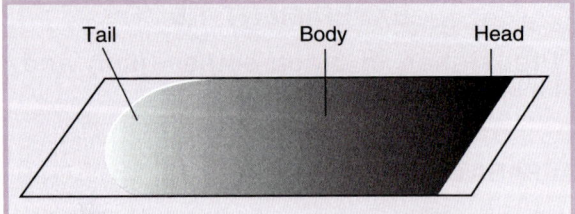

Fig. 1.6.2: A typical blood smear.

(B) Staining of Blood Smear

1. Place 3–4 good slides horizontally on the stand.
2. Add Leishman's stain drop by drop till it covers whole of the smear. Count the number of drops you have put.
3. Leave it for 1–2 minutes for fixation of the smear.
4. Add equal number of drops of buffered water (pH 6.8) on the slide. Mix the stain with water by blowing air with the help of a glass tube or with a dropper.
5. Wait for 8–10 minutes for staining to complete. During this period in the presence of buffered water staining is taking place because of formation of cations and anions of basic and acidic dyes respectively. Methyl alcohol is unable to ionise the stain so unable to stain the cells.
6. Wash the smear in slow running tap water or with the help of wash bottle till the smear becomes pink in colour. Clean the back of the slide to remove the stain from back side.
7. Let the slide dry and focus it under high power. If it is under stained, stain it again and if it is overstained wash it again.

(C) Examination of Smear under Oil Immersion Lens

Focus the slide under high power. Put a drop of cedar wood oil or liquid paraffin on the slide and shift the oil immersion lens by constantly looking from the side of the microscope so that it just dips in the oil.

Now focus with the help of fine adjustment screw and examine the various cells for their identification. (Identifying features of various cells are given in Table 1.6.1.) The various features of different cells are also shown in Fig. 1.6.3.

PRECAUTIONS

1. Slide should be clean and grease free.
2. Edge of the spreader should be smooth.
3. Do not take much time in making the smear once the blood has been taken on the slide.
4. Stain should not dry on the blood smear.
5. Assess the quality of blood smear both grossly and microscopically before staining it.

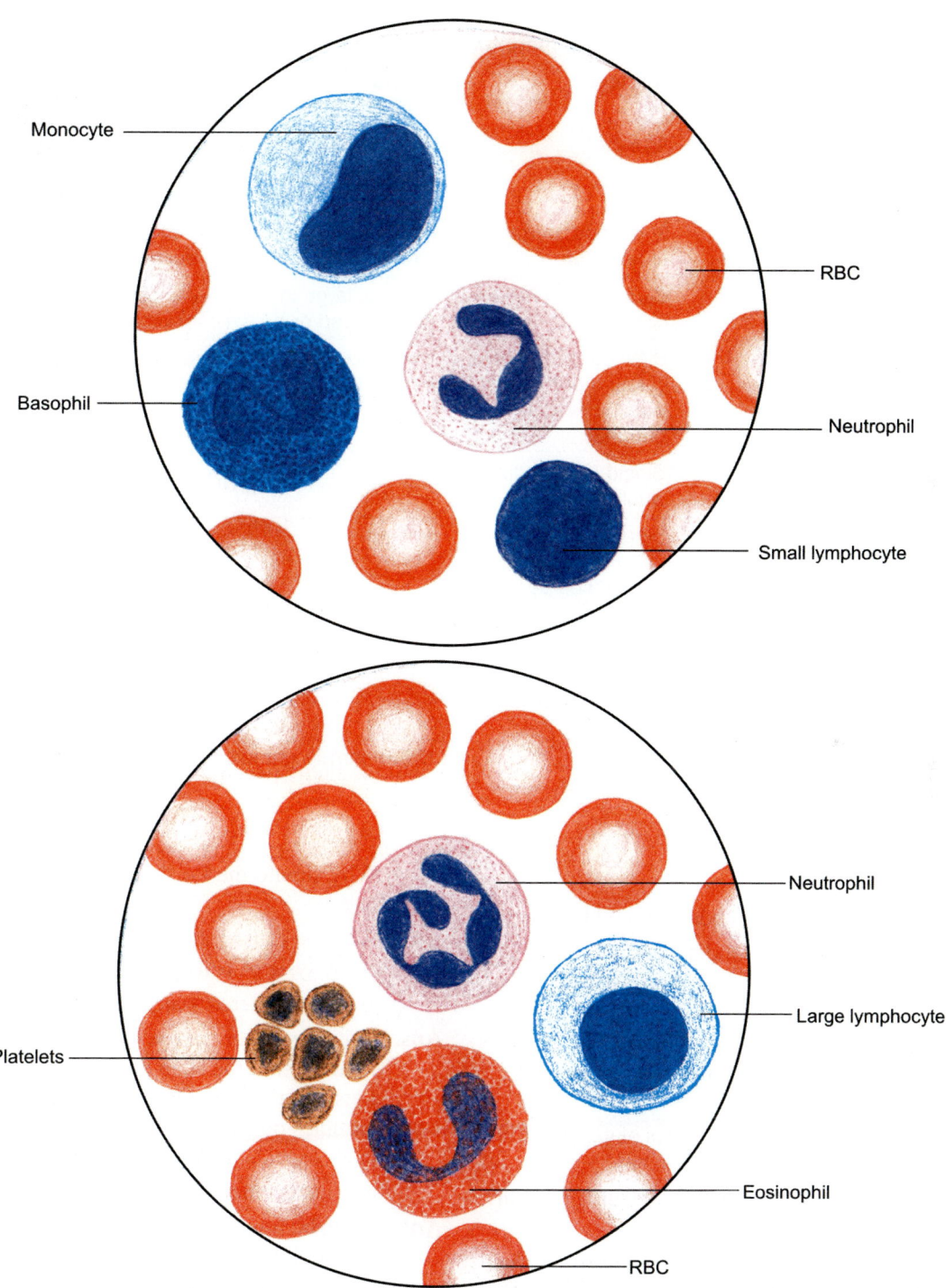

Fig. 1.6.3: Blood cells under oil immersion lens (Leishman's stain)

		Table 1.6.1: Identifying features of various cells in blood smear.		
Cells	Size (μm)	Nucleus	Granules	Cytoplasm
RBC	7–8	Absent	Absent	Pink or red colour, lighter in the centre as compared to periphery
Neutrophil	10–14	2–5 lobes, purple/ blue colour	Fine, few in number, pink/purple	Pink/purple in colour because of fine granules
Eosinophil	10–14	Bilobed, purple/blue colour	Coarse, large in number, red or brown	Almost not visible because of large number of granules
Basophil	10–14	Bilobled, purple/blue colour, not properly visible because of granules	Large number, dark blue colour	Almost not visible because of granules
Small lymphocyte	7–10	Single mass, filling whole of the cell	Absent	Almost absent
Large lymphocyte	10–14	Single mass covering 2/3rd of cell, blue or purple, coarse and lumpy	Absent	Ring of light blue or sky blue colour
Monocyte	10–18	Blue or purple colour, cine chromatin, indented from one side	Usually absent	Light blue/sky blue, more on one side
Platelets	2–4	Absent	Brown/purple granules	Pale cytoplasm

OBJECTIVES

At the end of the practical student should be able to:
  (i) make and stain a blood smear.
 (ii) identify RBCs, different types of WBCs and platelets.

QUESTIONS AND ANSWERS

1. Enumerate the characteristics of a good blood smear.
2. What are the constituents of Leishman's stain? Enumerate their functions.
3. Why the cells do not get stained in the first two minutes after adding the stain on the smear?

4. Why should the Leishman's stain be acetone free?

Ans. Acetone causes shrinkage of cells and it may cause lysis of cells.

5. What is buffered water and why we use it?

Ans. It is the water whose pH is 6.8. It causes ionization of the stain particles present in the Leishman's stain. Optimal ionization of stain particles occurs at pH 6.8.

6. How can we estimate size of a white blood cell under microscope?

Ans. It can be found by comparing these cells with RBCs. The size of RBC is about 7–8 μ.

7. Why the left ring finger is chosen for giving prick?

EXPERIMENT 1.7

To do the differential leukocyte count (DLC) of your own blood

APPARATUS

4–5 glass slides, Leishman's stain, compound microscope, cedar wood oil, buffered water and staining tray.

PRINCIPLE

Total 100 leukocytes are studied, identified and recorded from a blood smear.

PROCEDURE

1. Prepare, stain and examine a blood smear under oil immersion lens.
2. Draw one hundred squares on a paper.
3. Identify various types of leukocyte and enter them by first letter (N—Neutrophil, E—Eosinophil, B—Basophil, L—Lymphocyte, M—Monocyte) in all 100 squares.
4. Count the cells in a specific sequence to avoid repeated counting.
5. Cells are counted in one direction and then field is shifted and counting is done in opposite direction. Field is again shifted in the same direction and counting is done in same direction as in the beginning. Direction of counting is shown in Fig. 1.7.1.
6. Percentage of various types of white cells is calculated by counting the different cells in various squares.

Normal DLC

Neutrophil	40–70%
Eosinophil	1–4%
Basophil	0–1%
Lymphocyte	20–40%
Monocyte	2–8%

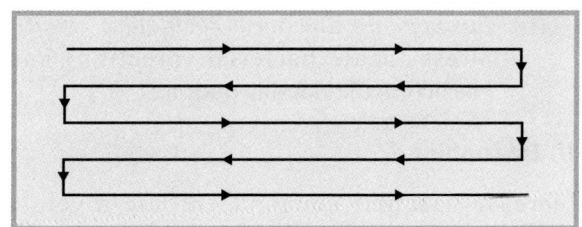

Fig. 1.7.1: Direction of shifting the field during counting of WBCs.

PRECAUTIONS

1. Same as in preparation of blood smear and identification of various cells.
2. We should not count the same cells twice.

VARIATIONS

A. Neutrophils

(a) *Neutrophilia*: Increase neutrophil count.
　　1. Severe muscular exercise, pregnancy and food in take.
　　2. Acute pyogenic infectious, e.g. abscess, boils, tonsillitis, etc.

(b) *Neutropenia*: Decrease neutrophil count.
　　1. Depression of bone marrow: Aplastic anaemia, bone marrow depressant drug, e.g. Chloramphenicol.
　　2. Typhoid, paratyphoid and malaria.

B. Lymphocytes

(a) *Lymphocytosis:* Increase lymphocyte count.
　　1. Newborn and infant lymphocytes are more.
　　2. Chronic infection, e.g. tuberculosis

(b) Decrease lymphocytes (lymphopenia) ACTH and steroid therapy.

C. Eosinophil

(a) *Eosinophilia (increase eosinophil count):* Allergy condition like pulmonary eosinophilia, worm infestation, Hay fever and urticaria.

(b) *Eosinopenia (decrease eosinophil count):* Stress (acute bacterial infection) and glucocorticoid administration.

D. Basophils

Increase basophil count in chronic myeloid laeukemia, small box and polycythemia. Decrease basophil count in acute Pyogenic injections.

E. Monocyte

Increase monocyte count in infection mononucleosis, kala azar and malaria.

OBJECTIVES

Student should know:

1. Method of counting of different cells.
2. Significance of DLC.

QUESTIONS

1. What are the physiological and pathological causes of increased neutrophil count?
2. What are the pathological conditions causing neutropenia?
3. What are the causes of increased eosinophil count?
4. What are the physiological and pathological causes of lymphocytosis?
5. What are the pathological conditions leading to increase in monocyte count?

EXPERIMENT 1.8

To determine bleeding time (BT) and clotting time (CT) of your own blood

PRINCIPLE

A. *Bleeding time*: Time elapse between skin prick and arrest of bleeding.

B. *Clotting (coagulation) time*: Time elapse between skin prick and formation of fibrin thread.

A. Duke Method of Bleeding Time

Apparatus

Pricking needle, spirit swab and filter paper.

Procedure

- Get 2–3 mm deep prick after cleaning tip of ring finger of left hand.
- Note down the time (zero time).
- Remove the blood every 15 seconds by touching the finger gently on a filter paper till bleeding stops.
- Note the time when no trace of blood on the filter paper.
- Count the stops of blood on filter paper and express bleeding time in minutes and seconds. Normal bleeding time: 1–4 min.

Other Methods

1. *Saline beaker method*
   - Prick is given in all sterile conditions and time is noted.
   - Finger is put in to the beaker containing normal saline at 37°C.
   - Time is noted when bleeding stops.
   Normal BT by this method: 2–6 min.

2. *Ivy method*
   - Sphygmomanometer cuff is tide on the left arm and pressure is maintained to 40 mmHg.

- About 3 mm deep prick is given on the left forearm after cleaning the area with spirit swab.
- Blood is absorbed by filter paper till bleeding stops.

Normal BT by this method: Up to 9 min.

B. Capillary Blood Clotting Time

Apparatus

Pricking needle, glass capillary tube, spirit swab.

Procedure

- Get a deep prick (3 mm) on the finger tip after cleaning it with spirit swab.
- Fill a capillary glass tube by dipping its one end in the blood drop on the finger.
- Note down the time as soon as blood starts to enter in the tube.
- Break off a small piece (1/2 to 1 cm) of capillary tube from one end of it.
- Capillary tube is held horizontally between palms.
- Break the tube at every 30 seconds till fibrin thread is seen between the broken ends.
- Note down the time again.

Normal clotting time: 2–5 min.

Precautions

1. There should be no air bubbles in blood column in capillary tube.
2. Hold the capillary tube horizontally between the palms when you are doing the test in winter.
3. Note down the time when blood starts to enter the capillary tube.

Other Methods

1. *Drop method*
   - This method is less and accurate.
   - Blood drop is taken on a clean dry glass slide.

- An all pin is drawn at an interval of 30 seconds till fibrin threads are seen.
- Time is noted.

Normal time: 2–4 min.

2. *Lee and White test tube method*
- Blood is collected by vene puncture and transferred in three clean and dry test tubes.
- Keep these tube in a beaker having normal saline at 37°C.
- Shifting of blood column is checked at the interval of one minute by tilting the test tube at an angle of 45°.
- Once the blood column is not shifting, second tube is inverted.
- Finally it is confirmed from the third tube.

- Time from collection of blood and staying of clotted blood in the inverted tube is noted.

Normal clotting time: 5–10 min.

Variations in bleeding and clotting time.

1. Bleeding time is prolonged in purpura not affected in haemophilia.
2. Clotting time is prolonged in haemophilia.

OBJECTIVES

Student should be able to:

1. perform these tests,
2. tell the clinical significance of these tests,
3. name the conditions in which bleeding and clotting times are prolonged.

QUESTIONS AND ANSWERS

1. What do you understand by bleeding and clotting time?
2. What is their clinical significance?
3. What is the effect of environment temperature on BT and CT?

Ans. With rise in temperature (in summer) there is prolongation of bleeding time (vasodilatation) and shortening of the clotting time (enzyme reactions become faster). With decrease in environment temperature (in winter) there is decrease in bleeding time (vasoconstriction) and prolongation of clotting time (enzyme reactions slow down)

4. Name the condition in which clotting time is prolonged and bleeding time remains normal.

Ans. Haemophilia.

5. What happens to BT and CT in purpura/haemophilia?

Ans. In case of purpura bleeding time increases and clotting time remains normal. In case of haemophilia bleeding time remains normal and clotting time increases.

EXPERIMENT 1.9

Determine your own blood group

APPARATUS

Normal saline, antisera A, antisera B, antisera D, prickling needle, porcelain tile/glass slides, dropper, application sticks, glass marking pencil, coverslips, microscope, prickling needle and spirit swab.

PRINCIPLE

Saline suspension of red cells is mixed with antisera A, antisera B, antisera D and agglutination looked for, presence or absence of agglutination may be confirmed by microscope examination of the sample.

PROCEDURE

1. Take 2 ml of normal saline in a watch glass or one ml in a pit of porcelain tile.
2. Add a drop of blood after prickling the finger in all aseptic conditions in saline.
3. Make A, B, D, and S near different pits on the tile or take two slides and mark A and B on one slide and D and S on other with the help of glass marking pencil as shown in Fig. 1.9.1.

4. Now put a drop of antisera A, antisera B, and antisera D in the pits or on the slide according to the respective markings from antisera vials.
5. Add one drop of saline suspension of cells with the help of dropper to different antisera without touching any antisera with dropper.
6. Add two drops of this saline suspension of cells where you have marked S on tile or on glass slide. It will act as a control to compare with agglutinated cells.
7. Mix the cells with antisera by using separate application sticks or by rocking the tile or glass slide to and fro.
8. Wait for 10 minutes and examine the mixture for agglutination (clumping of RBCs) with naked eye, if required confirm under low power of microscope.
9. With naked eye agglutination of RBCs appears as a coarse separation of red cells in isolated clumps (red precipitates of cells).
10. By rocking the tile or slide agglutinated cells do not make uniform/homogeneous mixture of cells.
11. Agglutination can be compared with saline mixture of cells which is taken as control.
12. Under low power of microscope RBCs are together in clumps.

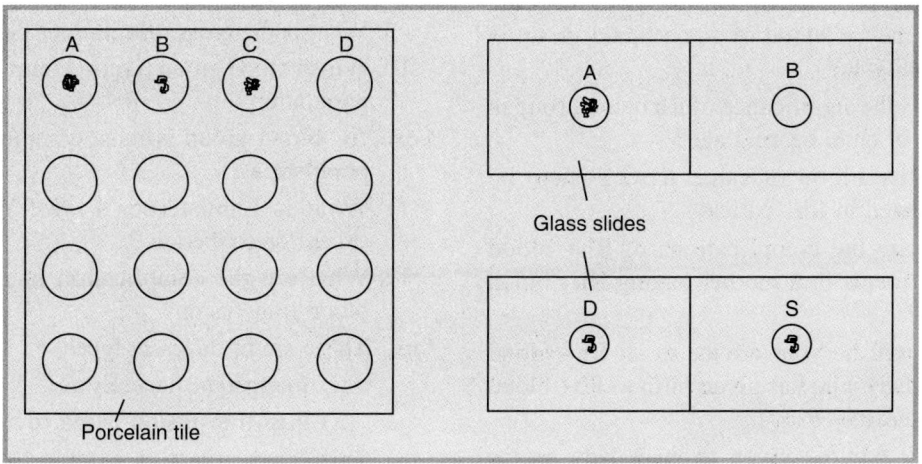

Fig. 1.9.1: Markings on porcelain tile and glass slides for determination of blood groups.

13. Blood group is determined as indicated in the table give below.

Antisera			Blood Group
A	B	D	
+	−	+ / −	A + / A −
−	+	+ / −	B + / B −
+	+	+ / −	AB + / AB −
−	−	+ / −	O + / O −

+ Indicates agglutination   − Indicates no agglutination.

Result

Blood group should be expressed in ABO system and Rh system, e.g. A$^+$ / A$^-$.

Precautions

1. Tile or slide should be clean and dry.
2. There should be no intermixing of the mixture put on different places on tile or on slide.
3. Any doubt in agglutination must be confirmed under low power of microscope.

Objectives

At the end of the practical student should be able to:

1. Determine the blood group,
2. Tell the principle underlying the determination of blood group,
3. Tell the clinical significance of the investigation,
4. Tell the difference between rouleaux formation and agglutination.

QUESTIONS AND ANSWERS

1. What is the status of antigen and antibodies in a person of particular blood group?
2. What is the significance of determination of blood groups?
3. Who are universal donor and universal recipient?
4. Which type of blood can be given in acute emergency if blood of same blood group is not available?
5. What is the significance of Rh blood group in a lady of child bearing age?
6. Can Rh+ blood of same ABO system be transferred in Rh− patient?
7. What are the complications of Rh+ blood group foetus in a mother having Rh− blood group?
8. What will be your advice to an Rh− blood group lady who has given birth to Rh+ blood group healthy baby?

Ans. Various advices given to such lady are as follows:

   (i) She should not have another pregnancy.
  (ii) She should be given a bolus dose of anti-D to destroy Rh+ cells just after delivery.
 (iii) She should come regularly for obstetrical check up if she still wants next pregnancy.

9. What is the cross matching of blood?
10. Which blood group is most common in Indian population?

Ans. 'B' blood group is most common in Indian population.

11. What is Landsteiner's law? What is the exception to the law?
12. What are the complication of mismatched blood transfusion?

Ans. These are of different types:

   (i) Inapparent haemolysis.
  (ii) Post-transfusion jaundice.
 (iii) Severe reaction leading to haematuria and renal failure.

13. What are the other complications of blood transfusion?

Ans. Other complications of blood transfusion are:

    (i) Pyrexia (post-transfusion fever).

    (ii) Transfer of infections, e.g. AIDS, malaria, hepatitis.

    (iii) Alkalosis (when large quantity of blood is transfused).

    (iv) Hyperkalemia.

    (v) Overloading of circulation.

14. What is the role of Rh antibodies (Anti-D) in an Rh– lady given after the birth of Rh+ baby?

Ans. They destroy Rh+ cells entered in mother's circulation from the placenta at the time of delivery so the further sensitization and production of antibody will stop.

15. Why we should wait for 10 minutes before looking for agglutination?

Ans. This time is given to complete the agglutination reaction.

16. Why are the antibodies in plasma of donor ignored?

Ans. Because antibodies of the donor get diluted in the recipient's blood but in case of repeated blood transfusion they may create problem.

17. Explain, why ABO incompatibilities rarely produce haemolytic disease of newborn?

Ans. ABO incompatibilities are rare because α and b antibodies are of IgM type and cannot cross the placenta.

18. What is the medicolegal significance of blood grouping?

Ans. With the help of blood group of child and a father we can say that he may not be the father of the child.

Determination of erythrocyte sedimentation rate (ESR)

APPARATUS

Westergren's tube with stand, Wintrobe's tube with stand, long nozzled capillary pipette (Pasture pipette), 3.8% sodium citrate solution, mixture of double oxalate, 2 ml disposable syringe with needle and spirit swab.

Westergren's Tube with Stand

(i) It is a thick walled glass tube of length 30 cm, open at both the ends with internal bore 2.5 mm (Fig. 1.10.1).

(ii) Tube is graduated along the lower 2/3 portion, 0–200 mm from up to down.

(iii) Westergren's stand: Tall stand for holding the Westergren's tube vertically with rubber pad at the bottom and screw at the upper end.

Wintrobe's Tube with Stand

(i) It is a thick walled glass tube of length 11 cm, closed at one end with internal bore of 2.5 mm (Fig. 1.10.1).

(ii) Lower 10 cm of the tube is graduated from 0 to 100 mm from top to bottom and bottom to upper end.

(iii) Markings from 0 to 100 mm from up to down are used for reading ESR and markings from bottom to upward are used for reading PCV (haematocrit).

(iv) Wintrobe's stand: It is a small stand as compared to Westergren's stand. It is used to keep the Wintrobe's tube vertically.

ERYTHROCYTE SEDIMENTATION RATE (ESR)

It is the rate at which RBCs settle down when anticoagulated blood is allowed to stand in a narrow tube for one hour. It is measured in terms of clear plasma above the settling RBCs.

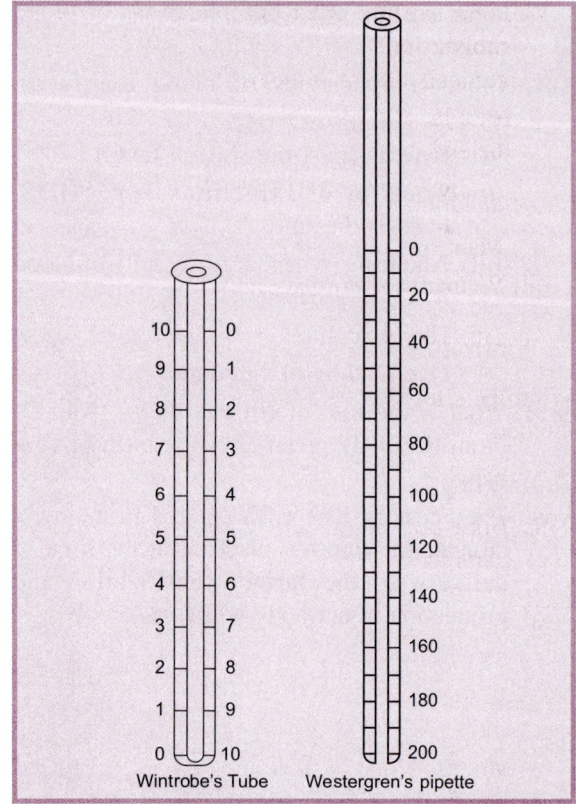

Fig. 1.10.1: ESR tubes

There are two methods for estimation of ESR.

I. Westergren's Method

Westergren's tube is used to measure ESR in this method.

Procedure

1. Take 0.5 ml of 3.8% sodium citrate solution in a clean and dry glass vial.

2. Withdraw 2 ml of blood from anticubital vein in all aseptic conditions. Remove the needle of the syringe and transfer the blood in vial containing sodium citrate solution. Immediately mix the content.

3. Suck citrated blood in Westergren's tube up to mark '0' and immediately close its upper opening with the help of index finger or thumb.

4. Press the tube after placing its lower end on rubber pad in the stand and fix the tube vertically in the stand with the help of screw.

5. Note the time and take the reading for ESR at the end of one hour of clean plasma column.

Normal Value

(i) Man: 0–4 mm at the end of one hour.

(ii) Woman: 0–8 mm at the end of one hour.

II. Wintrobe's Method

Wintrobe's tube is used to determine ESR by this method.

Procedure

1. Take powder mixture of double oxalate (Ammonium and Potassium in ratio of 3:2) in a clean and dry glass vial.

2. Draw 2 ml of blood from anticubital vein in all aseptic conditions and remove the needle of the syringe and eject the blood in glass vial.

3. Mix the blood with anticoagulant gently.

4. Fill this blood in pasture pipette and introduce the capillary tube of pipette up to the bottom of Wintrobe's tube.

5. Now apply the pressure on rubber teat and slowly take the pipette nozzle out so that tube will be filled up with the blood up to mark zero.

6. Note down the time and put the tube in the stand for one hour. Take the reading at the end of one hour of clean plasma column.

Normal Value

(i) Man: 0–4 mm at the end of one hour.

(ii) Woman: 0–6 mm at the end of one hour.

ESR value more than 20 mm is pathological.

Precautions

1. ESR tube should be clean and dry.

2. Blood sample must be collected in fasting state.

3. There should be no air bubble in ESR tube.

4. Single oxalate should not be used as anti-coagulant in Wintrobe's method.

5. Don't disturb the tube once kept in the stand for ESR.

Variations in ESR

Increase in ESR is seen in physiological and pathological conditions.

    (a) Physiological:

        1. Pregnancy

        2. Menstruation

        3. Increased temperature

        4. Higher in female

    (b) Pathological: Any destructive process.

        1. Acute infection – Pneumonia process,

        2. Chronic infections – Tuberculosis, rheumatic fever,

        3. Anaemia,

        4. Malignancy,

        5. Severe trauma.

Decrease in ESR is seen in

1. Infancy   2. Polycythemia

3. Afibrinogenemia   4. Spherocytosis

Clinical Significance

    (a) Diagnostic significance: It is non-specific investigation. In increases in the various pathological conditions when there is destruction of cells in the body.

    (b) Prognostic significance: It is a very important prognostic investigation. Repeated estimation is done during treatment period. Progressive decrease in ESR shows patient is improving and treatment is effective.

OBJECTIVES

At the end of the class student should be able to:

1. determine ESR,

2. tell normal value of ESR,

3. tell the significance of the investigation.

QUESTIONS AND ANSWERS

1. What is the normal value of ESR in adult male and female?

Ans. Because specific gravity of cells is more as compared to plasma and rouleaux formation further enhance this process.

2. Why cells settle down in anticoagulant mixed blood?

3. What is rouleaux formation?

4. Why ESR is less in infancy?

Ans. Because of high RBC count in infancy ESR is less.

5. Why ESR is higher in pregnancy?

Ans. Because of haemodilution ESR is higher in pregnancy and in later months of pregnancy there is increase in fibrinogen level in the blood which also increases ESR.

6. Why blood sample is taken in fasting for ESR?

Ans. Because water and food intake affect erythrocyte sedimentation rate.

7. Why ESR is higher in woman?

Ans. Because RBC count is less in woman.

8. Why double oxalate is used in Wintrobe's method?

Ans. Because double oxalate is not affecting the size of the blood cells as this method is used to measure PCV.

9. Name the pathological conditions in which ESR is raised.

10. Name the pathological conditions in which ESR is decreased.

11. Name the physiological conditions when ESR is decreased.

12. What are the various factors which effect ESR?

Note : Students are supposed to draw well-labelled diagram of Westergren's and Wintrobe's tubes.

EXPERIMENT 1.11

Determination of packed cell volume (PCV) and calculation of blood indices

APPARATUS

Wintrobe's tube with stand, 2 ml disposable syringe with needle, pasture pipette, mixture of double oxalate, centrifuge machine and spirit swab.

PRINCIPLE

Anticoagulant mixed blood is filled in a tube and centrifuged. Cells settle down towards the bottom because of their greater density leaving the clear plasma on upper side. Percentage of volume of cells in total blood is known as packed cell volume.

PROCEDURE

1. Take powdered mixture of double oxalate (ammonium oxalate 3 mg and potassium oxalate 2 mg) in a clean and dry glass vial.
2. Draw 2 ml of blood from the vein in all aseptic condition and eject the blood in the vial after removing the needle from the syringe. Mix the blood with anticoagulant gently.
3. Fill the Wintrobe's tube with the help of pasture pipette up to the mark 100 mm.
4. Centrifuge the blood in Centrifuge machine at 3000 revolutions per min for 30 minutes.
5. Three layers are formed:
   (i) Clear plasma in upper part of tube.
   (ii) Buffy coat (layer) (in between two layers).
   (iii) Red cells (red column) in lower part of tube.
6. PCV is read directly from the calibration of tube from bottom to upper end.
7. Buffy layer: Grayish white layer about 1 mm size on the upper end of red layer. It consists of WBC and platelets.

Normal Value

Adult man: 45% (40–50%)

Adult woman: 42% (37–47%)

Precautions

1. There should be no air bubble or froth of blood in the tube.
2. Always use double oxalate as anticoagulant.
3. Wintrobe's tube should be clean and dry.

Variation in PCV

(a) *Increase in PCV*

Physiological

1. Newborn and infant
2. High attitude
3. Higher in man as compared to woman

Pathological

1. Hypoxia
2. Polycythemia
3. Spherocytosis
4. Dehydration

(b) *Decrease in PCV*

Physiological

1. Less in woman than man
2. Pregnancy

Pathological

1. Anaemia
2. Bone marrow depression

OBJECTIVES

At the end of the practical the student should be able to:

1. Estimate PCV,
2. Tell significance,
3. Enumerate factor's effecting PCV.

CALCULATION OF BLOOD INDICES

1. Mean Corpuscular Volume (MCV)

It is the average volume of a single red blood cell.

$$MCV = \frac{PCV \text{ in ml per 100 ml blood}}{\text{Number of RBCs in 100 ml blood}}$$

$$= \text{in ml}$$

$$(1 \text{ ml} = 10^3 \text{ mm}^3 = 10^{12} \mu^3)$$

$$(100 \text{ ml} = 10^5 \text{ mm}^3)$$

$$MCV = \frac{PCV \text{ in ml per 100 ml blood in } \mu^3}{\text{Number of RBCs in 100 ml blood}}$$

$$= \text{in } \mu^3$$

$$MCV = \frac{PCV \% \times 10^{12}}{RBC \text{ in million} / mm^3 \times 10^6 \times 10^5}$$

$$MCV = \frac{PCV \% \times 10^{12}}{RBC \text{ in million} / mm^3 \times 10^{11}}$$

$$MCV = \frac{PCV \%}{RBC (\text{million} / mm^3)} \times 10$$

$$= \text{in } \mu^3$$

Normal: 78–94 μ^3

MCV Variation

Increased in

   1. Megaloblastic anaemia

   2. Spherocytosis

Decreased in

   Iron deficiency anaemia.

Clinical Significance

Useful in laboratory classification of anaemia.

   (i) Microcytic anaemia MCV < 78 cu μ

   (ii) Normocytic anaemia MCV = 78–94 cu μ

   (iii) Macrocytic anaemia MCV > 94 cu μ

2. Mean Corpuscular Haemoglobin (MCH)

It is an average quantity of Hb of a single RBC.

$$MCH = \frac{Hb \text{ in gm per 100 ml blood}}{\text{Number of RBCs in 100 ml blood}}$$

$$= \text{in gm}$$

$$(1 \text{ ml} = 10^3 \text{ mm}^3, 100 \text{ ml} = 10^5 \text{ mm}^3)$$

$$(1 \text{ gm} = 10^{12} \mu\mu \text{ gm or pg})$$

$$MCH = \frac{Hb \text{ in } \mu\mu \text{ gm 100 ml blood}}{\text{Number of RBCs in million} / mm^3 \times 10^6 \times 10^5}$$

$$= \text{in } \mu\mu \text{ gm}$$

$$MCH = \frac{Hb (\text{gm}\%) \times 10^{12}}{RBC (\text{million} / mm^3) \times 10^{11}}$$

$$= \text{in } \mu\mu \text{ gm}$$

$$MCH = \frac{Hb (\text{gm}\%)}{RBC (\text{million} / mm^3)} \times 10$$

$$= \text{in } \mu\mu \text{ gm}$$

Normal : 27–32 mm gm/pg (picogram)

MCH decreases in iron deficiency anaemia.

Clinical Significance

Useful in laboratory classification of anaemia.

   (i) Normochromic anaemia MCH = 27–32 pg.

   (ii) Hypochromic anaemia MCH < 27 pg

3. Mean Corpuscular Haemoglobin Concentration (MCHC)

It is a percentage of Hb in relation to packed cell volume.

$$MCHC = \frac{Hb \text{ gm} / 100 \text{ ml}}{PCV / 100 \text{ ml}} \times 100$$

$$MCHC = \frac{Hb (\text{gm}\%)}{PCV (\%)} \times 100$$

$$= \text{in } \%$$

Normal: 32–38%

Clinical Significance

Normochromic anaemia: MCHC = 32–38%

Hypochromic anaemia: MCHC < 32%

4. Colour Index

It is the ratio of Hb% with RBC%.

$$CI = \frac{Hb\,\%}{RBC\ count\,\%}$$

Normal: 0.85–1.15

It is clinically insignificant index, because of vide variation in 100% Hb and 100% RBC count.

OBSERVATIONS AND CALCULATIONS
Objectives
At the end of practical student should be able to:
1. Calculate various blood indices.
2. Tell clinical significance of various blood indices.

QUESTIONS AND ANSWERS

1. Why double oxalate is used as an anticoagulant in this test?

Ans. Ammonium oxalate responsible for increase in size of the cells and potassium oxalate decreases the size of the cells, this is why only mixture of these two oxalate (double oxalate) is used as an anticoagulant in this test.

2. What is the buffy coat? What is its normal thickness?

Ans. There is a white layer on the column of the blood cells in the Wintrobe's tube which is called as buffy coat. This contains WBCs and platelets. It is about one mm in thickness.

3. When does buffy coat size increase?

Ans. Its thickness increases in leucocytosis, leukaemia and marked thrombocytosis.

4. Is there any difference between PCV of arterial and venous blood?

Ans. Because of the phenomenon of chloride shift venous blood cells are slightly larger in size as compared to arterial blood. This is why the PCV of venous blood is about 3 % higher than that of arterial blood.

5. What is the significance of PCV?

6. Enumerate physiological and pathological condition which cause decrease or increase in PCV.

7. What do you mean by MCV, MCH, MCHC, and colour index?

8. What is the clinical significance of MCV?

9. What is the clinical significance of MCH and MCHC?

Ans. Both are used to classify the anaemia. If the MCH and MCHC are decreased it is called as hypochromic anaemia. The MCHC is a better indicator as compared to MCH because there are less chances of error in MCHC.

10. Name the cause of Microcytic hypochromic anaemia.

Ans. Most common cause of microcytic hypochromic anaemia is iron deficiency.

11. In which condition there is macrocytic anaemia seen?

Ans. Deficiency of cynacobalamin (vitamin B_{12}) or folic acid (vitamin B_6).

12. What is the cause of normocytic normochromic anaemia?

Ans. Haemorrhage induced anaemia.

13. Is there a possibility of hyperchromic anaemia?

Ans. No, because RBC cannot accommodate more Hb than its capacity.

EXPERIMENT 1.12A

Determination of specific gravity of a given sample of blood by copper sulphate method

APPARATUS

Stock solution of copper sulphate ($CuSO_4$), distilled water, wide mouth glass bottle, blood sample and dropper.

Stock Solution

159 gm $CuSO_4 \cdot 5H_2O$ is dissolved in one litre of distilled water, specific gravity (SG) of this solution is 1.100. It is used to make the $CuSO_4$ solutions of different specific gravity.

PRINCIPLE

The specific gravity of blood is compared with copper sulphate solution of known specific gravity.

PROCEDURE

1. Prepare 100 ml $CuSO_4$ solution of specific gravity from 1.050 to 1.066 in wide mouth glass bottles as shown in Table 1.12a.1.

2. Add a drop of blood in each bottle by keeping the dropper one cm above the surface of the solution. Blood remains in the form of drop because a layer of copper proteinate is formed around blood.

3. Observe the behaviour of the drop in solution within 15 seconds. There are three possibilities (Fig. 1.12a.1).

    (i) Blood drop sinks in the solution and goes towards the bottom. Because specific gravity of solution is less.

    (ii) Blood drop goes in and comes out towards the surface of solution. It shows specific gravity of solution is higher than blood.

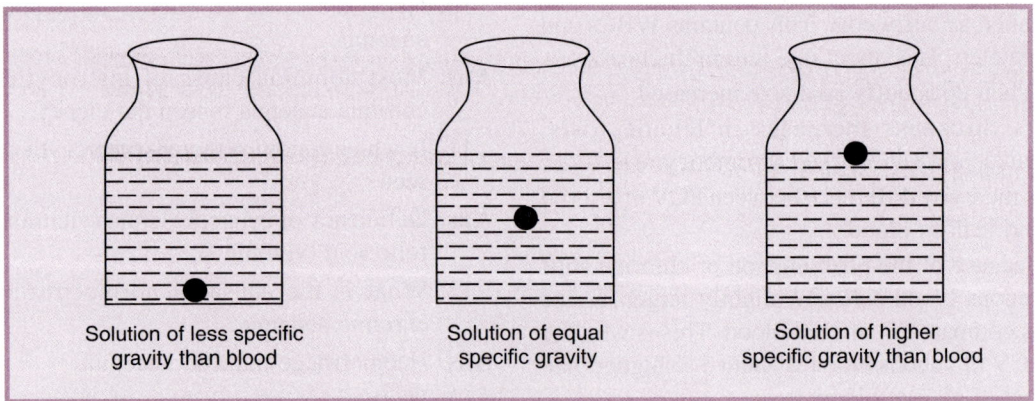

Fig. 1.12a.1: Position of blood drop in copper sulfate solution of different specific gravity.

Table 1.12a.1: Procedure to prepare CuSO₄ solution of different specific gravity.									
Bottle No.	1	2	3	4	5	6	7	8	9
CuSO₄ solution (ml)	49	51	53	55	57	59	61	63	65
DW (ml)	51	49	47	45	43	41	39	37	35
SG of solution	1.050	1.052	1.054	1.056	1.058	1.060	1.062	1.064	1.066

(iii) It goes in the solution and remains suspended in the solution. It is because specific gravity of solution is equal to that of blood. Note down the specific gravity of this solution. It will be the specific gravity of blood.

After 20 seconds all the drops in different bottles go towards the bottom in the solution because of formation of more copper proteinate and the drops become heavier.

Normal Value

Specific gravity of blood: 1.048–1.066

Specific gravity of plasma: 1.026–1.035
Specific gravity of RBCs: 1.092–1.095

Result

Precautions

1. Same size of blood drop should be added in each bottle. It can be done by using the same dropper.
2. Blood drop should be added from same height in each bottle.
3. Regarding position of blood drops observation should be made within 15 seconds.

QUESTIONS AND ANSWERS

1. What is the range of specific gravity of blood?
2. What are the physiological and pathological factors affecting SG of blood?

Ans. Factors affecting the specific gravity are:
   A. *Physiological factors:*
      (i) Sex: Less in female.
      (ii) Pregnancy: Less during pregnancy.
      (iii) Increase with high water in take.

   B. *Pathological factors:* Specific gravity increases when there is a loss of water from the body, e.g. vomiting and diarrhoea.
3. What determines the SG of blood?

Ans. RBC count, Hb concentration, plasma protein and water content are measure determinants of specific gravity of blood.
4. What change will be there in SG of blood in anaemia?

Ans. It will decrease.

EXPERIMENT 1.12B

To study the effect of hypotonic, hypertonic, isotonic saline, HCl and tanic acid

APPARATUS

Compound microscope, watch glass, few glass slides, 0.4% saline, 0.9% saline, 2% saline, N/10 HCl, tanic acid, pricking needle, and spirit swab.

PROCEDURE

1. Take 2 ml of 0.9% saline in a water glass.
2. Add a drop of blood after pricking the finger in all aseptic conditions.
3. Take a drop of suspended cells on a clean dry glass slide and cover it with coverslip.
4. Examine the cells first under low power and then in high power.
5. Take a drop of hypotonic saline (0.4%) on a glass slide and add a drop of cell suspension from watch glass. Wait for 5 minutes and examined under microscope after placing coverslip on it.
6. Similarly study the effect of hypertonic saline, 0.1 N hydrochloric acid, tanic acid, and alkali.

OBSERVATIONS

1. *Effect of normal saline:* Shape of RBCs is not disturbed.
2. *Effect of hypotonic saline:* Size of RBCs increases and burst RBCs can be seen.
3. *Effect of hypertonic saline:* Size of RBCs decreases and margin becomes crenated.
4. *Effect of N/10 HCl:* Haemolysed red cells are seen with brown acid haematin in the surrounding.
5. *Effect of alkali:* Lysed RBCs are seen.
6. *Effect of tanic acid:* Condensed Hb in the cell is seen.

EXPERIMENT 1.12C

Determination of osmotic fragility of erythro-cytes

APPARATUS

15 small test tubes, rack for holding tubes, long nozzle dropper, 0.5% NaCl solution and distilled water.

Osmotic Fragility

It is designed as the ease with which the cells are broken down in hypotonic solutions. It is expressed in terms of concentration of saline solutions in which cells are haemolysed.

Haemolysis begins at 0.42% saline solution and completes at 0.35% saline solution.

Indicator of haemolysis is appearance of red colour in mixture and when colour becomes saturated shows completion of haemolysis.

PROCEDURE

1. Take 15 small test tubes and keep them in rack.
2. Mark the test tubes W, 12, 13, 14 .... 23, 24 and S from 1st test tube to 15th.
3. Now add number of drops of 0.5% NaCl solution and distilled water as shown in Table 1.12c.1.
4. Add a drop of anticoagulant mixed blood with the help of a dropper in each test tube.
5. Shake each test tube gently to mix the blood and keep them for one hour.
6. After one hour check for haemolysis by observing the colour of mixture.
7. Note down the concentration of saline in which red colour just appears and concentration of saline in which intensity of colour becomes maximum (saturation of colour).
8. Just appearance of colour indicates beginning of haemolysis and saturation of colour indicates completion of haemolysis.

Table 1.12c.1: Procedure for preparation on increasing hypotonicity of NaCl solution.

No. of test tubes	Labelling of tube	No. of drops of 0.5% NaCl	No. of drops of distilled water	Concentration of saline
1	W	0	25	0
2	12	12	13	0.24
3	13	13	12	0.26
4	14	14	11	0.28
5	15	15	10	0.3
6	16	16	9	0.32
7	17	17	8	0.34
8	18	18	7	0.36
9	19	19	6	0.38
10	20	20	5	0.4
11	21	21	4	0.42
12	22	22	3	0.44
13	23	23	2	0.46
14	24	24	1	0.48
15	S	25	0	0.5

9. Residue at the bottom of tube can be used to see haemolysed cell under microscope.

OBSERVATIONS

Haemolysis starts at 0.42% saline solution.
Haemolysis completes at 0.35% saline solution.

RESULT

Osmotic fragility of RBCs ranges from 0.42% to 0.35% saline solution.

Precautions

1. Use the same dropper for adding 0.5% saline, distilled water and blood in all the test tubes.
2. Don't shake the tube vigorously for mixing blood drop in saline.
3. Take the reading exactly after one hour.

Clinical Significance

Test detects increased red cell fragility in patient with intrinsic or acquired red cells abnormality.

QUESTIONS AND ANSWERS

1. Define osmotic fragility of erythrocytes.
2. What are isotonic, hypotonic and hypertonic solutions?
3. What is haemolysis?
Ans. The haemolysis is the release of haemoglobin after breakdown of red blood cells.
4. What is the cause for haemolysis at lower concentration of saline solution?
5. What is the clinical significance of test?
6. Name some haemolytic agents.

Ans.   (i) Hypotonic saline.
    (ii) Acids and alkalies.
    (iii) Agglutinins.
    (iv) Snake venoms.

7. Name the conditions in which fragility of erythrocytes is increased?

Ans. Fragility of erythrocytes increases in hereditary spherocytosis and Glucose-6 phosphate dehydrogenase (G-6 PD) deficiency.

EXPERIMENT 1.13

Determination of reticulocyte count

APPARATUS

Glass slides, new methylene blue, 3% sodium citrate, 0.9% NaCl, incubator, compound microscope, cedar wood oil and pricking needle.

Vital stains used are:
1. 1 gm new methylene blue in
   100 ml citrate saline solution.
   (Citrate saline solution-1 volume of 3% sodium citrate solution + 4 volumes of 0.9% NaCl)
2. (i) Brilliant cresyl blue 1.0 gm
   (ii) Sodium citrate 400 mg
   (iii) 0.85 % NaCl 100 ml.

Reticulocytes

These are juvenile red cells. They contain ribosomes and ribonucleic acid (RNA) in their cytoplasm. Ribosomal material has the property of reacting with new methylene blue or brilliant cresyl blue to form a blue dots. This reaction takes place only in vitally stained unfixed preparations. Vital staining means the staining of cells after their somatic death but before their molecular death i.e. after their removal from the living body but before all cellular activity stops.

PRINCIPLE

Relative count of reticulocytes is done in relation to number of red cells after their identification among RBC. Reticulocytes are expressed as 1% age of RBCs.

PROCEDURE

1. Preparation of staining solution: Fresh mixture of new methylene blue is prepared citrate saline and filtered.
2. Preparation of blood film:
   - Take 2–3 drops of New methylene blue solution in a glass tube.
   - Add 4–8 drops of blood sucked in heparinised pipette on syringe.
   - Keep the tube in water bottle at 37°C for 15–20 min.
   - The red cells are then resuspended by gentle mixing and films are made on glass slides as usual way.
   - When dry films are examine under oil immersion objective.
3. Identification of reticulocytes and counting.
   - Reticulocytes contain blue coloured reticulum or blue dots in pale greenish blue cytoplasm.
   - RBCs are containing pale greenish blue cytoplasm without reticulum or dots.
   - For counting an area of film should be chosen where the cells are undistorted and staining is good. The reticulocytes are counted in 1000 RBC in different fields and entered in the following table.

Divide the total number of reticulocyte counted in 1000 cells by 10 to find percentage reticulocyte.

Absolute count (Reticulocyte/cu mm) can be calculated as follows:

Absolute count = % Reticulocyte ×
RBC count / cu mm

Observations

Field No.	Number of reticulocytes (1)	Number of RBC (2)	Total cell (1) + (2)
1.			$n1 = ...$
2.			$n2 = ...$
3.			$n3 = ...$
4.			$n4 = ...$
5.			$n5 = ...$
Total = $n1 + n2 + n3 + n4 + n5$		=	1000

Normal Value

Adult : 0.2 to 2.0%

Absolute count : 24000–84000 / cu mm

Newborn : 30–50 %

Increased reticulocyte count (Reticulocytosis) in:

1. Anaemia (During recovery).
2. After haemorrhage
3. Proliferation of bone marrow.

Decrease reticulocyte count in bone marrow depression

Objectives

At the end of the practical, the student should be able to:

1. Perform vital staining of reticulocytes with new methylene blue.
2. Prepare a slide with stained blood
3. Identify the reticulocytes in the film.
4. Perform and interpret relative reticulocyte count.

QUESTIONS AND ANSWERS

1. What is reticulocyte? What is its normal count in newborn and adult?
2. What are the physiological and pathological causes of reticulocytosis?
3. What is reticulocyte response?

Ans. When anaemia is treated with iron or folic acid reticulocyte count increases during recovery. This increase reticulocyte count is called as reticulocyte response.

4. What are the identifying features of reticulocytes?
5. What are the indications of doing reticulocyte count?

Ans. Indictions of reticulocyte count are:

(i) All conditions where reticulocytosis is suspected.

(ii) Aplastic anaemia.

(iii) Haemolytic anaemia.

6. What is vital staining? How it differs from supra vital staining?

Ans. Vital staining means the staining of cells after their somatic death but before their molecular death i.e. after their removal from the living body but before all cellular activity stops. Supra vital staining is the process *in vitro*, where stain reacts with the cells, when it is partly injured.

EXPERIMENT 1.14
Determination of platelets count

APPARATUS

Neubauer's chamber, RBC pipette, platelets diluting fluid (1.0% ammonium oxalate), compound microscope, coverslips, pricking needle, and spirit swab.

Function of platelets diluting fluid (1.0% ammonium oxalate):

1. Acts as anticoagulant.
2. Preserves the platelets.
3. Destroys RBCs and WBCs.

PRINCIPLE

Platelets are counted in diluted blood in Neubauer's chamber. Number of platelets counted then multiplied by dilution factor to calculate platelet count in undiluted blood.

PROCEDURE

1. Prick the finger under all septic conditions and suck the blood up to mark 0.5 in the RBC pipette.
2. After wiping off tip of the pipette, suck platelet diluting fluid up to mark 101.
3. Mix the solution and blood for 10 minutes so that there will be complete haemolysis of RBCs.
4. Discard first two drops of mixture and charge the Neubauer's chamber.
5. Wait for 15–20 min so that platelets will settle down.
6. Identify platelets and count them in 25 medium size RBC squares.

Platelets are 2–4 μm size non-nucleated cells. They are highly refractile in nature.

OBSERVATIONS

Enter the number of platelets counted in all RBC squares like $n1$, $n2$ ....$n24$, $n25$.

Total number of cells in all 25 RBC squares

$$= n1 + n2 + ... + n24 + n25 = N$$

CALCULATION

Volume of fluid in which cells are counted

$$= 1 \text{ mm} \times 1 \text{ mm} \times 0.1 \text{ mm}$$
$$= 0.1 \text{ cu mm}$$

Total number of cells in 0.1 cu mm

$$\text{Undiluted blood} = N$$

Number of platelets in 1 cu mm

$$\text{Undiluted blood} = N \times 10$$
$$\text{Dilution factor} = 200$$

Total number of platelets in undiluted blood

$$= N \times 10 \times 200 = N \times 2000$$

Result

Normal platelets count: 1.5– 4 lac / cu mm.

Variations in count:

1. Thrombocytosis: when platelet count is more than 4 lacs/cu mm.
2. Thrombocytopenia: when platelet count is less than 1.5 lac/cu mm

Objectives

At the end of the experiment student should be able to:
1. Fill the pipette with blood and diluting fluid.
2. Charge the Neubauer's chamber.
3. Identify the squares required for platelets count.
4. Identify and count the platelets.

Precaution

Same as in RBC count.

QUESTIONS AND ANSWERS

1. What are identifying features of platelets?
2. What is the composition of platelets diluting fluid?
3. What are the functions of ingredient of platelets diluting fluid?
4. What is the normal range of platelet count?
5. What are thrombocytosis and thrombocytopenia?
6. Enumerate the functions of platelets.

Ans. Platelets are playing role in:
  (i) Haemostasis (arrest of bleeding).
  (ii) Coagulation.
  (iii) Clot retraction.
  (iv) Storage of certain chemical substances, e.g. Histamine and 5 HT.
  (v) Phagocytosis of very small microorganisms (viruses) and particles.

7. What is purpura?

Ans. It is a condition in which there is a tendency to spontaneous bleeding usually beneath the skin, from the various mucous membranes and in internal organs. Purpura may be thrombocytopenic (when reduction in platelets count is decreased) or athrombocytopenic (platelets count normal).

8. What are the causes of thrombocytosis?

Ans. Common causes of thrombocytosis are:
  (i) After trauma, e.g. surgery and injury.
  (ii) Splenectomy.
  (iii) Haemorrhage.
  (iv) Injection of epinephrine (because of contraction of spleen).

9. What are the causes of thrombocytopenia?

Ans. Common causes of thrombocytopenia are:
  (i) Bone marrow depression.
  (ii) Hypersplenism.
  (iii) Leukaemia.
  (iv) Drug administration, e.g. Aspirin.

10. How platelets appear in Leishman's stain in peripheral blood smear?

Ans. In Leishman's stain platelets are seen in groups with light blue cytoplasm and reddish purple granules looking like nucleous, but no nucleus is present.

11. Name any other diluting fluid for platelet count.

Ans. Rees–Ecker fluid may also be used as a diluting fluid. It contains sodium citrate (anticoagulant), brilliant cresyl blue (staining platelets) and formaldehyde (fixative and lyses RBCs).

12. Explain that dilution factor is 200 in platelet count.

EXPERIMENT 1.15

Determination of absolute eosinophil count

APPARATUS

Eosinophil diluting fluid, WBC pipette, Neubauer's chamber, compound microscope, coverslips, pricking needle and spirit swab.

EOSINOPHIL DILUTING FLUID

1.0% solution of eosin in water = 5 ml

Acetone = 5 ml

Distilled water = 90 ml

Functions:

Eosin: Stains granules (red or pink)

Acetone: Lyses RBCs and other white cells

PRINCIPLE

Eosinophils are counted in diluted blood in Neubauer's chamber. Count is then multiplied by dilution factor to calculate eosinophil count in undiluted blood.

PROCEDURE

1. Get a prick in the finger under all aseptic conditions.
2. Discard first drop of blood and fill the WBC pipette up to mark 1.0 with blood from second drop.
3. Clean the tip of the pipette and suck eosinophil diluting fluid up to mark 11.
4. Mix the fluid and blood by rotating the pipette in between palms. Wait for 15–20 min for lyses of other cells.
5. Mix the fluid once again and discard two drops of fluid.
6. Charge the Neubauer's chamber.
7. Count the eosinophil in 4 WBC squares under low power. In case of doubt cell can be confirmed under high power.

OBSERVATION

Enter the cells in squares (Fig.1.15.1) as shown below:

Total number of cells counted in WBC squares

$= x_1 + x_2 + x_3 + x_4 = x$

No. of cells $= x_1$

No. of cells $= x_2$

No. of cells $= x_3$

No. of cells $= x_4$

CALCULATION

Dilution factor = 10

Volume of fluid in which eosinophils are counted

$$= (1 \text{ mm} \times 1 \text{ mm} \times 0.1 \text{ mm}) \times 4$$
$$= 0.4 \text{ cu mm}$$

Number of eosinophils in 0.4 cu mm volume $= x$

No. of eosinophils in 0.1 cu mm of diluted blood

$$= x \div 4$$

No. of eosinophils in 1.0 cu mm of diluted blood

$$= (x \times 10) \div 4$$

No. of eosinophils in 1.0 cu mm of undiluted blood

$$= (x \times 10 \times 10) \div 4 = x \times 25$$

Result

Absolute eosinophil count $= x \times 25$ /cu mm

Normal Eosinophil count: 10–400 /cu mm

Variation: Eosinophil count increases in allergic conditions and parasitic manifestations.

Precaution

Same as in total leucocytic count.

OBJECTIVES

At the end of the class student should be able to:

1. Identify the eosinophils.
2. Perform absolute eosinophil count.
3. Tell the clinical significance of the investigation.
4. Charge Neubauer's chamber.

No. of cells=x_1 No. of cells=x_2

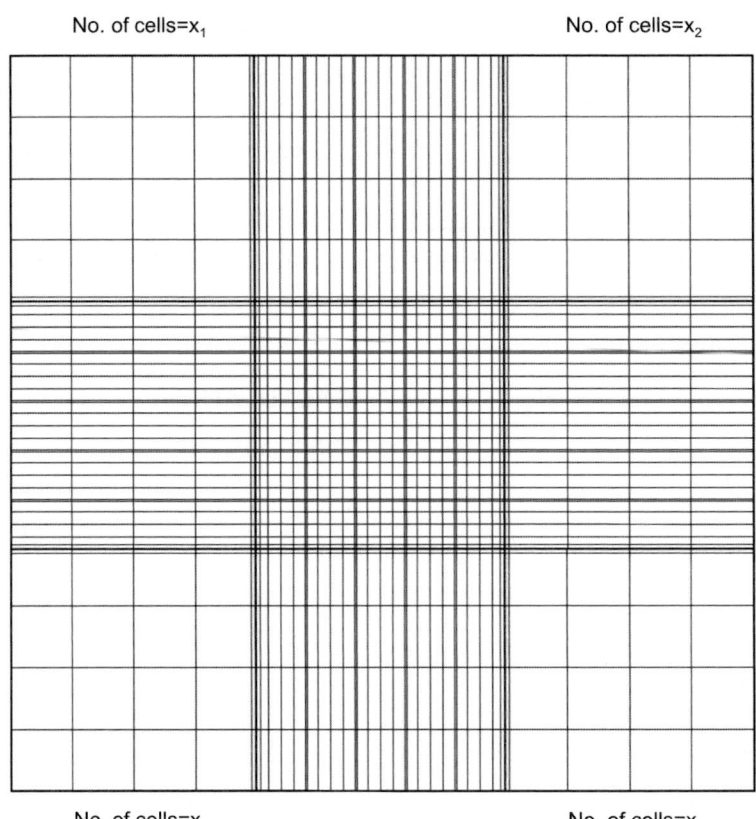

No. of cells=x_3 No. of cells=x_4

Fig. 1.15.1: Eosinophil counting squares (WBC squares).

QUESTIONS AND ANSWERS

1. What is the normal absolute eosinophil count?
2. Enumerate the conditions causing increase in eosinophil count.
3. Mention any other diluting fluid for eosinophil count.

Ans. Pilot's solution. It contains phloxine, propylene glycol, sodium carbonate and heparin.

4. What are the functions of eosinophils?

Ans. Functions of eosinophils are:
   (i) They are phagocytic but less motile.
   (ii) Their granules are lysosomal in character.
   (iii) There is a very high content of peroxidase enzyme (parasiticidal).
   (iv) It limits the effects of mediators of allergic reactions.

5. What is the clinical significance of test?

Ans. To find out whether patient is suffering from eosinophilia. Eosinophil count is increased in different allergic conditions, worm infestations and in pulmonary eosinophilia.

6. Why the diluting factor is 10 in eosinophil count?

<table>
<tr><td>

EXPERIMENT 2.1

General apparatus used in the amphibian experiments

</td></tr>
</table>

APPARATUS

Experimental physiology is concerned with the study of living tissues and their responses to various stimuli. So in the laboratory there is need of a living tissue, a stimulating device and a device to record the responses of a tissue.

1. Living Tissue

For nerve muscle experiment frogs are preferred because of

(i) Frog is a cold blooded animals so the survival of a preparation is better as compared to warm blooded animals.

(ii) Easily available and easy to handle.

(iii) Easy to dispose off after experiment.

2. Stimulating Device

Stimuli can be mechanical thermal, chemical, and electrical.

Electrical stimuli are usually used to stimulate the tissue because of:

(i) Its site, intensity, frequency, timing and duration can be easily and accurately controlled.

(ii) It is least injurious with threshold strength.

(iii) Electrical stimuli can be produced easily with the help of induction coil or with the help of student stimulation (electronic stimulator).

3. Recording Device

Responses of living tissue is recorded by using a writing lever (capillary per ink writer or a pointer) which writes on the white paper or smoked paper pasted on a kymograph drum or on physiograph.

1. Induction Coil

(i) It is used to convert direct current into induced current (Faradic current). Induced current is produced only at the time of make and break of the circuit.

(ii) It consists of two coils, primary and secondary (Figs 2.1.1 and 2.1.2). These are made of well insulated copper wire wound on a soft iron core. Number of turns in primary are about 250–500 and in secondary about 7000–8000.

(iii) Terminals of primary coil are connected to DC source of about 10 volts and terminals of secondary are connected to stimulating electrodes.

(iv) Primary coil is fixed and secondary coil slides on two metallic horizontal bars.

(v) Secondary coil can also be adjusted at different angles ($0°$–$90°$) in relation to primary coil.

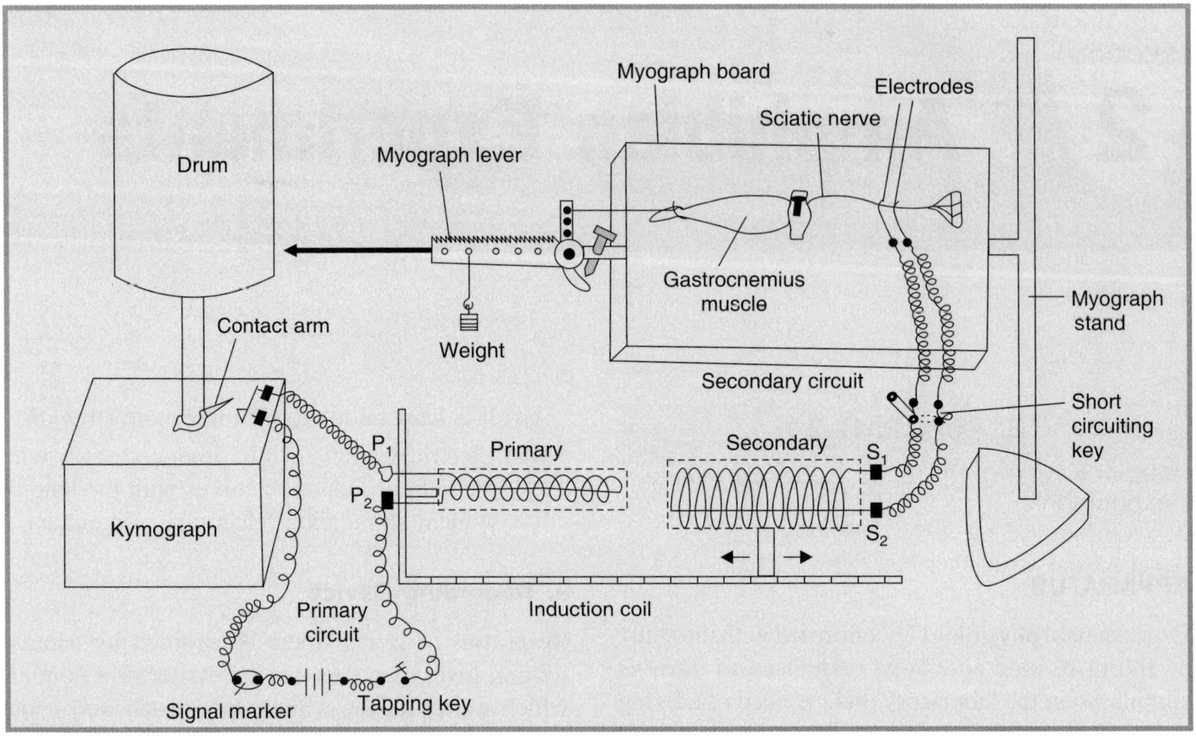

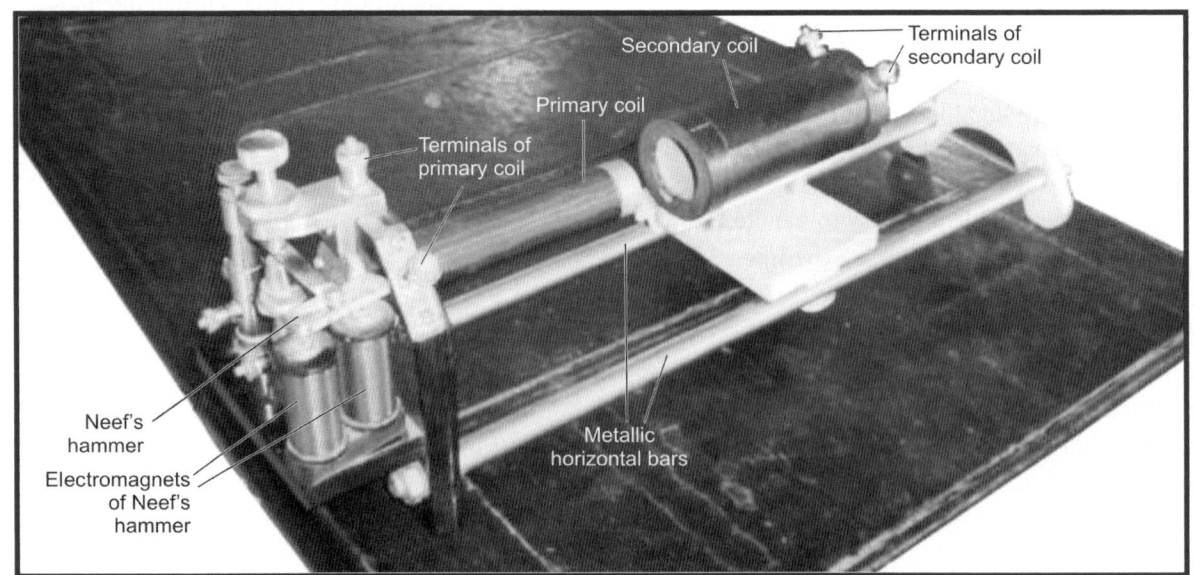

Fig. 2.1.1: Connections and arrangement to record simple muscle twitch from gastrocnemius muscle and sciatic nerve of frog.

Fig. 2.1.2: Induction coil.

(vi) Almost no current is produced in secondary coil, when the angle between primary and secondary coil is 90°. With decrease in angle, strength of current produced in secondary increases and it is maximum when angle is 0° (when it is parallel) at particular distance from the primary coil.

(vii) Strength of induced current further increases when distance between two coils decreases and it is maximum when secondary coil is overlapping the primary coil.

(viii) At the time of make (on) induced current in the secondary coil is in the opposite direction which tries to resist the change in the magnetic flux (rate of change of magnetic flux is lesser) around the secondary coil.

(ix) At the time of break (off) induced current produced in the secondary coil is in the same direction which does not resist the fall of magnetic flux around the secondary coil (rate of change of magnetic flux is higher). This why at the time of break the strength of induced current is greater than at the time of make.

2. High Volume Mains

It is a routine domestic electricity supply of 220 volt. It is used only in kymograph and student stimulator. (No other stimulator used in amphibian experiment, is connected to it.)

3. Low Voltage DC

Its strength varies from 4 to 10 volt, supplied by step down transformer (central transformer) working at 220 volt AC routine supply of electricity. Two terminal of primary coil of induction coil are connected to low DC supply. Other instruments like signal marker (time marker) and various keys are connected with this low voltage supply.

4. Simple Key and Tap Key (Fig. 2.1.3)

Used in low voltage DC supply to put the circuit on and off.

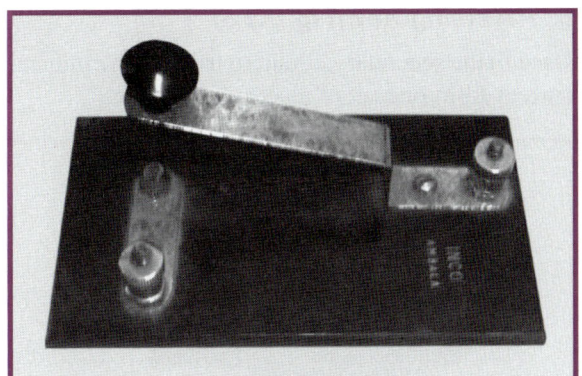

Fig. 2.1.3: Tap key.

5. Short Circuiting Key (Fig. 2.1.4)

It is used in the secondary circuit to make the circuit short, when we do not want to stimulate the tissue. It protects the tissue from unwanted damage because of accidental passage of induced current. It is normally kept closed and open only at the time of stimulation.

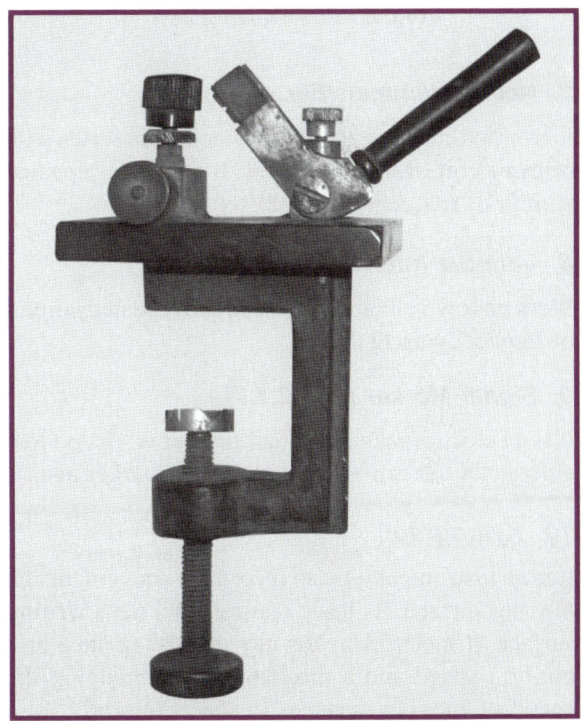

Fig. 2.1.4: Short circuiting key

6. Reversing Key (Fig. 2.1.5)

Used in the secondary circuit to transfer the induced current from one set of electrodes to other.

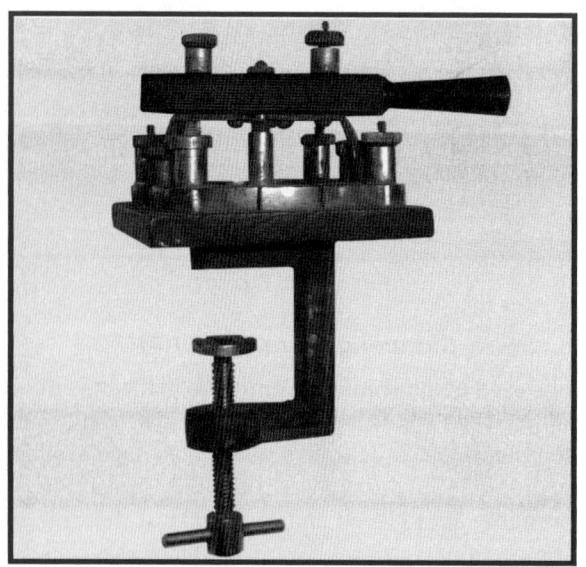

Fig. 2.1.5: Reversing key.

7. Neef's Hammer (Fig. 2.1.2)

It is an automatic interrupter connected in series with primary coil of induction coil. It provides repeated stimuli of frequency 40–100/sec.

8. Variable Interrupter (Fig. 2.1.6)

Work on low voltage DC to produce repeated stimuli of frequency up to 25/sec.

9. Signal Marker (Fig. 2.1.7)

It is an electromagnetic signal marker works on low voltage DC. It can be used as a time marker also.

10. Kymograph

It is an instrument used to record the movements on moving surface. Its basic features include a writing surface, a mechanism for moving the surface at a uniform speed and a mechanism for changing the speed of moving surface. In the commonly used kymographs, there is a cylindrical drum mounted

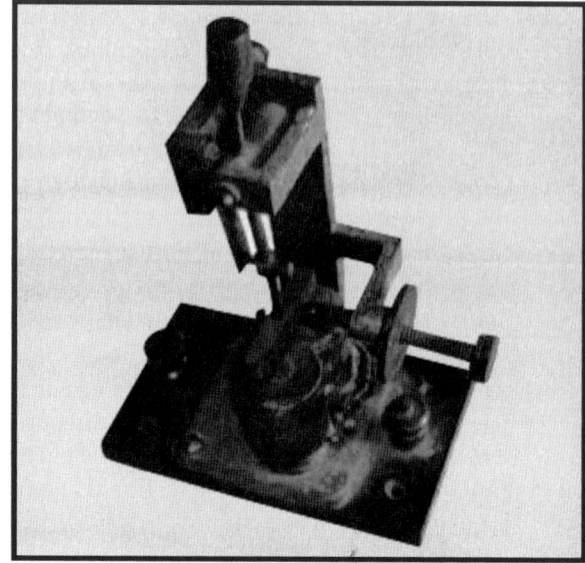

Fig. 2.1.6: Variable Interrupter.

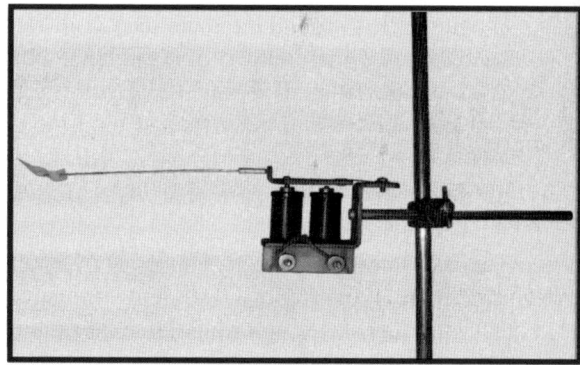

Fig. 2.1.7: Signal marker.

on a vertical shaft, which is run by an electric motor (Figs 2.1.1 and 2.1.8). This electrical motor runs on 220 volt AC. Speed at which drum moves varies from 0.12 mm to 640 mm/sec. It is adjusted with the help of clutch and gears. There are two metallic strikers (contact arms) at the base of the shaft which can be made to separate widely or brought together to coincide with each other. On rotating the shaft they strike against a contact point (contact knob) which is pressed and the circuit is completed (Primary circuit). Two contact arms are used to give the two stimuli at different time intervals in a single revolution of drum.

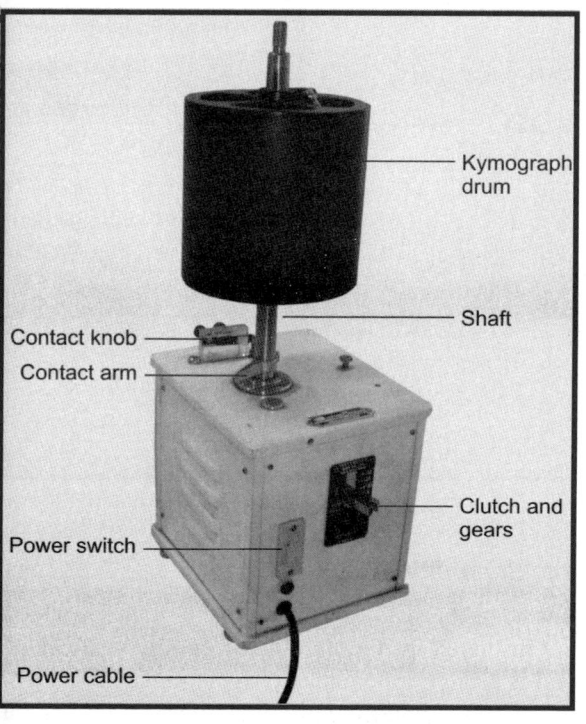

Fig. 2.1.8: Kymograph.

General instructions for use of kymograph

(i) Place the recording lever to the right of the kymograph so that the paper on the revolving drum slides from under the pen and not against it.

(ii) The writing point should lightly touch the recording surface and at a tangent to it.

(iii) Start writing from a point about a centimeter to the right of the joint in the paper.

(iv) Avoid spilling of ringer solution or saline over the kymograph as it is liable to spoil the electric wiring. If there is any spilling, wipe it promptly.

(v) Levelling of the kymograph must be done with help of levelling screws present at the base.

(vi) Always use clutch when ever you rotate the drum manually.

11. Myograph Board and Myograph Stand

Myograph board is a rectangular wooden board with a cork sheet is fixed on it (Fig. 2.1.9). Board is fixed on myograph stand with one end and at the opposite end of the board myograph lever is fixed.

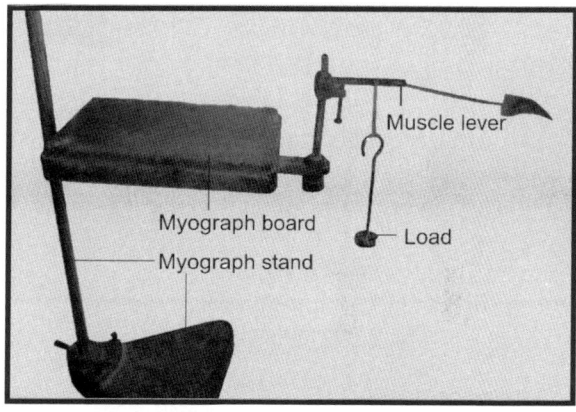

Fig. 2.1.9: Myograph board and stand.

12. Muscle Trough/Lucas Chamber

It is a rectangular porcelime chamber with outlet in the bottom which is guarded with a rubber tube and a clamp. A cork is also fixed it the bottom for fixing the muscle/tissue. A pair of electrode is fixed on the wall of the chamber. Myograph lever is fixed in the chamber.

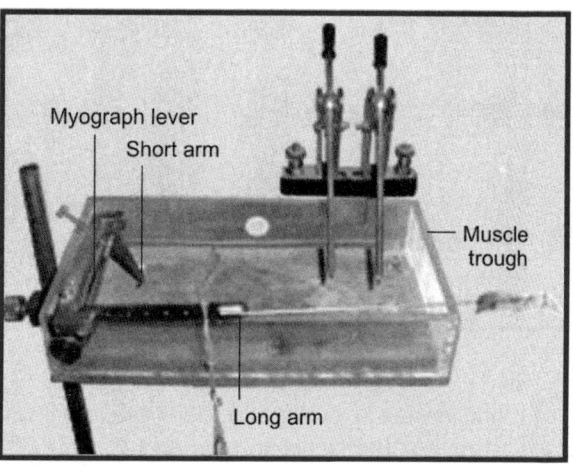

Fig. 2.1.10: Muscle trough and myograph lever.

13. Recording Levers

Muscle lever: It is isotonic liver. It is fixed with myograph board (Fig. 2.1.11).

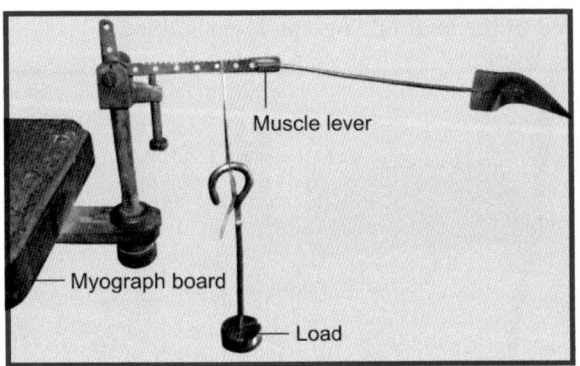

Fig. 2.1.11: Muscle lever.

Myograph lever (Fig. 2.1.10) is used to record the mechanical respond of muscle stimulation. It has two arms: short arm and long arm. Short arm is used to tie the tendon of the muscle and long arm is used to record the contraction. It is isotonic lever.

Starling Heart Lever (Fig. 2.1.12): It is used to record weak contractions like mechanical activity of the heart. It is isotonic lever.

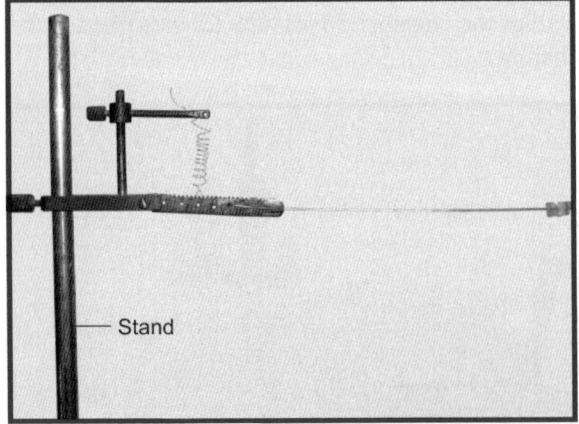

Fig. 2.1.12: Starling heart lever.

Frontal writing lever (Fig. 2.1.13): Isometric lever used to record intestinal movements and frog's mechanical cardiogram.

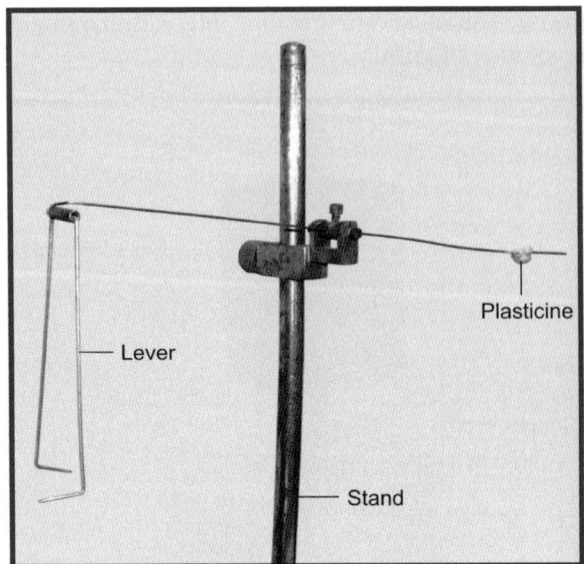

Fig. 2.1.13: Frontal writing lever.

14. Stimulating Electrode

These are basically two thick metallic wires which are insulated from each other. It has two ends. One end is brought in contact to tissue to be stimulated. Other end is connected to induction coil or student stimulator.

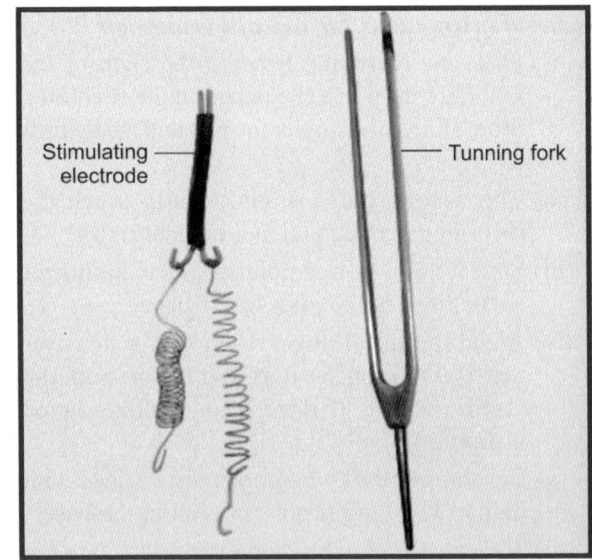

Fig. 2.1.14: Stimulating electrode and tunning fork.

15. The Student Physiograph

The student physiograph is a complete system design with couplers, matching transducers and pick-ups. It comprises of the following parts:

- The main console
- Couplers
- Transducers
- Accessories like electrodes, junctional boxes, etc.

The Main Console

This is the main body of the physiograph (Figs 2.1.15a to c). It has:

1. Main 'on' and 'off' switch of the motor which moves the paper.
2. Speed range selector for different speeds.

3. Speed selector push button for selecting the desired speed out of mentioned speeds above these buttons.
4. Pen lift knob.
5. Window for paper feeding.
6. Ground terminal for grounding the physiograph.
7. Sensitivity selector: To select desired sensitivity.
   Sensitivity selector: Used to calibrate the system (Fig. 2.1.15c).
8. Knob for pen position: To adjust base line of recoding.
9. Switch of 50 Hz filter for filtering the artifacts of this frequency.
10. Ink wells contain ink for recording.

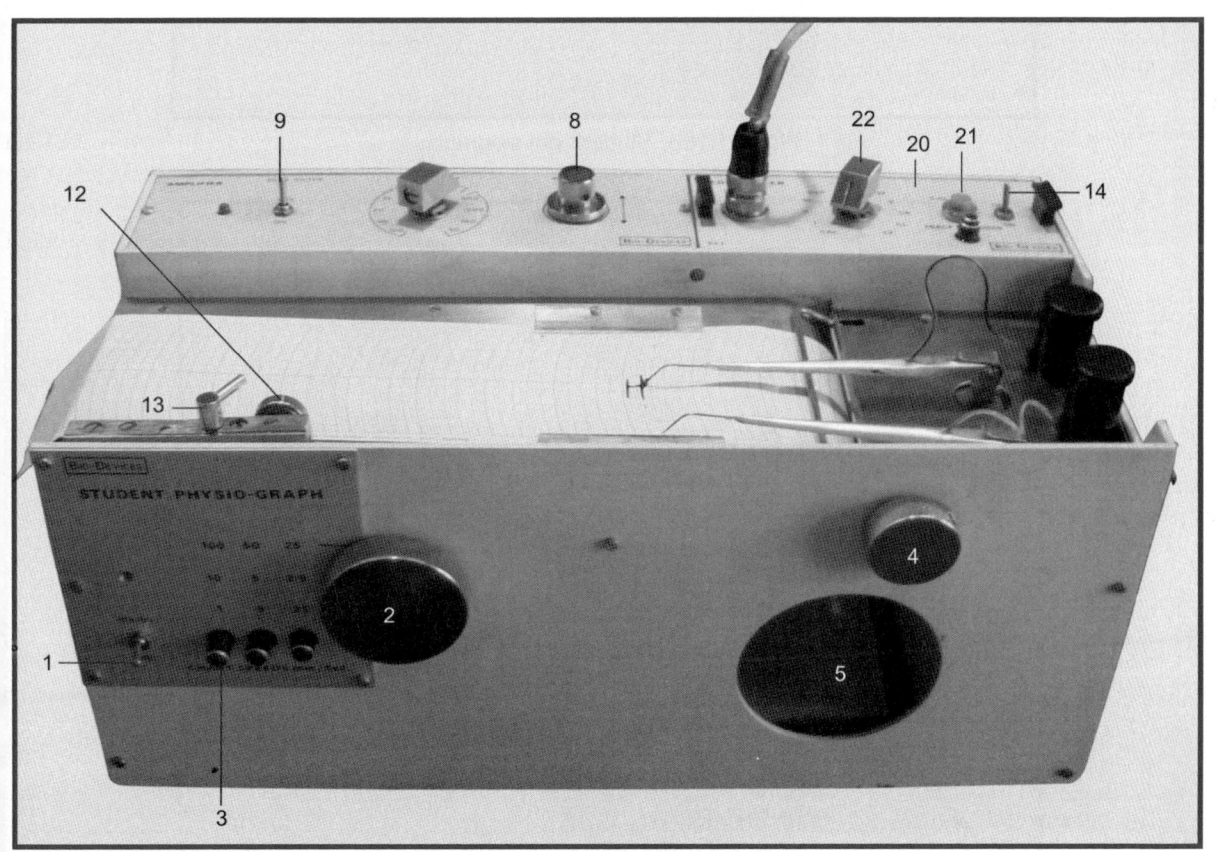

Fig. 2.1.15a: Student physiograph.

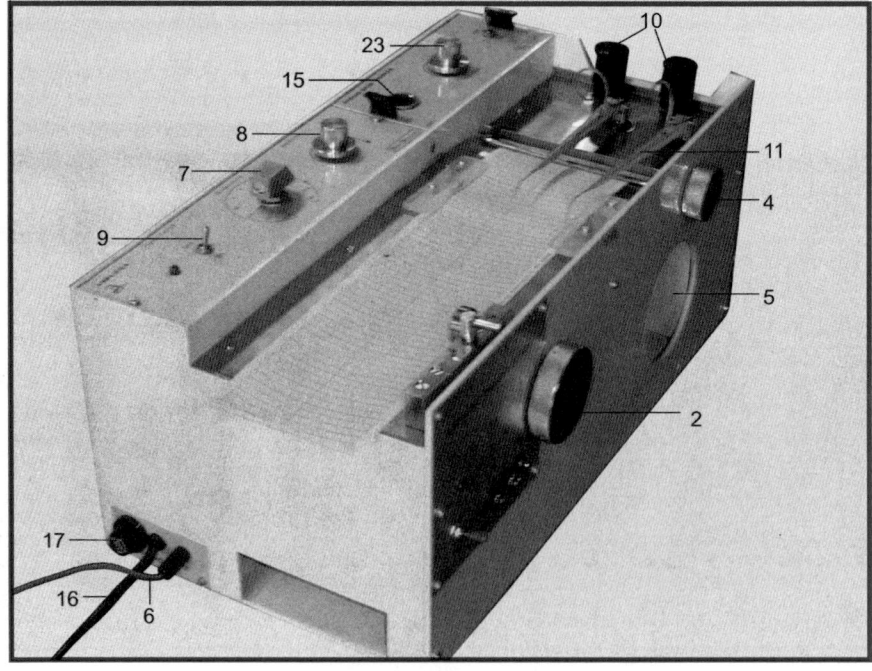

Fig. 2.1.15b: Student physiograph.

Fig. 2.1.15c: Student physiograph.

11. Pen: For recording the parameter.

12. Paper drive bearing: For movement of the paper.

13. Thumb screw: Screw for 'on' and 'off' of the speed of the paper during recording.

14. 'on' and 'off' switch on coupler.

15. Input socket: To connect the transducer to the coupler.

16. Power cable: 220 volt AC current.

17. Fuse.

18. Stimulator socket: To connect electronic/student stimulator.

19. Input and output socket: To connect more than one physiograph to show the same recording simultaneously at different places.

20. EKG coupler: To record ECG.

21. Calibration switch.

22. Lead selector: To select leads for ECG recording

23. Respiration coupler.

Couplers

Different types of couplers are there for recording different types of activity. Main couplers are:

1. *Biopotetial coupler:* For recording electro-cardiogram (ECG), electromyogram (EMG), electroencephalogram (EEG) and electro-retinogram (ERG).

2. *Strain gage coupler:* Used to record various parameters like blood pressure, arterial and venous pulse, heart sounds, plethysmography, all experiments of frog and experiment with isolated tissues.

3. *Pulse respirator coupler:* To record pulse and respiratory movements and volumes.

4. *Temperature coupler:* To record temperature experimental animal.

Transducers

This is a device which converts different forms of energy in electrical energy so that it can be recorded.

There are different types of transducers to record different types of activity. Main transducers are:

1. Force transducer

2. Pressure volume transducer

3. Volume transducer

4. Pulse transducer

5. Respiration transducer

6. Temperature transducer

16. Student Stimulator

Student stimulator (electronic stimulator): It works at 220 volt AC. This is designed for use with Physiograph. It is used to provide stimuli of different duration, strength and frequency. It is also used for marking the events (Time as well as other events). It can also give twin stimuli.

Electrical Circuits

When induction coil is used to stimulate the tissue, there are two circuits primary and secondary as shown in Figs 2.1.16.

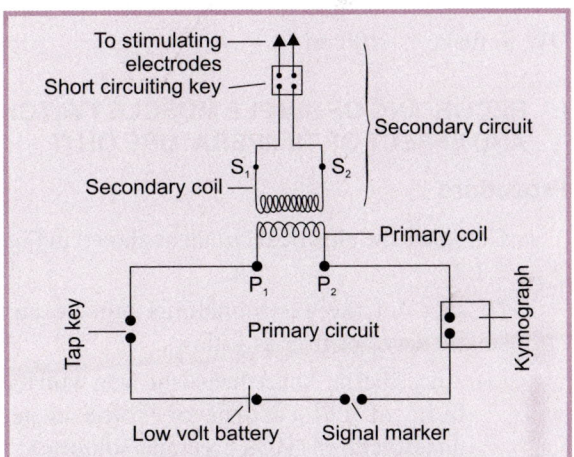

Fig. 2.1.16: Primary and secondary circuit. S_1, S_2: Terminals of secondary coil. P_1, P_2: Terminals of primary coil.

EXPERIMENT 2.2

Demonstrate the following with gastrocnemius muscle and sciatic nerve preparation of frog
  I. Recording of simple muscle twitch and effect of temperature on it.
  II. Effect of strength of stimulus on muscle contraction.
  III. Conduction velocity of sciatic nerve.

APPARATUS

Kymograph with drum, myograph lever, myograph board, tapping key, ringer solution or isotonic saline (0.6%), induction coil, thermometer, weights, tunning fork (100 Hz) and cotton swabs.

Composition of Ringer Solution:

NaCl	:	0.65 gm (maintains isotonicity).
KCl	:	0.014 gm (excitation and contraction).
$CaCl_2$	:	0.012 gm (excitation and contraction).
$NaHCO_3$	:	0.020 gm (maintain pH)
NaH_2PO_4	:	0.001 gm (maintain pH)
Dextrose	:	0.1 gm (provide nutrition)
DW to make	:	100 ml

I. RECORDING OF SIMPLE MUSCLE TWITCH AND EFFECT OF TEMPERATURE ON IT

Procedure

1. Complete the electrical circuit as shown in Fig. 2.1.1.
2. Dissect out the gastrocnemius muscle and sciatic nerve of frog as follows:
   (a) Anaesthesia: Anaesthetise the frog with the help of chloroform or some other anaesthetic (5–10% urethane solution).
   (b) Pithing:
      • Using a cotton cloth hold the frog in your hand, keeping its head flexed in such a way that your index finger lies just at external nares and thumb below the forelimbs on the dorsal surface of the frog; rest of the fingers lie on ventral surface below the forelimbs.
      • Take a pithing needle in your right hand and hold it firmly and place its pointed end at the midline at an angle of about 30° between the eyes of the frog and pull it up to the lower level of the tympanic membrane where you feel the depression.
      • Push the needle at this point into the skull of the frog and destroy the brain by giving the circulatory movements to its pointed end.
      • Pull back the needle and change its direction to about 180° towards the vertebral canal and push it into the canal; it leads to contraction of muscles of the trunk and hindlimbs.
      • Destroy the spinal cord by giving the axial movement to the pithing needle. When the spinal cord is destroyed hindlimbs hang limply and loosely; this shows that pithing is over.
   (c) Dissection:
      • Cut through the skin with scissors completely around the trunk just below the forelimbs.

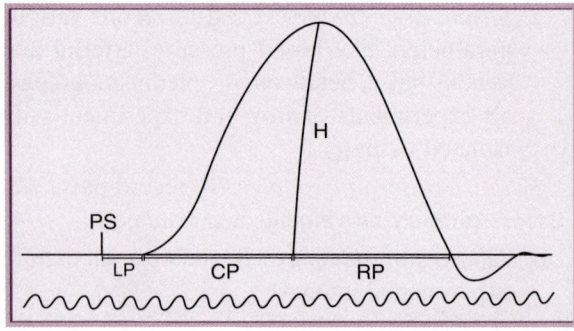

Fig. 2.2.1: Simple muscle twitch with various time periods. (PS: point of stimulus, LP: latent period, CP: contraction period, RP: relaxation period, H: height of contraction).

- Hold the frog below the forelimbs with the help of thumb and fingers of left hand firmly.
- Seize the skin in between the thumb and fingers of right hand with the help of piece of cloth and strip off the skin up to the toes of hindlimbs.
- Place the frog on its ventral surface.
- Lift the urostyle with the help of a forceps and give a cut just below it.
- Cut the muscles attached on its both the sides with the help of a scissor; take care that you should not damage the nerves just underlying the urostyle.
- Extend these lateral cuts forward and cut through the hopp gridle on either side with a bone cutter. As the urostyle is lifted, sciatic nerves can be seen emerging from the vertebral column.
- Cut the vertebral column above and below the exit of sciatic nerves.
- Divide this piece of vertebral column in two halves at midline with a bone cutter.
- Lift up each piece and free the attached tissues. Cut off the nerve fibres going to the nearby structures taking care not to injure the sciatic nerve. Observe that sciatic nerve is entering in the thigh muscles.
- Cut the fascia covering the thigh muscles and separate the muscles with the help of thumb and fingers; now sciatic nerve becomes visible.

- Further separate these muscles very carefully with the help of a blunt glass rod; pass the glass rod below the nerve and separate it out of the muscles up to the knee joint.
- Cut the various branches of the nerve going to the thigh muscles.
- Cut the thigh bone (femur) just above the knee joint with the help of bone cutter and cut the thigh muscles also at the same level.

3. Transfer the preparation and fix on myograph board (Frog board) as shown in Figs 2.1.1 and 2.1.9.
4. Apply the load about 10 gm (according to need) for proper recording of muscle twitch.
5. Find out threshold strength of stimulus by adjusting the distance between primary and secondary coils.
6. Mark the point of stimulus manually by moving lever up when contact arm just touches the contact knob.
7. Now record the simple muscle twitch on fast moving drum (640 mm/sec).
8. Take time tracing with help of vibrating tunning fork (100 cycle/sec) at the base of the twitch.
9. Take the marking on the twitch with the help of writing lever by bringing the pointer at the top of the twitch up to the base line on stationary drum (Fig. 2.2.1).
10. Record the two more twitches after pouring warm and cold ringer solutions (Fig. 2.2.2).

OBSERVATION AND RESULT

S.No.	Temperature of ringer (Degree C)	Latent period (m sec)	Contraction period (m sec)	Relaxation period (m sec)	Height of contraction (cm)
1	Room temp. (25 °C)				
2	Warm ringer (40 °C)				
3	Cold ringer (10 °C)				

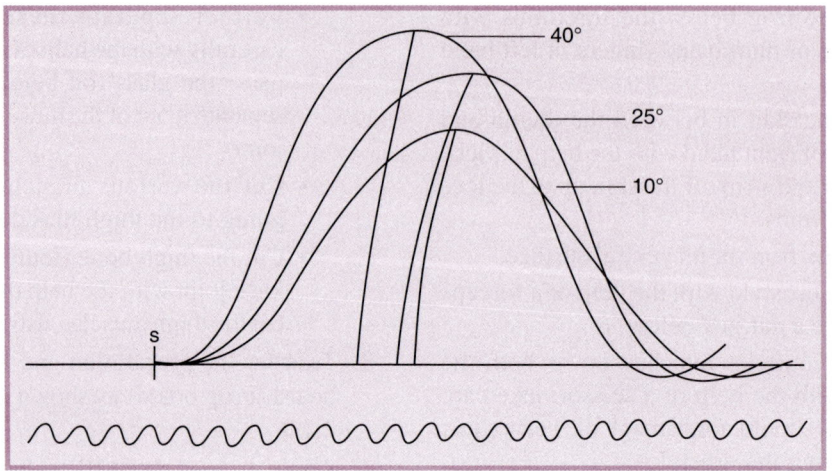

Fig. 2.2.2: Three different twitches taken after pouring ringer solution of different temperatures.

Precautions

1. Must note the temperature of ringer solution.
2. Keep pouring ringer solution to prevent during the preparation.
3. Pour ringer solution for 1–2 min of different temperature then record the twitch.

II. EFFECT OF STRENGTH OF STIMULUS ON MUSCLE CONTRACTION

Procedure

1. Kymograph is replaced by signal marker in the primary circuit. Rest of the circuit is same as shown in Fig. 2.1.1.
2. Adjust the secondary coil from primary at maximum distance and try to record simple muscle twitch on stationary drum.

3. Decrease the distance by 1.0 cm each time and record the response by rotating the drum 1.0 cm manually.
4. Continuously record the response till get maximum response and there is no further increase in height of contraction.
5. Mark the distance carefully on the drum in relation to stimulus applied (Fig. 2.2.3).

Precautions

1. Give 1–2 minutes gap between two stimuli to avoid beneficial effect.
2. Keep the preparation wet by pouring ringer solution repeatedly.
3. Avoid unnecessary stimulation to prevent fatigue.

RESULT AND DISCUSSION

S.No.	1	2	3	4	5	6	7	8
Distance between primary and secondary coils (cm)								
Height of twitch (cm)								

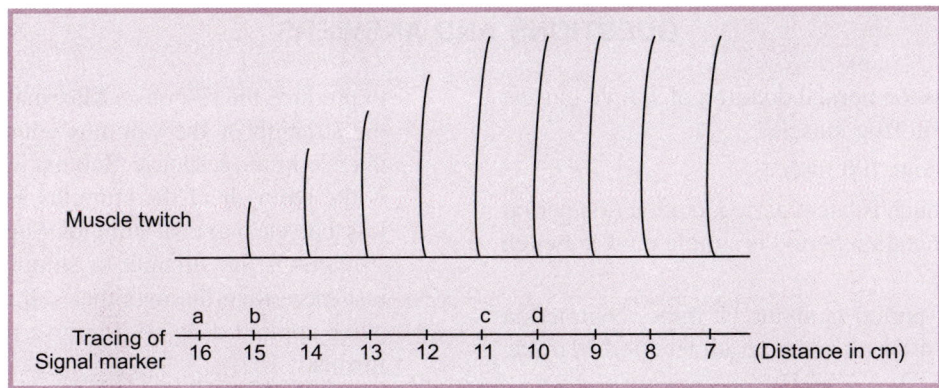

Fig. 2.2.3: Muscle twitch on stationary drum with increase in strength of stimuli. (a—Subthreshold, b—Threshold, c—Maximal, d—Supramaximal).

III. CONDUCTION VELOCITY OF SCIATIC NERVE

Procedure

1. Electrical circuit and fixing of preparation is same as in simple muscle twitch.
2. Record the simple muscle twitch by stimulating sciatic nerve at muscular end and mark the twitch ME.
3. Record the another twitch with same point of stimulus by stimulating nerve at vertebral end and mark the twitch VE.
4. Take time tracing with the help of tunning fork (100 cycles/sec).
5. Measure the length of nerve between two points where electrodes were placed to record two twitches.
6. Find out the latent periods of both the twitches (Fig. 2.2.4).

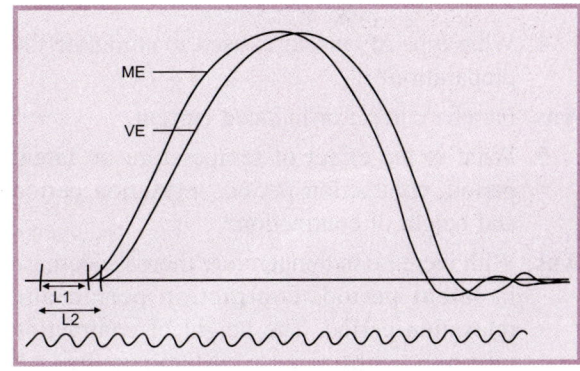

Fig. 2.2.4: Two simple muscle twitches when stimulated at muscular end (ME) and at vertebral end (VE). L_1 and L_2 are latent periods in respective twitches.

CALCULATION AND RESULT

Difference between latent periods of two twitches $(L1 - L2) = t$ sec.

Length of the nerve between two points where electrodes applied = d meters.

$$\text{Conduction velocity} = \frac{\text{Distance travelled}}{\text{Time taken by stimulus from vertebral end to muscular end}}$$

$$= \frac{\text{Length of nerve between two points (m)}}{\text{Difference in latent periods (sec)}}$$

$$= \text{m/sec}$$

Precautions

1. Remove the ringer solution or saline from frog board with the help of cotton swab.
2. Electrode should be placed as close as possible at muscular end and vertebral end.

QUESTIONS AND ANSWERS

1. What is the normal duration of simple muscle twitch in frog muscle?

Ans. It is about 100 msec.

2. How much is latent period, contraction period and relaxation period is simple muscle twitch of frog?

Ans. Latent period is about 10 msec, contraction period 40 msec and relaxation period 50 msec.

3. What is the strength of normal saline for frog tissue?

Ans. Strength of normal saline for frog's tissue is 0.65%.

4. What type of current is used to stimulate the preparation?

Ans. Faradic current or induced current.

5. What is the effect of temperature on latent period, contraction period, relaxation period and height of contraction?

Ans. With increase in temperature there is decrease in latent period, contraction period and relaxation period. The height of contraction increases with increase in temperature. All these effects are produced because of stimulation of various enzymes which responsible for increase in conductance of various ions and increase in metabolism.

6. What is the effect of temperature on velocity of contraction of muscle?

Ans. Velocity of contraction of muscle increases with increase in temperature. It is because of decrease in viscosity and increase of force of contraction.

7. Define threshold, subthreshold, submaximal, maximal and supramaximal stimuli.

Ans. Threshold stimulus is the minimum strength of stimulus which produces the response when applied for a sufficient time. Subthreshold stimulus is the strength of the stimulus just less than the threshold stimulus which is not able

to produce the response. Maximal stimulus is the strength of the stimulus which produces the maximum response. Submaximal stimulus is the strength of the stimulus which is just less than the maximal stimulus. Supra-maximal stimulus is the strength of stimulus which is just more than the maximal stimulus. Which when applied does not improve the response further.

8. Why with increase strength of stimulus height of contraction increases?

Ans. With increase in strength of the stimulus there is recruitment of more and more motor units having higher threshold. This is why with increase in strength of stimulus there is increase in height of contraction. At maximal stimulus there are firing of all the motor units and there is a maximum height of contraction.

9. Why does supramaximal stimulus not increase height of contraction?

Ans. At maximal stimulus there are firing of all the motor units and there is a maximum height of contraction. This is why further increase in strength of stimulus to supramaximal there is a no more increase in height of contraction.

10. What is motor unit?

Ans. A motor unit is consisted of a single motor neuron and the number of muscle fibres supplied by it.

11. How is power increased in muscles in infact body?

Ans. It is done by increase in the discharge in motor neurons leading to more and more recruitment of motor units.

12. Does motor unit follow all or none law?

Ans. Yes, motor unit follows all or none law.

13. What is the normal conduction velocity of sciatic nerve in frog?

Ans. It is about 10 m per second.

14. What are the factors affecting conduction velocity of nerve?

Ans. Conduction velocity of a nerve is affected by following factors:

   (i) Diameter of nerve fibres present in the nerve.

   (ii) The myelination of the fibres.

   (iii) Temperature, with increase in temperature there is increase in velocity.

15. What is the clinical importance of conduction velocity of nerve in human?

Ans. It is helpful to find out whether defect in nerve or some other tissue during trauma or in recovery phase of it. Other pathological factors are there which affect the conduction velocity of the nerve.

EXPERIMENT 2.3

Demonstrate the following on gastrocnemius muscle and sciatic nerve preparation of frog
- I. Effect of two successive stimuli applied at different time intervals.
- II. Genesis of tetanus.

I.   EFFECT OF TWO SUCCESSIVE STIMULI APPLIED AT DIFFERENT TIME INTERVALS

Apparatus

Same as in simple muscle twitch.

Procedure

1. Record a simple muscle twitch as described in Experiment 2.2.

2. Separate the contact arm (strikers) in such a way that second stimulus will fall in early part of latent period of first stimulus and record the simple muscle twitch.

3. Repeat the same procedure in such a way that second stimulus falls.
   - (i) In second fall of latent period.
   - (ii) In contraction period.
   - (iii) In relaxation period.
   - (iv) Immediately after relaxation period of first twitch.

Result and Discussion

Precautions

Same as in simple muscle twitch.

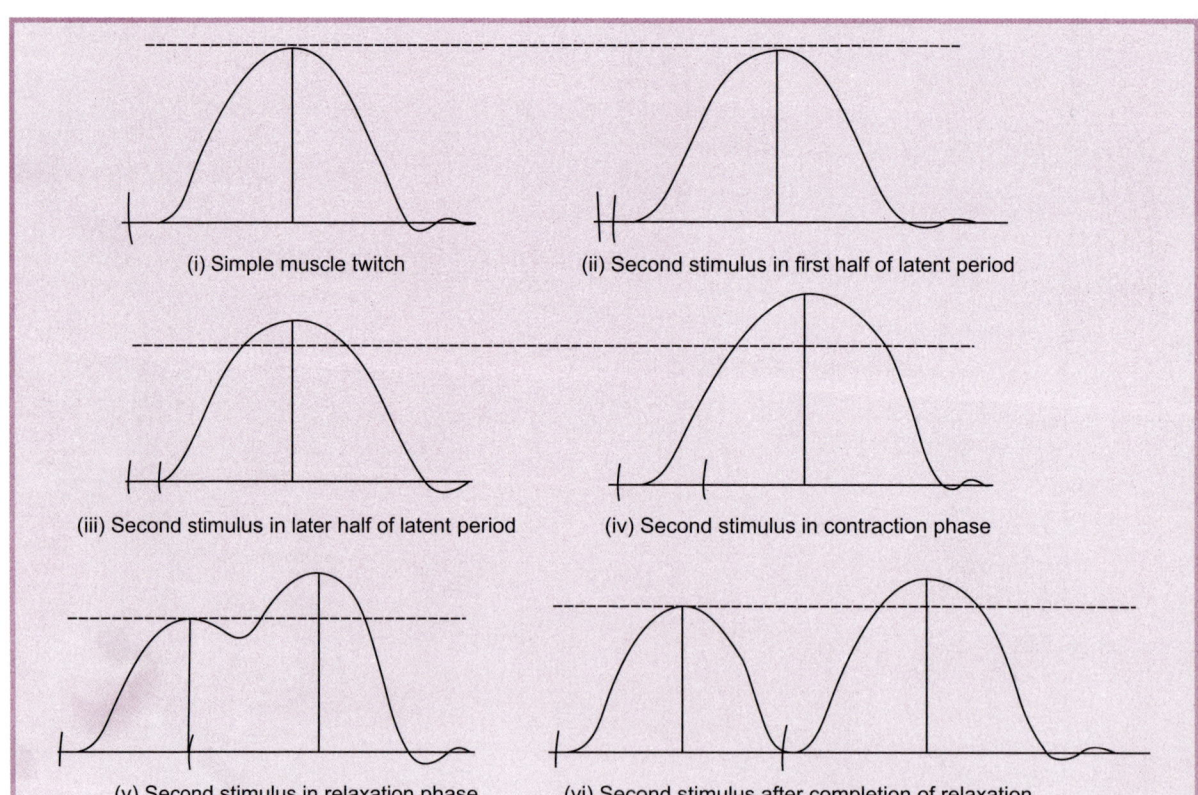

(i) Simple muscle twitch

(ii) Second stimulus in first half of latent period

(iii) Second stimulus in later half of latent period

(iv) Second stimulus in contraction phase

(v) Second stimulus in relaxation phase

(vi) Second stimulus after completion of relaxation

Fig. 2.3.1: Simple muscle twitch with two successive stimuli.

II. GENESIS OF TETANUS

Apparatus

Same as in simple muscle twitch except variable interrupter and signal marker.

Procedure

1. Arrange the muscle nerve preparation as for simple muscle twitch.
2. Remove kymograph from the primary circuit and add variable interrupter in the circuit.
3. Now record simple muscle twitches at slow speed (12.5 mm/sec) with frequency of stimuli above 5/sec.
4. Increase the frequency of stimuli 10 and 20 per second and take the record.
5. Now remove the variable interrupter from primary circuit and include Neef's hammer of induction coil in the primary circuit and adjust frequency of stimuli 30 and 50/sec and take the recording again. Nerve can be stimulated with the help of student stimulation (Electronic stimulation) with different frequency of stimuli (variable interrupter gives low frequency of stimuli up to 25–30/sec and Neef's hammer gives higher frequency of stimuli 40–100/sec).

Precautions

1. Prevent drying of preparation.
2. Avoid unnecessary stimulation of the preparation.

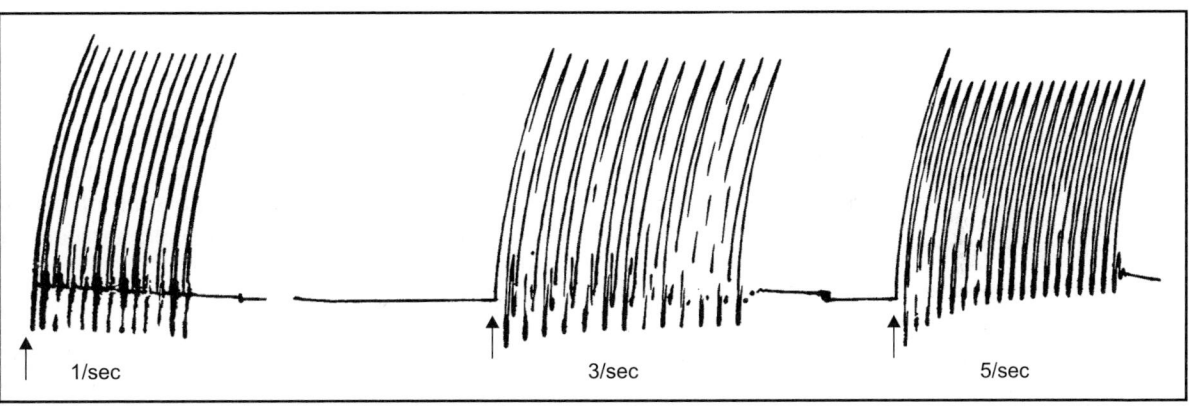

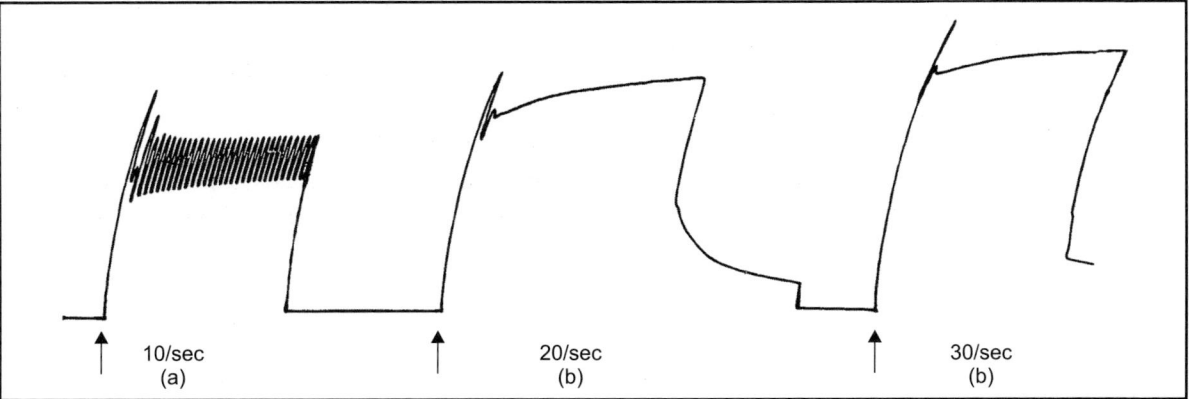

Fig. 2.3.2: Effect of frequency of stimuli on gastrocnemius muscle contraction. (a) clonus (b) complete tetanus.

QUESTIONS AND ANSWERS

I. Effect of Two Successive Stimuli Applied at Different Time Intervals

1. What is beneficial effect?

Ans. There is a gradual rise in the height of first three or four contractions when stimulated successively just after relaxation of muscle each time. The important reasons underlying the phenomenon are:

   (i) Available of more Ca^{++} at actin-myosin site because of incomplete withdrawal of these ions during relaxation.

   (ii) Increase in the temperature of muscle.

   (iii) Decrease in internal viscosity of muscle.

2. What is summation of effect?

Ans. When the second stimulus is given to the tissue after the refractory period of the first is over it leads to further development of tension.

3. What is summation of stimuli?

Ans. When preparation is stimulated repeatedly with sub-threshold stimuli it produces response. This is called as summation of stimuli.

II. Genesis of Tetanus

1. What do you understand by incomplete and complete tetanus?

Ans. In incomplete tetanus there is slight relaxation in between the contractions. In complete tetanus there is no relaxation at all.

2. What type of activity is involved in maintenance of posture?

Ans. Incomplete tetanus type of contractions are present in maintaining the posture. The asynchronous discharge of nerve fibers causes smooth muscle contractions.

3. What is clonus?

Ans. It is a state of incomplete tetanus.

4. Can you calculate tetanizable frequency for a given simple muscle twitch?

Ans. Yes. It can be calculated by dividing one second by contraction period of that muscle. E.g. Contraction period of a muscle = 0.04 sec or 40 m sec. Tetanizable frequency for that muscle = $1 \div 0.04 = (1000 \div 40) = 25$ per sec.

5. How does tetanus differ from tetany?

Ans. Tetanus is a state of sustain contraction because of repeated stimulation and tetany is because of deficiency of calcium ions in the body which causes hyperexcitability of neural tissue.

6. What is pathological tetanus?

Ans. It produced because of toxins of certain anaerobic bacteria.

7. What is physiological contracture?

Ans. When fatigue sets in, the muscle is unable to relax fully and remains in a state of partial contraction called physiological contracture or contraction remainder.

8. What is rigor?

Ans. Removal of calcium ions from actin-myosin site is a active process, a decrease in ATP during fatigue not allowing the muscle to relax and there is state of muscle contraction called rigor. When it occurs after death it is called as rigor mortis.

9. Why the cardiac muscle cannot be tetanized?

Ans. Cardiac muscle is having a long refractory period this is why it cannot be tetanised.

EXPERIMENT 2.4

Demonstrate the following on gastrocnemius muscle and sciatic nerve preparation
   I. Effect of load on muscle performance.
   II. Phenomenon of fatigue.

APPARATUS

Same as in simple muscle twitch.

I. Effect of Load on Muscle Performance

Load can act on muscle in two situations—after load and free (pre) load.

- After load means load acts on muscle after contraction.
- Free load (pre-load) means load acts on muscle even before contraction and it exert stretch on muscle.

Effect of load in both the situation can be studied on fast moving drum and also on stationary drum.

PROCEDURE

A. *Recording on Fast moving Drum*

1. Arrange the nerve muscle preparation as for simple muscle twitch.
2. Add 10 gm weight to lever about 1 cm from fulcrum.

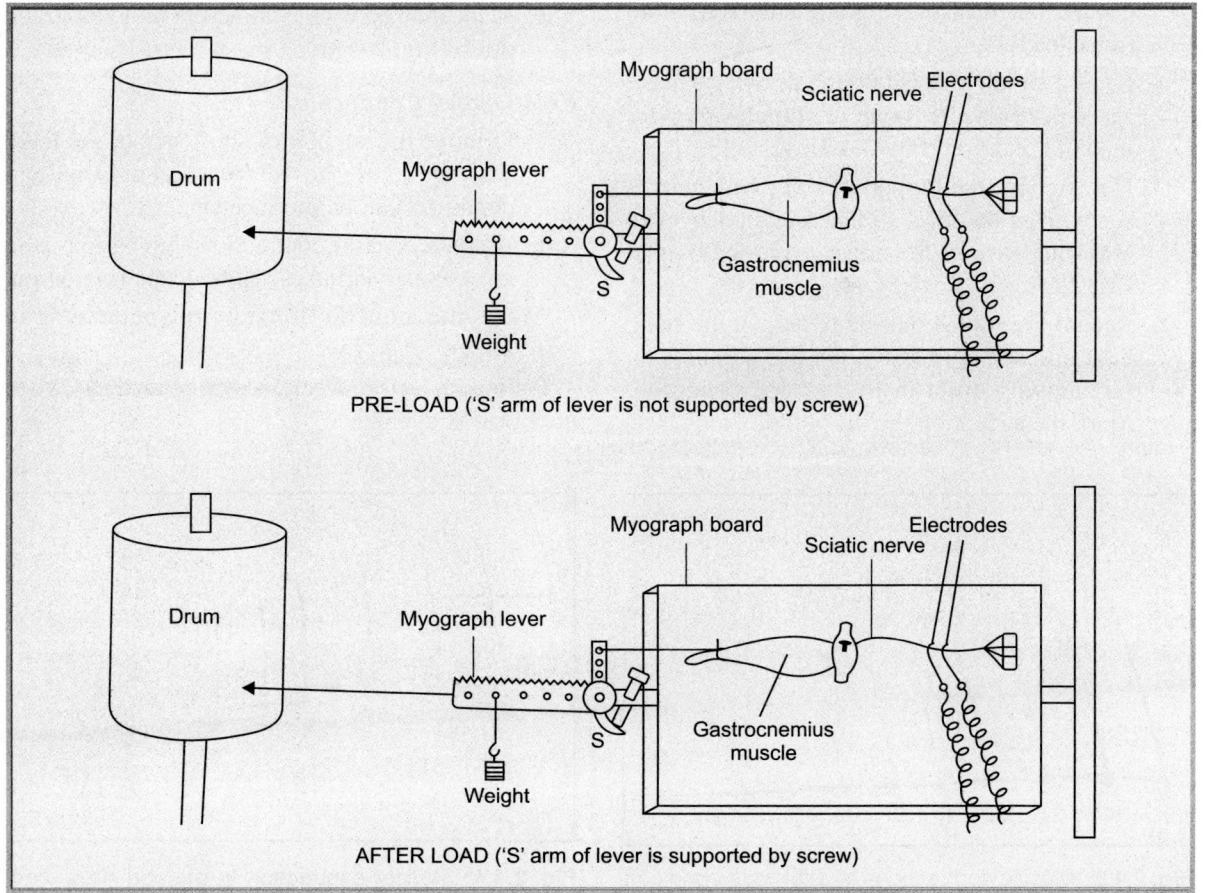

Fig. 2.4.1: Myograph lever in preload and after load condition.

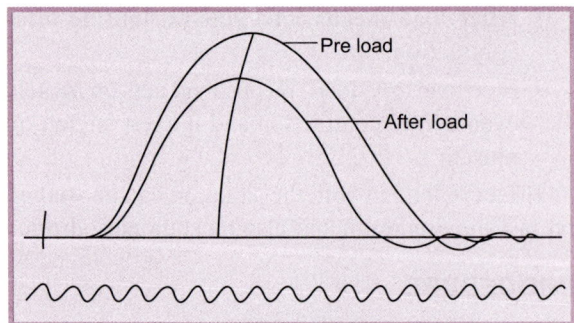

Fig. 2.4.2: Simple muscle twitches in preload and after load condition on fast moving drum.

3. Support the myograph lever with the help of the screw shown in Fig. 2.4.1 so that load will not act on muscle at resting (relaxed) state (after load).

4. Record simple muscle twitch at 640 mm/sec. speed of drum after point of stimulus, in after load of condition (Fig. 2.4.2).

5. Now remove the support of lever with help of screw from the level so that weight acts even at resting state of the muscle (pre-load) as in Fig. 2.4.1.

6. Record the simple muscle twitch on the same base line and with same point of stimulus on fast moving drum in free loaded condition. Mark the switch on the drum free.

B. Recording on Stationary Drum

After Loaded Condition

1. Exclude the kymograph from the primary circuit.

2. Support the myograph lever with screw to produce after loaded condition.

3. Record the contraction of muscle with adding any load on lever on stationary drum.

4. Move the drum manual 1 cm and add a load of 10 gm on lever and record the contraction.

5. Now goes on increasing the load on lever 10 gm each time and record the contraction on stationary drum till load goes up to 90–100 gm.

6. Mark load on each contraction on kymograph drum (Fig. 2.4.3).

Free Loaded Conduction

1. Remove the support of short arm of the lever with help of the screw so the free load condition can be produced.

2. Again record the contraction with various load on stationary drum as in after loaded condition.

Mark the contractions with specific load (Fig. 2.4.4).

As load is acting freely base line changes when next load is applied.

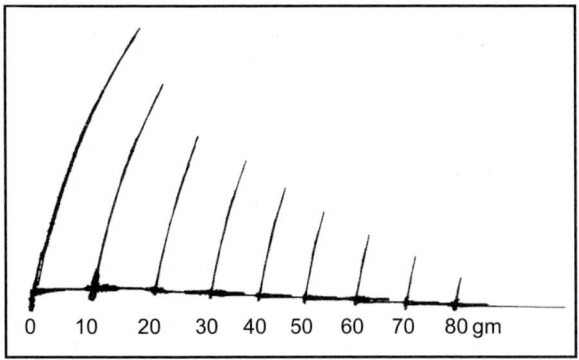

Fig. 2.4.3: Muscle contractions in after load condition with different loads in gm (on stationary drum with ink writer).

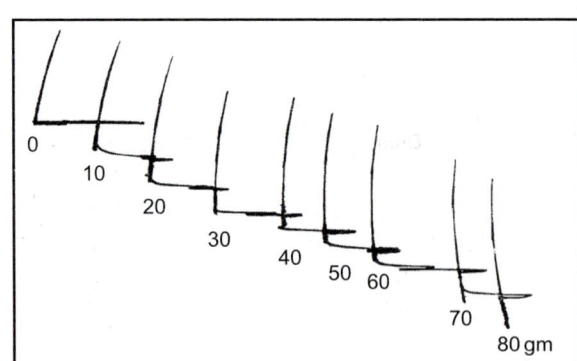

Fig. 2.4.4: Muscle contraction in preload (free load) condition with different loads in gm (on stationary drum with ink writer).

Calculation of Work Done

Height which is recorded is not the actual height to which weight is lifted.

To find out actual height we have to measure (Fig. 2.4.5):

1. Length of the lever (from fulcrum to writing point) = L
2. Distance between fulcrum and point where load added to the lever = l

3. Height of contraction on kymograph = H
4. Actual height to which load is lifted (h)
   = $(l \times H) \div L$ (Fig. 2.4.5)
5. Work done = Force × Distance
   = Load × actual height to which
     load is lifted
   = W × h   gm cm/kg m
   = m × g × h
   (Ergs = gm × 981 × cm)

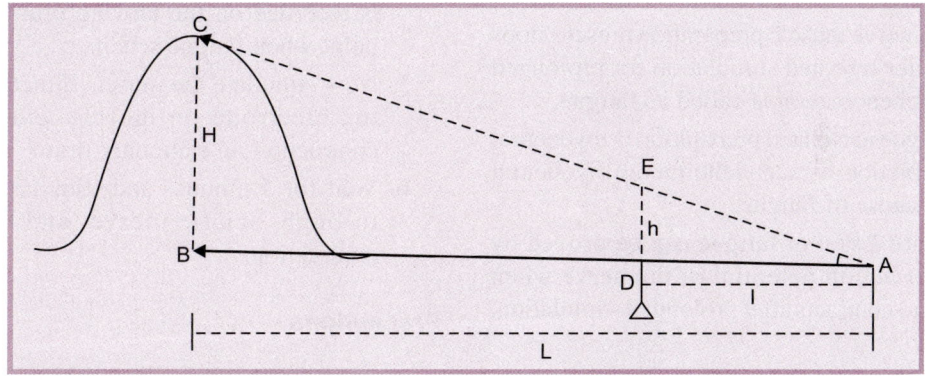

Fig. 2.4.5: Similar triangles ABC and ADE to calculate actual height (h) to which the load is lifted (A fulcrum).

RESULT AND DISCUSSION

Tabulate your data as follows

	After loaded condition	Free loaded condition
A. Simple muscle twitch:		
I. Latent period		
II. Contraction period		
III. Relaxation period		
IV. Height of cont.		
B. Work done (ergs) 90-100		
Load		
10 gm		
20 gm		
30 gm		
40 gm		
50 gm		
60 gm		
70 gm		
80 gm		
90 gm		

Precautions

1. Same as in simple muscle twitch recording.
2. Wait for one minute before recording the next contraction with different load to avoid beneficial effect.
3. Do not alter the strength of stimuli once adjusted.

II. PHENOMENON OF FATIGUE

Fatigue

In an isolated nerve muscle preparation muscle stops to contract after repeated stimulation for prolonged period. This phenomenon is called as fatigue.

Site of fatigue in isolated preparation is myoneural junction. Depletion of acetylcholine at myoneural junction is a cause of fatigue.

Nerve is not a seat of fatigue can be proved by recording the action potential of the nerve when muscle stops to contracts after prolonged stimulation.

Procedure

1. Arrange the nerve muscle preparation as for recording simple muscle twitch.

2. Repeatedly stimulate the nerve and record 1st, 2nd, and 3rd contraction by keeping the point of stimulus same. Mark these twitches on the drum.
3. Keep the point of stimulus same and move the writing point away from the drum for above 10 contraction and then record the 11th contraction by bringing the writing point closer to the drum (Fig. 2.4.6).
4. Repeat the same procedure till no contraction is recorded on the moving drum. This is the point when fatigue sets in.
5. Now stimulate the muscle directly by putting the electrode on muscle and record the contraction on stationary drum.
6. Wait for 5 minutes and stimulate the muscle through sciatic nerve and record the contraction.

Precautions

1. Same as in simple muscle twitch recording.
2. After appearance of fatigue stimulate the muscle immediately.

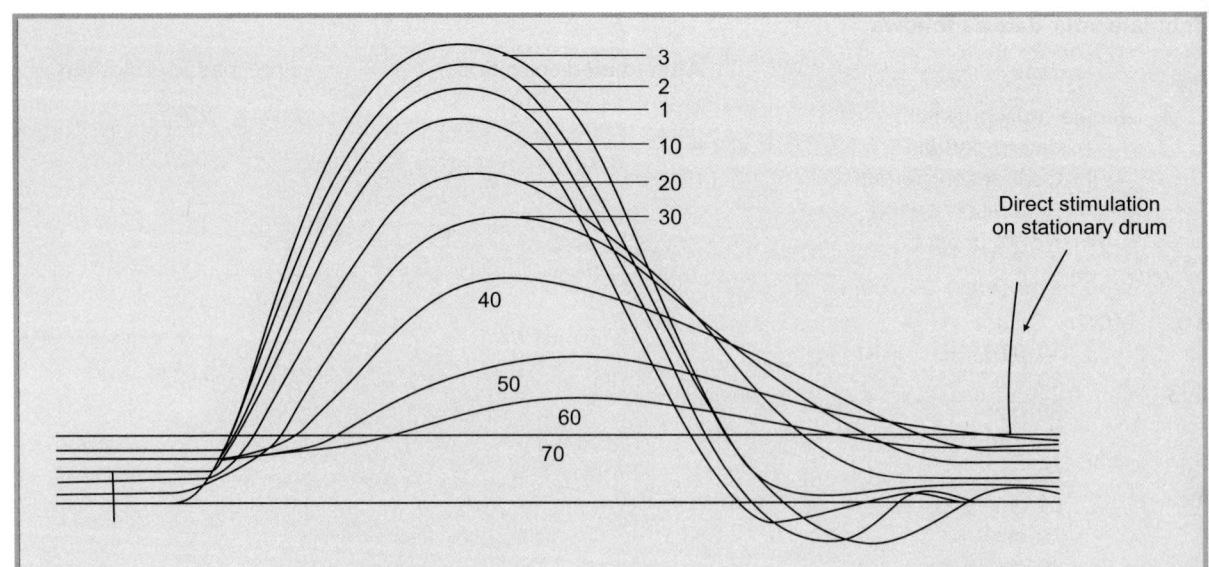

Fig. 2.4.6: Muscle curves show fatigue as a result of repeated stimulation on fast moving drum

RESULT AND DISCUSSION

Tabulate the observations as follows

S. No. of contraction	Latent period	Contraction period	Relaxation period	Amplitude of contraction
1				
2				
3				
10				
20				
30				
40				
50				
....				
....				

QUESTIONS AND ANSWERS

I. Effect of Load on Muscle Performance

1. What do you understand by free loaded and after loaded conditions?

Ans. *Free loaded (pre-loaded) condition:* This is the condition in which load acts on the muscle even before its contraction. In this situation muscle remains stretched at resting state.

After loaded condition: In this condition load is not acting on muscle in resting state, it acts only when muscle contracts.

2. What is optimum load in after loaded conditions?

Ans. Optimum load is a load at which tension developed is maximum or work done is maximum.

3. Why the performance of muscle is better in free loaded condition than after loaded condition?

Ans. In pre-loaded condition better performance of muscle is because of:

(i) The muscle is stretched in pre-load condition. The length of muscle is more in preload as compared to after load so the number of cross linkages between actin and myosin are more in this condition. In after load condition muscle is not stretched.

(ii) With further increase in load there is increase in length of the muscle in pre-load condition. In after load condition there is no change in the length of muscle with increase in the load.

(iii) Elastic component of muscle remain stretched in pre-load condition not in after load.

4. Why work done increases in free-loaded condition up to optimum level and after this work done decreases?

Ans. When the muscle is taken out of the body its length decreases and this length is called equilibrium length. With increase in load sarcomere length increases which leads to increase in number of cross bridges so work done by the muscle increases. It goes on increasing till maximum number of cross bridges are achieved at optimum length. After this number of cross bridges decreases again and work performance decreases.

5. What is the length tension relationship is skeletal muscle?

Ans. Tension developed in the skeletal is directly proportional to its initial length. It becomes maximum at optimum length. After optimum length it decreases.

6. Define resting length, equilibrium length, initial length, and optimum length.

Ans. *Resting length:* It is the muscle length at which it is present under natural conditions in the body in relax state. It is also called as optimum length, at this length active tension developed in the muscle is maximum.

Equilibrium length: It is the length of the relaxed muscle cut free from its bony attachments.

Initial length: It is the muscle length before it begins to contract.

7. What is the relevance of this experiment to medical physiology?

Ans. To understand the concept that muscles are present in the body in free-loaded condition and show the maximum performance.

II. Phenomenon of Fatigue

1. Define fatigue.
2. What is the site of fatigue in isolated preparation of nerve and muscle?
3. What is the site of fatigue in intact body?

Ans. Possible sites of fatigue in intact body are:
   (i) Central nervous system—probably at synapse level.
   (ii) Muscle itself—accumulation of various metabolites, and deficiency of oxygen and nutrients.

4. What are the factors responsible for fatigue in intact body?

Ans. The factors responsible for fatigue in intact body are:
   (i) Load acting on muscles.
   (ii) Frequency of muscle contractions.
   (iii) Pause in between contractions.
   (iv) Venous occlusion.
   (v) Arterial occlusion.

5. What is contraction remainder (physiological contracture)?

6. How can you prove that nerve is not a site of fatigue?

Ans. Induce the fatigue in nerve muscle preparation and record the action potential in the nerve on Cathode ray oscilloscope. The nerve is still able to produce and conduct the action potentials. This shows that nerve is not a site of fatigue.

7. How can you prove the muscle is not a site of fatigue in isolated preparation?

Ans. Induce the fatigue in a nerve muscle preparation and put the stimulating electrode directly on the muscle and stimulate it. Contraction of muscle shows that it is not a site of fatigue.

EXPERIMENT 2.5

Demonstrations

I. Recording of normal cardiogram of frog and to study effect of temperature on it.

II. To study the effect of adrenaline, acetyl choline and atropine on frog's heart.

III. To study the effect of stimulation of vago-sympathetic trunk and white crescentic line (WCL).

I. RECORDING OF NORMAL CARDIOGRAM OF FROG AND TO STUDY EFFECT OF TEMPERATURE ON IT

Apparatus

Kymograph, frog board, recording lever (Starling heart lever/Frontal writing lever), instruments for dissection, time marker, alpin, thread and ringer solution.

Procedure

1. Pith the frog after anaesthetising it with urethane solution (5–10%).

2. Give 'V' shaped incision after lifting the xiphisternum with the help of forceps on ventral surface.

3. Extend the incision up to jaw in 'V' shape manner and remove a triangular flap of skin and anterior wall of thorax.

4. Remove the pericardium and expose the heart.

5. Transfer the frog on frog board and fix the base of the heart.

6. Pass a hooked alpin through apex of the heart which is already tied with heart lever.

7. Record the normal cardiogram on slow moving drum (2.5 mm/sec).

8. With help of dropper pour about 2 ml of warm ringer (40°C) on heart and record the cardiogram (Fig. 2.5.1).

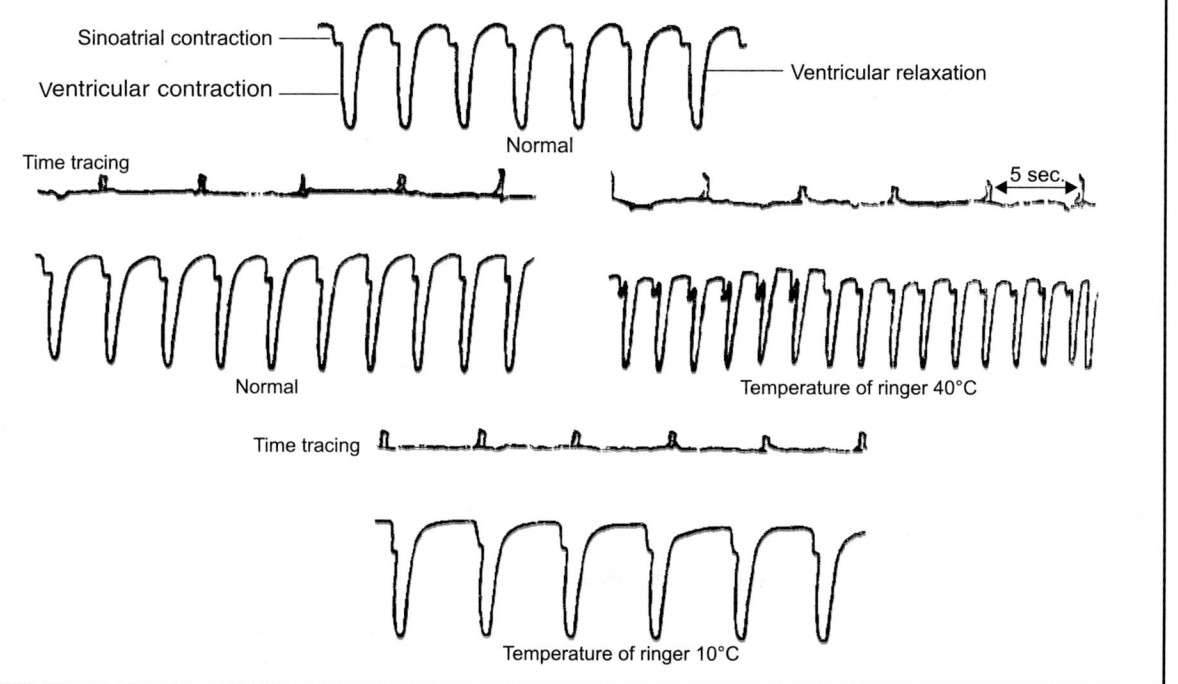

Fig. 2.5.1: Normal cardiogram of frog and effect of temperature on it (with starling heart lever and ink writer on a white chart paper).

9. Stop the drum and pour ringer of room temperature wait for heart beat return to normal.

10. Now pour 2 ml of cold ringer (10°C) solution and record cardiogram.

11. Take time tracing at the base of cardiogram.

Note: With starling heart lever systole is downward movement and diastole is upward but with frontal writing lever systole is upward movement and diastole downward.

Precautions

1. Pour ringer solution at regular intervals to avoid drying of heart.
2. Temperature of warm ringer should not exceed 42°C.
3. First record the effect of warm ringer and then cold.
4. Do not puncture the ventricle while passing a pin through apex.

II. TO STUDY THE EFFECT OF ADRENALINE, ACETYLCHOLINE AND ATROPINE ON FROG's HEART

Apparatus

Same as in normal cardiogram, except drug solutions.

Procedure

1. Same as in normal cardiogram.
2. After recording normal cardiogram add 0.5 ml 1:10000 solution of adrenaline on heart with the help of dropper and take the record.
3. Wait for normal record after pouring ringer solution for 1–2 min.
4. After getting normal cardiogram again, add 0.5 ml 1:1000000 acetylcholine solution with the help of dropper on heart and record the cardiogram.
5. Wait for normal record after pouring ringer solution for 1–2 min.

6. Add 0.5 to 1 ml of 1% solution of atropine and now add 0.5 ml of acetylcholine solution and record the cardiogram (Fig. 2.5.2).

Precautions

1. Same as in normal cardiogram recording.
2. Wash the effect of first drug before adding the other.
3. Record the effect of adrenaline before acetylcholine.

RESULT AND DISCUSSION

S.No.	Drug	Heart rate	Amplitude of contraction
1	Adrenaline		
2	Acetylcholine		
3	Atropine + Ach		

III. TO STUDY THE EFFECT OF STIMULATION OF VAGOSYMPATHETIC TRUNK AND WHITE CRESCENTIC LINE (WCL)

Apparatus

Same as in normal cardiogram recording, induction coil, signal marker, and wire electrodes.

Procedure

1. Expose the heart in the same manner as in normal cardiogram recording.
2. Cut the platysma muscle and remove the tissue running from the angle of the jaw to expose the thin petrohyoid muscle running from the base of the skull to the posterior cornu of hyoid bone. The glossopharyngeal and hypoglossal nerves are seen superficially crossing the petrohyoid muscle.
3. Along the lower border of the petrohyoid muscle run from above downwards.
   (i) Laryngeal nerve.
   (ii) Carotid artery.
   (iii) Vagus nerve (vagosympathetic trunk).

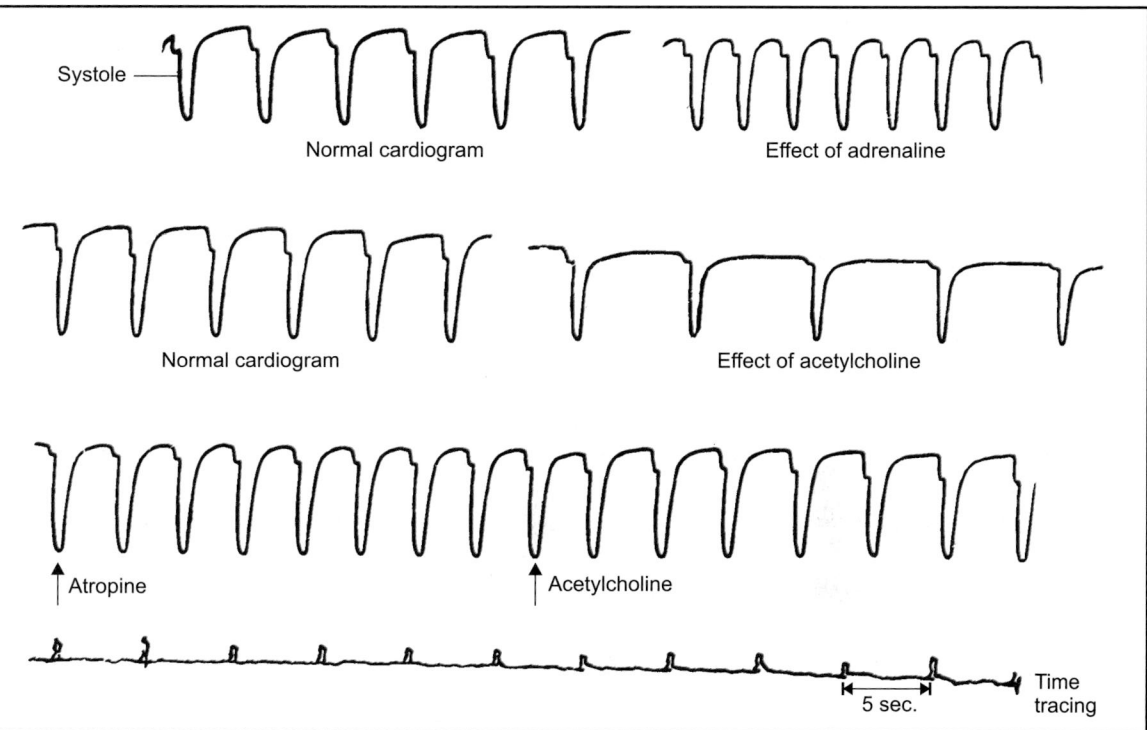

Fig. 2.5.2: Effect of various drugs on frog heart (with starling heart lever with ink writer on a white chart paper).

Isolate the vagus nerve carefully with the help of glass rod and pass a thread beneath the nerve.

4. Keep the electrical connection ready for multiple stimulation (Neef's hammer and signal marker in the primary circuit).

5. Confirm the vagus nerve by stimulating it before transferring it on the frog board. If heart stops, it confirms it is vagus nerve if not, isolate the nerve on opposite side and again confirm.

6. Transfer the frog on frog board and record the normal cardiogram after fixing the base of the heart.

7. Stimulate the vagosympathetic trunk with high frequency stimuli. There will be decrease in the heart rate and force of contraction.

8. Further increase the strength of stimulus and stimulate continuously. There will be arrest of the heart and ventricular contractions appear in spite of continuous stimulation. This phenomenon is called as vagal escape (Fig. 2.5.3).

9. Record the normal cardiogram and stimulate white crescentic line and record its effect. White crescentic line (WCL) is present at the junction of sinus venosus and auricles. It is pale or whitish line between two structures. It has preganglionic parasymphathetic fibres and the body of postganglionic parasympathetic neurones. This synapse is blocked by nicotine (nicotinic receptors). Postganglionic cholinergic fibres are blocked by atropine (muscarinic receptors) (Fig. 2.5.4).

10. Pour 0.5 ml 7% solution of nicotine with the help of dropper and record the effect of stimulation of vagus and white crescentic line separately.

11. Add 0.5 ml of 0.5% atropine solution on the heart and record the effect of stimulation of vagus and white crescentic line.

Precautions

Same as in recording of normal cardiogram.

Normal
Signal marker
Ventricular escape
Signal marker

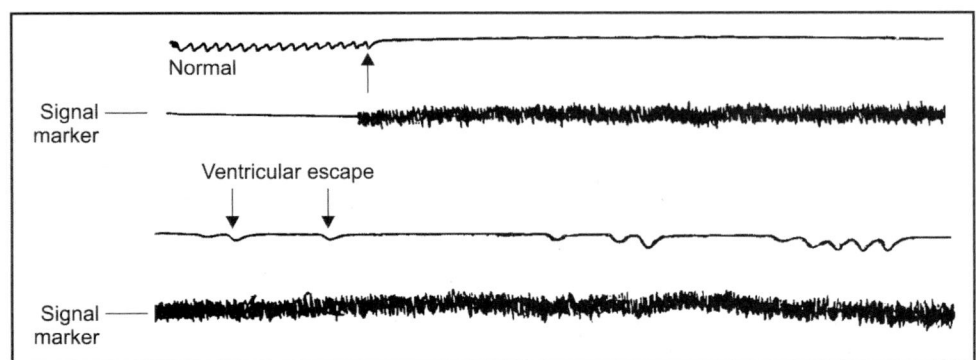

Fig. 2.5.3: Effect of vagosympathetic trunk stimulation on frog's heart (lower part of graph is continuous recording of upper graph) on white chart paper with frontal lever and ink writer.

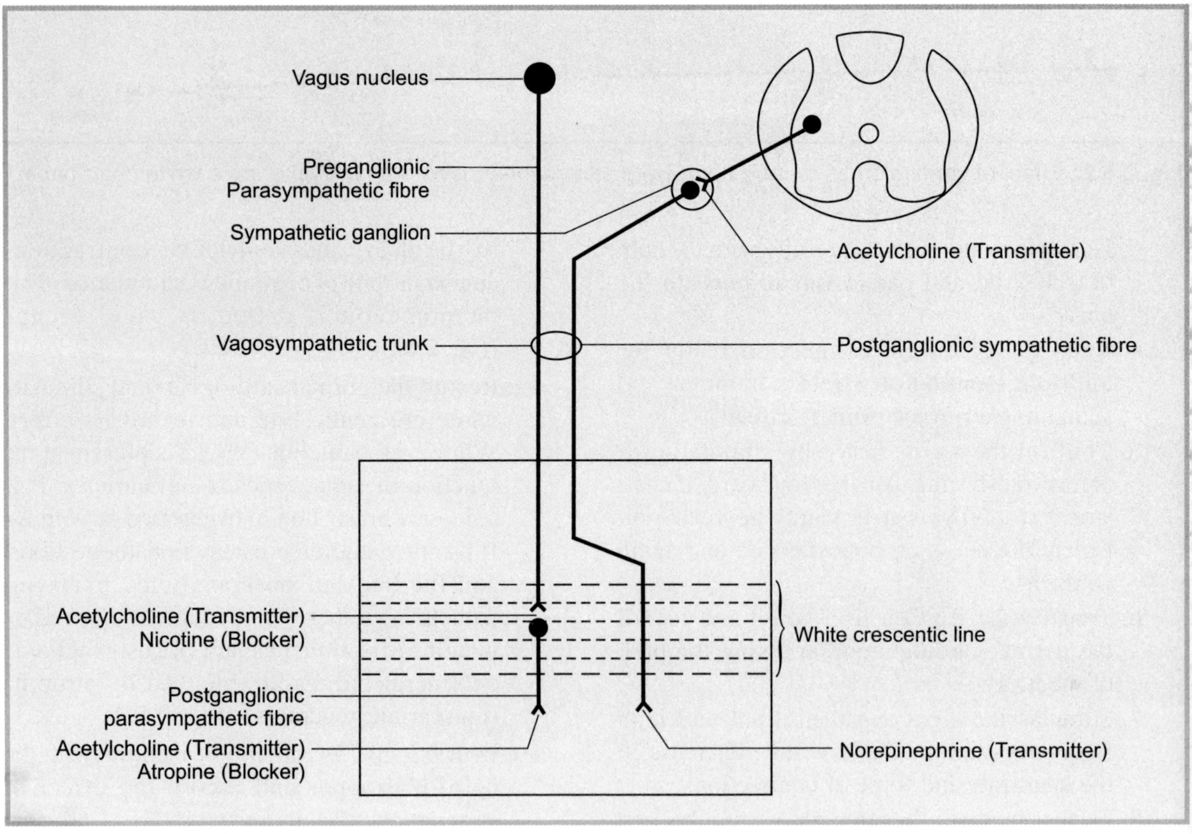

Vagus nucleus
Preganglionic Parasympathetic fibre
Sympathetic ganglion
Acetylcholine (Transmitter)
Vagosympathetic trunk
Postganglionic sympathetic fibre
Acetylcholine (Transmitter)
Nicotine (Blocker)
White crescentic line
Postganglionic parasympathetic fibre
Acetylcholine (Transmitter)
Atropine (Blocker)
Norepinephrine (Transmitter)

Fig. 2.5.4: Site of action of nicotine and atropine as blocker.

QUESTIONS AND ANSWERS

I. Recording of Normal Cardiogram of Frog and to Study Effect of Temperature on it

1. Identifying the various components of frog cardiogram.

2. What is the effect of warm and cold ringer on rate and force of construction of heart?

3. What is mechanism of action of increase or decrease in temperature on frog heart?

II. To Study the Effect of Adrenaline, Acetylcholine and Atropine on Frog's Heart

1. What type of nerve endings are present in white crescentic line?

Ans. Postganglionic sympathetic and preganglionic parasympathetic fibres are present in white crescentic line. It also contains postganglionic parasympathetic neurons.

2. What is the effect of stimulation of white crescentic line after atropine and nicotine?

Ans. If WCL is stimulated after adding atropine heart will not be inhibited because it blocks postganglionic parasympathetic fibres. If WCL is stimulated after adding nicotine heart will be inhibited because it blocks preganglionic parasympathetic fibres.

3. What is the effect of stimulation of vagosympathetic trunk after atropine and nicotine?

Ans. The heart will not be inhibited in both the cases.

4. What is vagal escape? What are its causes?

Ans. In spite of continuous stimulation of vagosympathetic trunk ventricle starts to contract it is called vagal escape. There are two probable causes of vagal escape.

(i) Depletion of acetyl choline at postganglionic parasympathetic fibres.

(ii) Stimulation of postganglionic sympathetic fibres.

5. What are the differences between preganglionic and postganglionic fibres?

Ans. The fibres which synapse on autonomic ganglion are called preganglionic fibres and the fibres originate from autonomic ganglion called postganglionic fibres.

EXPERIMENT 2.6

Demonstrate the following

I. Phenomenon of extrasystole, compensatory pause and refractory period in frog's heart.

II. Cardiac properties after tying stannius ligatures.

I. PHENOMENON OF EXTRASYSTOLE, COMPENSATORY PAUSE AND REFRACTORY PERIOD IN FROG'S HEART

Procedure

Same as in normal cardiogram recording.

Apparatus

1. Apply wire electrodes one around auriculo-ventricular groove and other to hooked pin passing through the apex of the heart.

2. Signal marker is placed in the primary circuit.

3. Record the normal cardiogram at slow moving drum (2.5 mm/sec).

4. Now stimulate the ventricle at different phases of cardiac cycle (Fig. 2.6.1)

    (i) Stimuli falling in systole do not show response.

    (ii) Stimulus falls in later part of diastole shows premature contraction (Extrasystole). It is followed by the compensatory pause (Fig. 2.6.1).

Note: With tension transducer on physiograph direction of systole and diastole recording may be adjusted with the help of polarity knob if available in the physiograph.

Precautions

Same as in normal cardiogram.

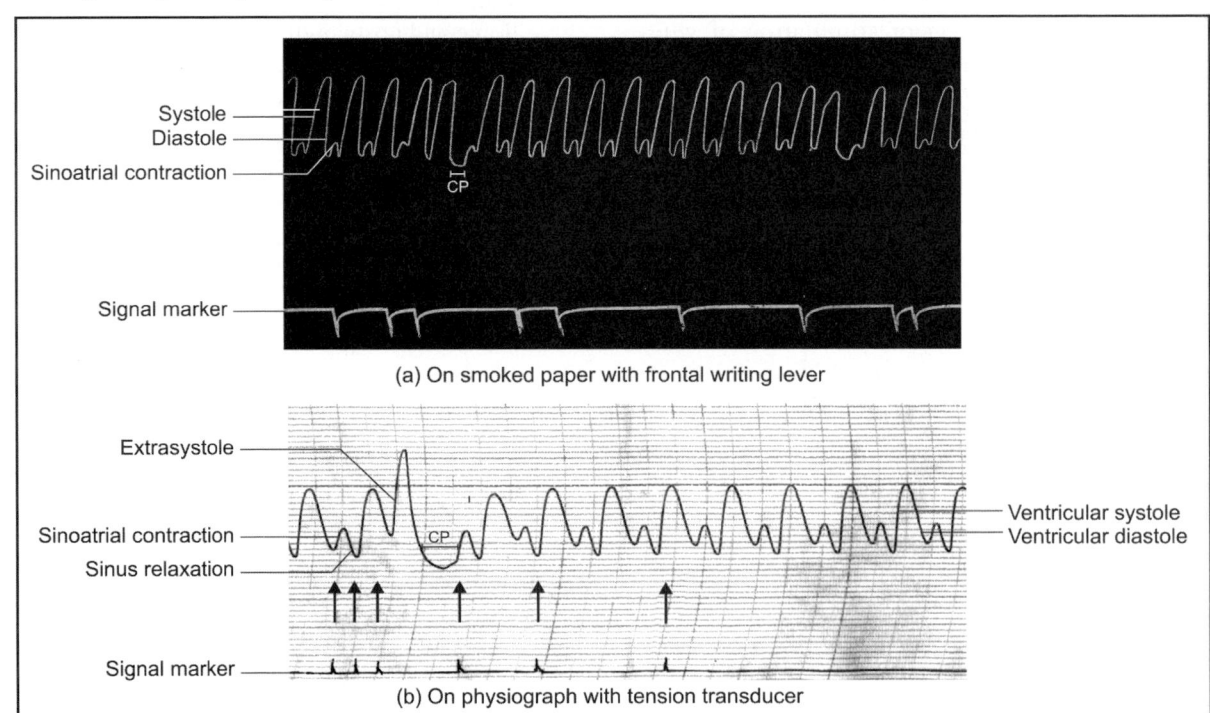

(a) On smoked paper with frontal writing lever

(b) On physiograph with tension transducer

Fig. 2.6.1: Frog cardiogram shows refractory period, extrasystole and compensatory pause (CP compensatory pause).

II. CARDIAC PROPERTIES AFTER TYING STANNIUS LIGATURES

Apparatus

Same as in normal cardiogram, induction coil, signal marker and wire electrodes.

Procedure

(i) Expose the heart as in recording of normal cardiogram.

(ii) Pass a thread with the help of fine forceps posterior to the trunks asteriosus and make a loop posteriorly at white crescentic line (Fig. 2.6.2).

(iii) Arrange the frog in the same way as in normal cardiogram.

(iv) Record the normal cardiogram on slow moving drum (2.5 mm/sec). Now record the following cardiac properties.

1. Conductivity

After recording normal cardiogram, apply a knot to the loop of the thread passed around white crescentic line. This is called first stannius ligature (Fig. 2.6.2). Impulses from sinus venosus are blocked and heart become quiescent for variable period of time (few minutes). After few minutes heart may start to contract again, this is because of atrial rhythm. In this case heart rate is less than sinus rhythm. Apply second stannius ligature around auriculoventricular groove with the help of a thread (Fig. 2.6.2). Heart becomes quiescent again for variable period of time (5–30 minutes). This shows the property of conductivity of impulses from pace make to ventricle.

2. Excitability and Summation of Subminimal Stimuli

Stimulate the quiescent heart with threshold strength of stimulus and second ventricular contraction. This is the property of excitability if cardiac tissue.

Decreases the strength of stimulus by slightly increasing the distance between primary and secondary coils of induction coil, there is no contraction. Apply this stimulus repeatedly, ventricle contracts. This is the summation of subminimal (subthreshold) stimuli.

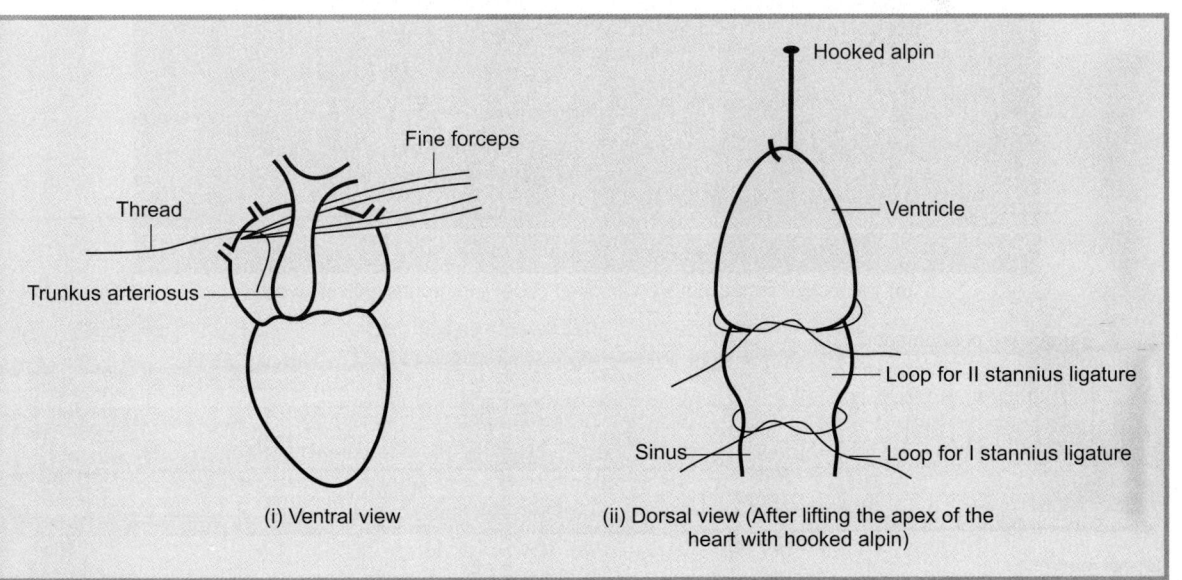

(i) Ventral view

(ii) Dorsal view (After lifting the apex of the heart with hooked alpin)

Fig. 2.6.2: (i) Passage of thread behind trunkus arteriosus for first stannius ligature. (ii) I stannius ligature at WCL and II stannius ligature at auriculoventricular groove.

3. All or None Law

Stimulate the ventricle by subthreshold stimulus, there is no response. Increase the strength of stimulus to threshold there will be ventricular contraction. Increase the strength of stimulus further and wait for 30 sec to one minute. Stimulate the heart with this stimulus, amplitude of contraction remains same. Further increase the strength of stimulus and record the response after one minute. Repeat same procedure 3–4 time by increasing the strength of stimulus (Fig. 2.6.3). Either there will be no response with subthreshold stimulus or with threshold or more strength of stimulus there will be same response. Time gap of 30 second to one minute is given to avoid beneficial effect of previous contraction.

4. Staircase Phenomenon

Adjust the strength of stimulus to suprathreshold and stimulate the ventricle repeatedly (each time just after diastole) and record the effect. First 3–4 contractions shows gradual increases in amplitude

contraction. This is called staircase phenomenon or beneficial effect (Fig. 2.6.3).

5. Idioventricular Rhythm

After some time heart starts to beat again in spite of II stannius ligature but rhythm is neither sinus nor atrial. Sinus, auricles and ventricle contract independently and it is called as idioventricular rhythm. Contraction waves will be different according to their own rhythm (Fig. 2.6.4).

Precautions

1. Pour ringer solution off and on to avoid drying of heart.
2. Do not puncture the ventricle while passing hooked pin through apex of the heart.
3. Use short circuiting key to avoid unnecessary electrical damage to the heart.
4. In case of all or none law wait for one minute before next stimulation.

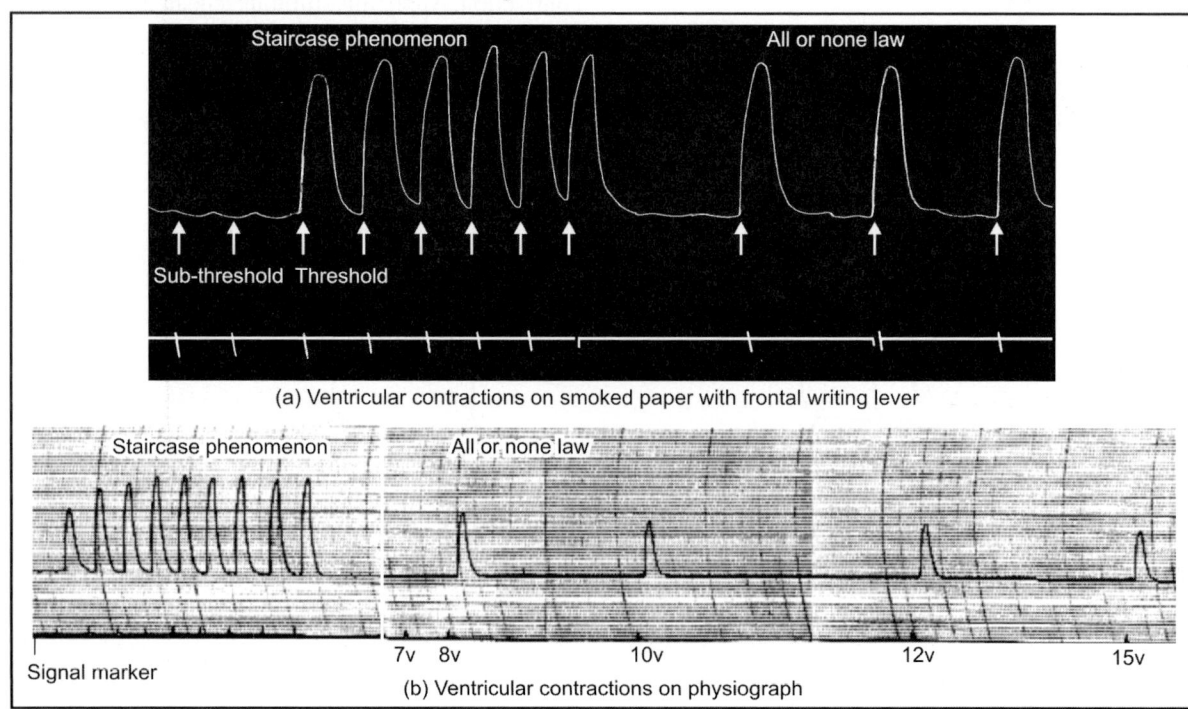

(a) Ventricular contractions on smoked paper with frontal writing lever

(b) Ventricular contractions on physiograph

Fig. 2.6.3: Records show cardiac properties of frog.

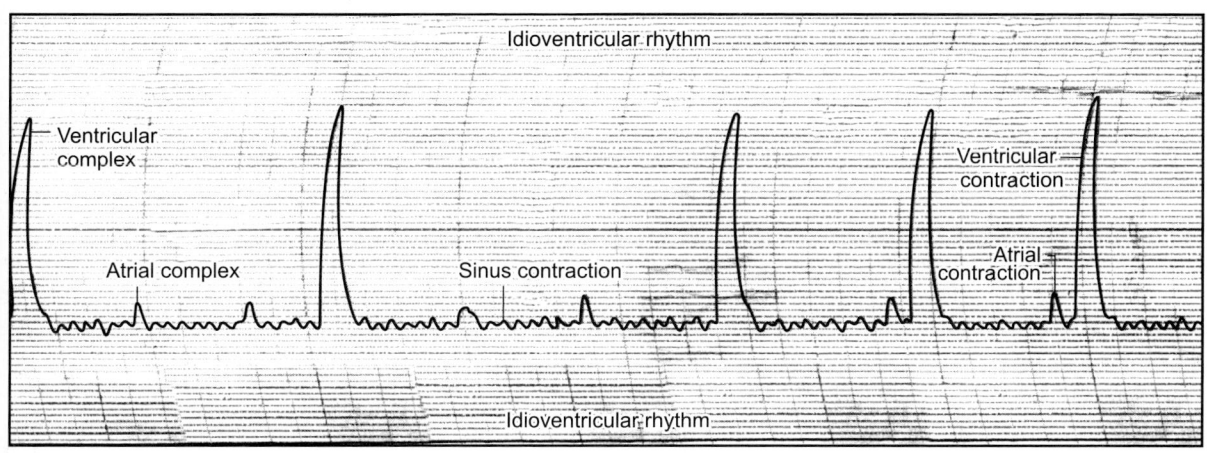

Fig. 2.6.4: Graph shows idoventricular rhythm after II stannius ligature in frog's heart (on physiograph with tension transducer).

QUESTIONS AND ANSWERS

I. Phenomenon of Extrasystole, Compensatory Pause and Refractory Period in Frog's Heart

1. Define extrasystole and compensatory pause.

Ans. When the heart is stimulated in non refractory period it shows premature ventricular contraction, it is called as extrasystole. Now next impulse coming from sinus venosus finds the ventricle in absolute refractory phase. For the next contraction it has to wait for the next impulse, coming from sinus venosus. This delay in next natural contraction is called as compensatory pause. The time of extrasystole and compensatory pause is equal to the duration of two normal cardiac cycles.

2. What is refractory period, which parts of cardiac cycle are absolute refractory and relative refractory periods?

Ans. Refractory period of heart is the phase of cardiac cycle in which cardiac tissue dose not show response when stimulated. The absolute refractory period starts from the beginning of cardiac depolarization to the early half of the repolarization (200 m sec.) in this phase heart does not show response what ever the strength of stimulus is. The relative refractory period is the later half of the repolarization (50 m sec.) in which higher strength of the stimulus is able to produce the response. The systole is absolute refractory and early part of diastole is relative refractory.

3. What is the cause for compensatory pause?

Ans. During extra systole natural impulse from sinus venosus finds it in refractory phase and it is wasted. So the cardiac tissue has to wait for next impulse from sinus venosus. This delay is the cause of compensatory pause.

4. What is the significance of refractory period in cardiac cycle?

Ans. Because of the property of refractory period cardiac tissue cannot be tetanised.

II. Cardiac Properties After Tying Stannius Ligatures

1. What is summation of subminimal stimuli?

Ans. Normally subthreshold stimulus is not able to produce the response. When it applied repeatedly it is able to produce the response. This is called as summation of subminimal stimuli.

2. Define All or None law and staircase phenomenon?

Ans. *All or None law:* This is in relation to the strength of stimulus and response of the tissue. With subthreshold stimulus there will be no response and with threshold or higher strength of stimulus there will be maximum response. *Staircase phenomenon:* It is also called beneficial response. There is a gradual rise in the height of first three or four contractions when stimulated successively just after relaxation of muscle each time. The important reasons underlying the phenomenon are:

   (i) Available of more Ca^{++} at actin-myosin site because of incomplete withdrawal of these ions during relaxation.

   (ii) Increase in the temperature of muscle.

   (iii) Decrease in internal viscosity of muscle.

3. What is idioventricular rhythm? How will you identify the different contraction waves from sinus venosus, atria, and ventricle?

Ans. When transmission of cardiac impulses is stopped from the pacemaker, different parts of the heart (sinus, atria, ventricle) start to contract independently at their own rhythm. This is called idioventricular rhythm. It happens after I and II stannius ligatures in frog heart.

4. What is the cause of all or none law?

Ans. The cardiac tissue is acting as a functional syncytium because of low resistance bridges among the myocardial fibers. This is the cause of all or none law.

5. What are the causes of staircase phenomenon?

Ans. The important reasons underlying the phenomenon are:

   (i) Available of more Ca^{++} at actin-myosin site because of incomplete withdrawal of these ions during relaxation.

   (ii) Increase in the temperature of muscle.

   (iii) Decrease in internal viscosity of muscle.

Human Experiments

EXPERIMENT 3.1

To study the phenomenon of fatigue and the effect of various variables on it by Mosso's ergograph

THEORY

The concept of human fatigue is very complex. It may be subjective i.e. a sensation of tiredness or objective i.e. a measurable decrease in performance. The question whether fatigue is central or peripheral is by no means settled. The basis of the extensive literature available on the subject, Earnest Somonsons conclusion is that the fatigue developing in maximal voluntary muscular effort is, to a large degree located in central nervous system.

Blood flow to exercising muscles not only supplies oxygen but also removes metabolites and heat. Therefore, restricting blood flow to exercising muscles accelerates the onset of fatigue. Venous occlusion impedes only drainage while arterial occlusion affects both supply and removal. Therefore, the later hastens the onset of fatigue more effectively.

During muscular contraction, the blood vessels supplying the muscles are squeezed by high extramural pressure. In case of isotonic contraction muscle gets a chance for liberal blood during relaxation, but in case of isometric contraction blood flow to muscle remains restricted throughout its activity. Therefore, there is no scope for further impairment of circulation if the blood flow is occluded by some other means. That is why, circulatory occlusion hastens the onset of fatigue to a much greater extent in case of isotonic exercise that in case of isometric exercise.

APPARATUS

Mosso's ergograph, metronome, kymograph, sphygmomanometer and weights.

Mosso's Ergograph

It is used for isotonic exercise. It is made up of

1. A wooden board tilted with two pairs of clamps for fixing the forearm of the subject and a pair of finger holders for fixing the index and ring fingers in position.
2. A hook attached to a cord for suspending the weights, is made to hang over the pulley. The

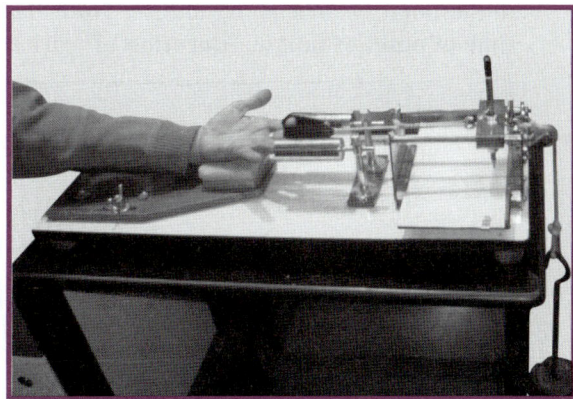

Fig. 3.1.1: Mosso's ergograph

other end of cord is attached to a sliding plate which moves to and fro.

3. The sliding plate carries a lever system to record the movements on a kymograph. The other end of the plate is connected through a sling to the middle finger of the hand.

4. Alternatively, the sliding plate is fitted with a chart holder. A pencil or a ballpoint pen can be tilted vertically over the chart paper so as to record the movements of chart holder when it moves.

PROCEDURE

1. The kymograph is laid on side and arrange the writing lever to write on a smoked paper on a slow moving drum. Alternatively fix a pencil or ballpoint pen in the chart holder and a paper on the platform underneath.

2. Fix the forearm on the ergograph by means of clamps. Put the middle finger in the loop to be pulled and the fingers on either side of into the finger holder provided in the ergograph. Adjust the subjects position and various adjustable points in the ergograph in such a way that forearm is properly fixed and at the same time the subject is comfortable.

3. Suspend a weight of 2 kg on the hook of ergograph. Adjust the metronome to the frequency of 30/min will serve as the control in the experiment. Work with this combination to the point of unbearable fatigue. **Note the time of onset of fatigue (duration of work).**

4. Repeat the experiment at frequency of 60/min with load remaining 2 kg.

5. Repeat the experiment with load of 3 kg frequency 30/min.

6. Repeat the experiment with frequency 30/min load 2 kg and a pause (rest) of 10 sec during work.

7. Wrap the armlet of sphygmomanometer round the arm and raise the pressure in the cuff to about 40 mm Hg to achieve venous occlusion. Repeat the experiment with frequency 30/min and load 2 kg with venous occlusion.

8. Raise the pressure in the cuff to 20 mm Hg more than systolic BP of the subject to achieve and repeat the experiment with frequency arterial occlusion of 30/min and load 2 kg.

9. Work done in each of the above case may be calculated from the weight lifted and the total distance moved as revealed by the lines on the paper (by measuring the individual height/ tracings and adding them up). Express the work done in kg meter.

$$W = D \times F$$

W = Work done

D = Distance to which load is lifted

F = Load

Note:

At the time of drawing the upper line of the rectangle and oblique line of triangle, the line must touch the maximum number of peaks in rectangle and triangle (Fig. 3.1.2).

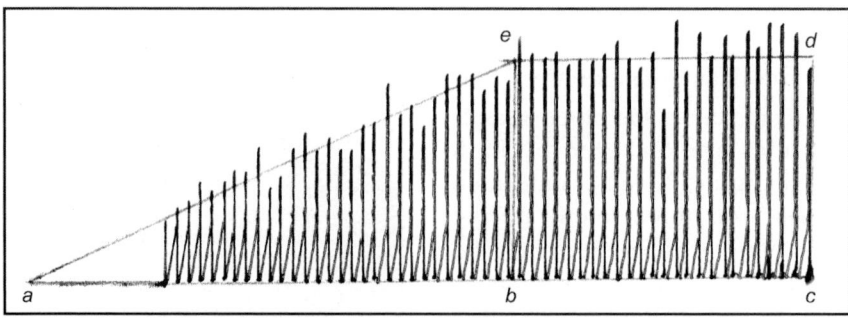

Fig. 3.1.2: Recording of finger movements by Mosso's ergograph.

When the graph recorded is lengthy then alternative method can be used for calculating average height to which the wait is lifted. This is an only alternative method, accurate method is by measuring the individual height. By this method we can calculate the average height as follows:

$$= \frac{\text{Area of the triangle} + \text{Area of the rectangle}}{\text{Total length of the base}}$$
$$\frac{(\frac{1}{2} \text{ base} \times \text{altitude}) \quad (\text{length} \times \text{height})}{\text{Total length of the base}}$$

RESULT AND DISCUSSION

Tabulate the result as follows:

S. No.	Weight (kg)	Frequency (per sec)	Onset of fatigue duration of work (min)	Work done (kg meter)
1.	2	30		
2.	2	60		
3.	3	30		
4.	2	30 (with pause)		
5.	2	30 (venous occlusion)		
6.	2	30 (Arterial occlusion)		

Relevance to Medical Physiology

In the competitive world of today, the doctor's opinion is being increasingly sought to increase production in industry and to improve performance in sports. This makes sound knowledge of work physiology essential for doctor. The phenomenon of fatigue is an important aspect of work physiology.

QUESTIONS AND ANSWERS

1. What is the effect of load and frequency on appearance of fatigue?

Ans. With increase in load there is increase in performance up to optimum load after that fatigue appears earlier and performance decreases. Similar fact is also observed with frequency of muscle contraction.

2. What is the effect of pause during work on fatigue?

Ans. The pause provided during work improves the performance and delays the appearance of fatigue.

3. How does fatigue of isolated nerve muscle preparation differ from that of intact body?

Ans. In case of isolated nerve muscle preparation site of fatigue is myoneural junction and in intact body it is central nervous system and muscle itself.

4. How and why do venous and arterial occlusion affect isotonic exercise?

Ans. In case of venous occlusion there is accumulation of various metabolites because of stoppage of drainage of blood which responsible for early appearance of fatigue and deterioration of performance. In case of arterial occlusion the drainage and the supply of blood both stop. It leads to accumulation of metabolites and deficiency of oxygen and nutrients.

There is further deterioration of performance and fatigue sets in very early.

5. What is the effect of venous and arterial occlusion on isometric exercise?

Ans. There is not much effect of venous and arterial occlusion on isometric exercise.

6. What is endurance? Do isometric and isotonic endurance correspondence with each other?

Ans. The endurance is the ability to do the work continuously. The isometric and isotonic endurance do not correspond each other. The isotonic endurance is more as compared to isometric endurance.

7. Name one condition each in which muscle performance gets impaired due to venous occlusion and arterial occlusion.

Ans. *Venous occlusion:* Venous thrombosis (thrombophlebitis).

Arterial occlusion: Buerger's disease.

EXPERIMENT 3.2

To study the phenomenon of fatigue in human by dynamometer

APPARATUS

Handgrip dynamometer, sphygmomanometer and stop watch.

PROCEDURE

1. Exert and measure maximal tension by handgrip dynamometer. Wait for one minute (max 1).
2. Repeat step 1 and wait for one minute (max 2).
3. Repeat step 1 again (max 3).
4. Take mean of the two closet reading call it maximal tension. Alternatively, two readings may be taken and higher one of the two be considered the maximal tension (T max).
5. Measure the endurance time for 60–80 % of maximal tension (T max). Wait for 5 minutes.
6. Occlude the veins by raising BP 40 mm Hg in the cuff and measure the endurance time for T max.

7. Occlude the arteries by raising the BP in the cuff 20 mm Hg more than systolic BP of the subject. Now measure the endurance for T max.
8. Compare the endurance time of without occlusion of circulation with that of venous occlusion and arterial occlusion. (Steps 5 with 6 and 7). Find out percentage decrease in endurance time in venous occlusion and arterial occlusion.

Relevance to medical physiology: In the competitive world of today, the doctor's opinion is being sought to increase production in industry and to improve performance in sports. The phenomenon of fatigue is an important aspect of work physiology.

QUESTIONS AND ANSWER

1. Which type of exercise is done by handgrip dynamometer?
Ans. Isometric exercise.
2. Do venous and arterial occlusion affect isometric exercise? If your answer is no, give reasons for your answer.
3. How fatigue of intact body differ from that of isolated nerve muscle preparation?

RESULT AND DISCUSSION

(i) Tabulate the tension developed as follows:

S. No.	1	2	3	4	5
Tension developed kg	Max 1	Max 2	Max 3	T max	60% T max

(ii) With 60% of T max tabulate the result as follows:

S. No.	Blood circulation	Endurance time	Percentage decrease in endurance time
1.	Intact	......	......
2.	Venous occlusion	......	......
3.	Venous + arterial occlusion	......	......

EXPERIMENT 3.3A

To record electromyogram (EMG)

THEORY

An electromyogram is a recording of electrical activity from a muscle during its activity. Procedure of recording EMG is called electromyography.

Normally skeletal muscle is electrically silent when at rest. It is because of slow asynchronous discharge in motor units. Excitation of muscle fibres voluntarily or by electrical stimulation of motor nerve cause a change in the membrane potential which sets up a current field in the neighbouring tissue. In normal human the skeletal muscle fibres do not contract individually. The functional unit of neuromuscular activity is the motor unit comprising the spinal motor neuron, its axon and all the muscle fibres supplied by it. Electrical disturbances produced by the excitation of an individual motor unit is called motor unit potential.

A slight voluntary contraction requires the activation of a small number of motor units but with increasingly vigorous contraction, more and more units are recruited by asynchronous valley of impulses along many axons. The rate of discharge along each axon is also augmented. The potentials run into one another and resulting composite picture is the interference pattern.

APPARATUS

Student's physiograph/polyrite/CRO, electrodes (silver chloride coated small discs or needles), preamplifier, spirit and cotton swabs.

PROCEDURE

1. The skin overlying the biceps muscle or thenar muscle is cleaned with spirit. Small area of skin is also cleaned on anterior surface of forearm.
2. Two disc electrodes acting as exploring electrode and indifferent electrode are fixed by using electrode paste on a small area of skin over biceps muscle. Third ground electrode is fixed at forearm.
3. The electrodes are connected to physiograph or CRO through amplifier (biopotential couples physiograph). Sensitivity of the physiograph is adjusted at 200 or 100 millivolt. Physiograph has to be earthed properly. Physiograph is calibrated at specific sensitivity.
4. Subject is asked to flex the forearm, then subject is asked to flex the forearm against resistance. Graph is recorded in both the situations. (Fig. 3.3a.1) at the speed of paper 25 mm/sec.

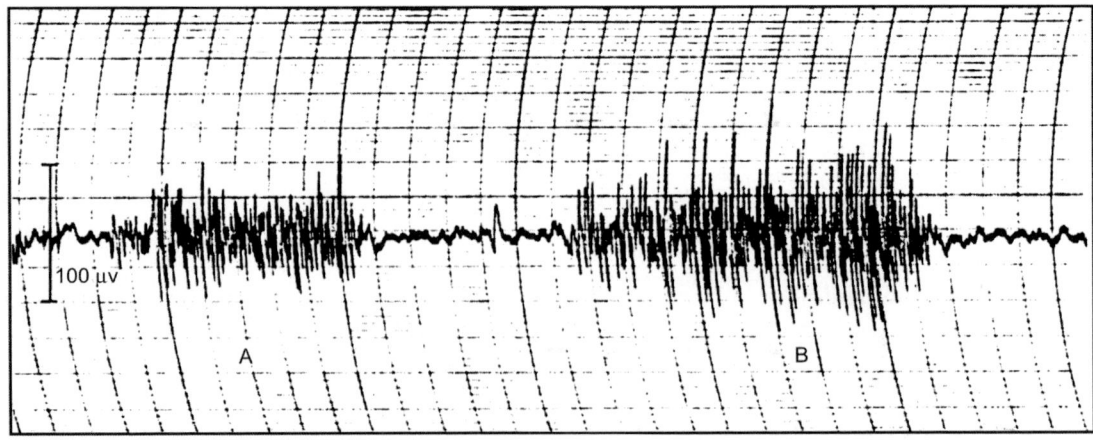

Fig. 3.3a.1: Electromyogram from biceps muscle. (A) less powerful contraction, (B) more powerful contraction).

QUESTIONS AND ANSWERS

1. What is motor unit?

2. What is motor unit potential?

3. What do you understand by recruitment of motor units?

Ans. The recruitment of motor units means more and more unit coming into action.

4. Why there is no potential in a muscle under resting condition?

5. What are the factors, which determine the gradation of muscle response?

Ans. Gradation of muscle response depends on:

   (i) Number of motor units involved in the response (recruitment of motor units).

   (ii) Frequency of discharge in the nerve fibre.

   (iii) Duration of discharge in nerve fibre.

EXPERIMENT 3.3B

Determination of conduction velocity of human ulnar nerve

THEORY

The conduction velocity of a nerve fibre is defined as the distance travelled by an action potential by the time taken to travel this distance.

The conduction velocity of a nerve fibre is determined by the fibre diameter and its myelination. In general, larger the diameter of the fibre, the higher is the conduction velocity.

The conduction velocity in human nerve can be determined by stimulating a peripheral nerve by placing an electrode over the skin in the vicinity of a nerve at two points along its course. Action potential of the muscle supplied by nerve is recorded. The difference in latencies in the two responses is the time taken by the nerve impulse to travel the distance between the two points of stimulation along the length of the nerve.

Thus velocity of conduction of the nerve can be calculated.

APPARATUS

Cathode ray oscilloscope (action potential recording instrument), stimulating electrodes, recording electrodes, preamplifier, electrode paste and spirit swabs.

PROCEDURE

1. Clean the skin overlying hypothenar muscle and fix the recording electrode over there with the help of electrode paste.
2. Ulnar nerve is stimulated with the help of stimulating electrode, posterior to medial epicondyle of humorous (posterior to elbow joint on medial side) after cleaning the area with spirit. Action potential is recorded from the hypothenar muscle.
3. Stimulate the ulnar nerve on the writ on medial side after cleaning the area with the help of stimulating electrodes. Muscle action potential from hypothenar muscle is recorded again.
4. Distance from one stimulating electrode to other stimulating electrode is measured with the help of measuring tape.
5. Find out latent periods (latency) at two muscle action potential recorded from hypothenar muscle.

CALCULATION AND RESULT

Distance between two stimulating point of ulnar nerve (D) = ...

Latent period of one muscle action potential (S1)
    = ...

Latent period of other action potential S2 = ...

Difference of two latent periods = (S1 – S2) = ...

Conduction velocity =

$$\frac{\text{Distance}}{\text{Difference in latent periods}} =$$

Normal conduction velocity 50 – 60 m / sec.

QUESTIONS AND ANSWERS

1. Define the conduction velocity of a nerve.
Ans. This is the speed at which impulse (action potential) can pass through a nerve.
2. What are the factors affecting conduction velocity?
Ans. Factors which affect the conduction velocity are:
    (i) Diameter of the nerve fibres present in a nerve.
    (ii) Myelination or unmyelination of the fibres present in the nerve.
    (iii) Temperature.
3. What is the clinical significance of conduction velocity of nerve?
Ans. The conduction velocity of a nerve is affected by certain physiological and pathological factors. It is having diagnostic as well as prognostic significance.

EXPERIMENT 3.4

Determination of blood pressure in man

PRINCIPLE

The principle of the experiment involves the balancing of air pressure against the pressure of blood in brachial artery, the air pressure being estimated by a mercury or air (aneroid) manometer.

APPARATUS

Sphygmomanometer, stethoscope and chair or couch.

SPHYGMOMANOMETER (Fig. 3.4.1)

It consists of a mercury manometer and inflatable cuff. The cuff is called a "Riva Rocci" cuff. The manometer is a U-shaped tube. One limb being broader than the other. The broader limb is the reservoir for mercury and the narrow limb is graduated from 0 to 300 mm, with the smallest division corresponding to a reading of 2 mm.

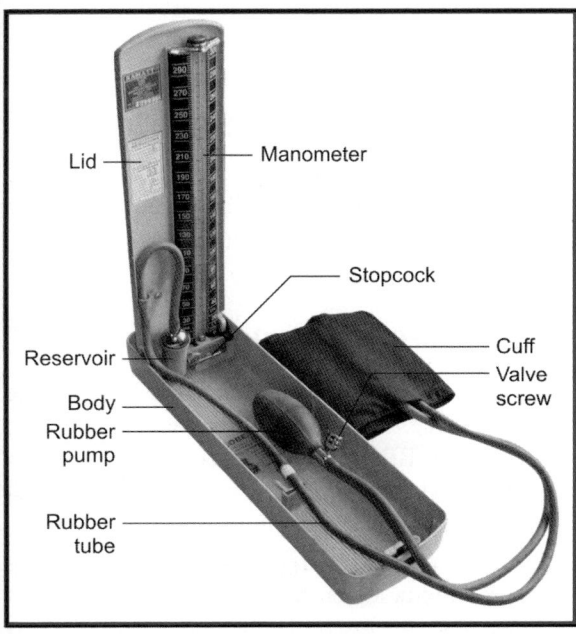

Fig. 3.4.1: Sphygmomanometer.

Cuff consists of an inflatable rubber bag covered by a non-distensible cotton fabric. The cuff is connected to the manometer and to a hand bulb (rubber pump) by rubber tubing. The cuff can be inflated to any desired pressure with the help of rubber pump permits the reduction in cuff pressure. To overcome tissue resistance the width of cuff should be 20% more than the diameter of the arm. Width of a cuff for adults is 12.5 cm, for children below 8 years is 8 cm, below 5 years is 5 cm and for infants below 1 year is 2.5 cm. Wider cuffs have to be used to record the blood pressure in obese individuals and in the lower limb to overcome tissue resistance. Length of rubber cuff should be 23 cm (It should cover 2/3 of arm circumference.).

PROCEDURE

Blood pressure is recorded by two method.

Direct Method

It is possible in experimental animals because it is unsafe. In this method artery is cannulated and other end of cannula is connected to mercury manometer. By this method we record end pressure which is slightly higher than lateral pressure measured by indirect methods.

Indirect Method

By this method lateral pressure exerted by the column of blood on arteries is recorded.

Subject is asked to sit comfortably in a chair or made to lie down supine on the couch and the arm (brachial artery) is kept at the level of the heart to obtain a pressure that is uninfluenced by gravity. The arm is exposed and cuff is tied in such a way that the mid point of the cuff overlies the brachial artery and the lower edge of the cuff is one inch above cubital fossa. Now the BP is recorded by palpatory method first and then by auscultatory method.

Palpatory Method

Rubber bag is inflated until the air pressure within it overcomes the arterial pressure and obliterates the arterial luman. This can be confirmed by feeling the radial pulse which will disappear when pressure is raised a little beyond the point, by about 30–40 mmHg and then slowly reduced again so that the pressure falls at the rate of 2–3 mmHg per second. Pulse starts reappearing at a point when pressure in the artery is equal to the pressure of air in the cuff and blood escapes beyond the cuff into the peripheral part of the artery. Manometer reading is taken when radial pulse is first felt at the wrist. It is the index of systolic BP.

Disadvantage

1. Pressure recorded is about 6–10 mm Hg less than that recorded by auscultatory method.
2. Only systolic blood pressure can be recorded by this method.

Auscultatory Method

Place the chart piece of stethoscope over the arm medial to the tendons of biceps where pulsations of brachial artery are felt.

Then inflate the cuff till the pressure is 30–40 mm Hg more than the reading obtained by palpatory method. Now gradually lower the pressure till a sharp light tapping sound (in the rhythm with the heart beat) is heard.

When the pressure in the cuff is further lowered, sound undergoes a series of changes in quality and intensity, which were first described by Korotkoff, a Russian Scientist in 1905.

This sound was labeled as Korotkoff sounds.

There are 5 phases of these sounds:

Phase I: Sudden appearance of a clear but faint tapping sound growing louder during the succeeding 10 mm Hg fall in pressure.

Phase II: The sound takes murmur like quality during the next 15 mm fall in pressure.

Phase III: Sound changes little in quality but become clearer and louder during next 15 mm fall in pressure.

Phase IV: Muffled quality lasting throughout the next 5–6 mmHg fall in pressure.

Phase V: Complete disappearance of the sound.

The appearance of the sound indicates the systolic BP. Disappearance of sound (Phase V) indicates diastolic BP. If sound does not disappear muffling of the sound (Phase IV) is taken as diastolic BP. It happens in case of hyperdynamic circulation.

Take three reading to reach the conclusion regarding blood pressure.

Precautions

1. The subject should be quiet and comfortable for 5–10 minutes before measurement of BP.
2. Arm, with the cuff wrapped around it should be at the level of the heart.
3. The cuff should not be tied too light or too loose.
4. The cuff should not be left inflated for long period, specially in persons suffering from purpura or tetany.
5. In the suspected hypertensive individuals, cuff pressure should be well above 200 mmHg (or above estimated BP by palpatory method) to avoid auscultatory gap.

Result

Concordant reading:
Systolic BP/Diastolic BP mmHg.
Normal value:
   Average value in adult = 120/80 mmHg
   Systolic BP range = 100–140 mmHg
   Diastolic BP range = 60–90 mmHg

Factors Affecting BP in Normal Subjects

1. *Age*: Both systolic and diastolic BP increase with age. Systolic BP increases more than diastolic BP. This is because of loss of elasticity of blood vessels (atherosclerosis) with age. (It is roughly 100 + age in years.)
2. *Sex*: In female before menopause blood pressure is lower than male.
3. *Body built*: Overweight individuals have higher values.

4. *Sleep*: BP falls during sleep due to generalised relaxation of blood vessels.

5. *Posture*: Described in separate practical (Experiment 3.5).

6. *Gravity*: BP increases in arteries below heart and decrease in arteries above heart.

7. *Exercise*: Described in separate practical (Experiment 3.6).

RESULT AND OBSERVATIONS

Blood pressure by palpatory method = I reading .... II reading ....

Readings	SBP mmHg	DBP mmHg	Pulse pressure mmHg	Mean pressure mmHg
1.				
2.				
3.				

QUESTIONS AND ANSWERS

1. Define blood pressure.

Ans. It is the lateral pressure exerted by the column of blood on blood vessels.

2. Define Systolic BP, diastolic BP, pulse pressure and mean pressure.

Ans. Systolic blood pressure is the maximum pressure exerted during systole. Diastolic pressure is the minimum pressure exerted during diastole. Pulse pressure is the difference between systolic and diastolic pressure. Mean pressure is the average pressure remains throughout the cardiac cycle. It is equal to the diastolic pressure plus one-third of pulse pressure.

3. What is the average value of BP in adult?

4. What is the range of SBP and DBP in adult?

5. What is end pressure?

Ans. End pressure is the pressure recorded from end of the vessel not from its walls. End pressure is slightly higher than the lateral pressure.

6. What is the mechanism for Korotkoff sounds?

Ans. Turbulence in blood flow in brachial artery because of slow release of pressure responsible for production of Korotkoff sounds.

7. Which phase of Korotkoff sound is considered end-point for diastolic BP?

Ans. Phase IV (muffling of sound) of Korotkoff sound is considered as end-point for diastolic BP.

8. Give merits and demerits of palpatory method of recording BP.

Ans. *Merits:*

(i) Simple method and not requires stethoscope.

(ii) It helps in detecting auscultatory gap.

Demerits:

(i) Rough method, value of systolic BP is about 6 to 10 mmHg is less than the auscultatory method.

(ii) Diastolic BP cannot be measured.

9. Why the arm (tied with cuff) should be placed at the level of heart?

Ans. To avoid the effect of gravity on the blood pressure.

10. What is the auscultatory gap? How can it be avoided?

Ans. It is seen in hypertensive patients while recording of blood pressure by auscultatory method. In such patients occasionally sound may disappear temporarily during phase I and II, covering a range of 40 to 50 mmHg pressure and reappear again. Cause of this gap is not known. This gives falls low value of BP in such patients. It can be avoided by first estimating the BP by palpatory method.

11. What are the factors affecting BP in normal individuals?

12. What is hyper and hypotension?

Ans. When the systolic BP and diastolic BP are more than 140 and 90 mmHg respectively it is called as hypertension. When systolic BP and diastolic BP are less than 100 and 60 mmHg respectively, it is called as hypotension.

EXPERIMENT 3.5

To study the effect of posture on BP in human

THEORY

Immediately after changing the posture from lying to standing blood pressure falls which persists for 20–30 seconds. It is because of venous pooling in lower parts of the body, which responsible for decreased venous return leading to decreased cardiac output. Fall in systolic BP is more as compared to diastolic BP. The fall in BP responsible for decreased baroreceptor discharge which leads to increased sympathetic discharge. It is responsible for increased heart rate, increased force of contraction of heart and increase in peripheral resistance. All these compensatory changes leading to increase in blood pressure. The rise in systolic BP is more as compared to diastolic BP. This reflex rise in BP takes about 30 seconds to one minute after change in the posture. This rise in BP further gets normalised in about 2–3 minutes. It fall in BP, after lying to standing posture persists for longer duration, it is called as orthostatic or postural hypotension.

APPARATUS

Sphygmomanometer, stethoscope and couch.

RESULT AND OBSERVATION

Tabulate your result as follows:

Posture	Systolic BP		Diastolic BP
Lying	1.		....
	2.		....
	3.		....
Sitting	1. Immediately	....	....
	2. After 1 min	....	....
	3. After 2 min	....	....
	4. After 3 min	....	....
Standing	1. Immediately	....	....
	2. After 1 min	....	....
	3. After 2 min	....	....
	4. After 3 min	....	....

PROCEDURE

1. Ask the subject to lie supine quietly on a couch.
2. Record the systolic BP by palpatory method and than by auscultatory method. Take three reading by auscultatory method.
3. Ask the subject to sit up on the couch and record the BP immediately, than after one minute, two minutes, and three minutes of sitting.
4. Similarly ask the person to stand and record the blood pressure.

PRECAUTIONS

1. BP should be recorded by keeping the arm at heart level.
2. To avoid loss of time don't untie the cuff after recording the BP in lying posture.

QUESTIONS AND ANSWER

1. What happens to BP when person stands up from lying?
2. What is postural hypotension?

Ans. When fall in the blood pressure from lying to standing persists for longer period and leads to fainting or darkness in front of the eyes it is called as postural hypotension.

EXPERIMENT 3.6

To study the effect of exercise on blood pressure

THEORY

To study the effect of exercise on BP, it is very important to know the severity of exercise. The grading of exercise is done depending up on percentage of O_2 used in relation to VO_2 max during exercise (VO_2 max is the rate of O_2 consumption during severest exercise by the individual).

Fortunately heart rate shows direct relationship with O_2 consumption during exercise and it is easy to measure pulse rate, this is why practically we are grading the exercise depending up on heart rate.

The changes in blood pressure during exercise depends up on the type of exercise an individual performing. During isometric exercise there is increase in SBP as well as DBP in all grades of exercise. During isotonic exercise effect on BP varies with severity of exercise. During mild grade of exercise there is increase in SBP and no change or light rise in DBP. During moderate exercise the more rise in SBP and no charge or slight fall in DBP. In heavy and very heavy exercise there is further rise in SBP and no charge or slight fall or slight rise in DBP. There is increase in pulse pressure during isotonic exercise. Blood pressure comes to normal in about 5–7 minutes.

APPARATUS

Sphygmomanometer, stethoscope and wooden step or bicycle ergometer.

PROCEDURE

1. Measure the radial pulse of the subject in comfortable sitting posture.
2. Record the blood pressure first by palpatory method and then by auscultatory method. Take three reading of blood pressure.
3. Disconnect the manometer of BP apparatus from rubber bag and give stepping exercise on wooden step or on bicycle ergometer to the subject for about 3–5 minutes.
4. Stop the exercise in 5 minutes or when the subject is not able to continue the exercise. Note down the pulse at this movement and record the blood pressure immediately after stopping the exercise.
5. Further record the BP after 1,2,3, and 4 minute of exercise.

PRECAUTIONS

1. Same as in recording blood pressure.
2. Don't give the exercise to the subject having resting pulse rate below 60/min and more than 90 min. (First find out cause for so low or so high pulse rate.)

WHO classification of grades of exercise		
	Heart rate (per min)	% of VO$_2$ max
I. Mild	< 100	< 25%
II. Moderate	100–125	25–50%
III. Heavy	126–150	51–75%
IV. Very heavy	> 150	> 75%

RESULT AND DISCUSSION

Tabulate your result as follows:

S.No.	Time of BP recording		SBP	DBP	Heart rate
1.	Resting state	(i)			
		(ii)			
		(iii)			
2.	Immediately after exercise				
3.	After one min				
4.	After two min				
5.	After three min				
6.	After four min				
7.	After five min				

QUESTIONS AND ANSWERS

1. What is the effect of isometric exercise on BP?
2. What is the effect of isotonic exercise on BP?
3. What are the causes for increase in heart rate and SBP during exercise?

Ans. There is increase in sympathetic discharge during exercise which responsible for increase in heart rate (positive chronotropic effect) and increase in force of contraction (positive inotropic effect) of cardiac tissue.

4. Why DBP do not show much change during isotonic exercise?

Ans. Diastolic BP mainly depends on peripheral resistance. In case of mild exercise there may be slight increase or no change in peripheral resistance which leads to slight increase or no change in BP. In case of moderate, heavy and very heavy exercise there may be slight decrease in peripheral resistance and accordingly BP may show slight fall or no change. An increase in diastolic BP more than 10 mmHg represents an unstable form of hypertension (Kelley et. al. 2000).

EXPERIMENT 3.7A

Recording of body temperature

APPARATUS

Clinical thermometer.

PROCEDURE

To record body temperature, when taking the temperature, the following points must be remembered.

1. The thermometer must be accurate.
2. Clinical thermometer should be kept in position for 1 or 2 minutes to record the body temperature.
3. In conscious adults the temperature is taken in the mouth or in the axilla. In young children the thermometer should be placed in the fold of the groin and the thigh is fixed on the abdomen or it may be inserted into rectum.

4. The temperature of the mouth and rectum is generally at least half a degree Celsius higher than that of the groin or axilla.
5. Before inserting the thermometer, make it an invariable rule to wash it in antiseptic or in cold water and see that mercury is well skendown (below the normal).

The temperature of the body depends on a balance between heat production and heat loss.

Sources of heat production are:
1. Basal metabolic processes.
2. Food intake (specific dynamic action).
3. Muscular activity.

Heat loss occurs through:
1. Radiation and conduction of heat from body surfaces.
2. Vaporisation of sweat from skin.
3. Respiration.
4. Urination and defecation,
5. Cutaneous vasodilatation.

TEMPERATURE RANGES

	Centigrade (C)	Fahrenheit (F)
1. Normal	36.6–37.2°	98–99°
2. Subnormal	< 36.6°	< 98°
3. Hypothermia	< 35°	< 95°
4. Febrile	> 37.2°	> 99°
5. Hyperpyrexia	> 41.6°	> 107°

Average normal temperature 37°C/98.6 °F

QUESTIONS AND ANSWERS

1. Why the thermometer is placed at different places in adult and child.
2. What are the various types of temperature depending upon the site of recording the temperature from various body part.

Ans. It is of different types:

(i) Oral temperature—from mouth.

(ii) Axillary temperature—from axilla.

(iii) Groin temperature—from groin.

(iv) Rectal temperature – from rectum.

3. What is core temperature?

Ans. It is internal body temperature. It can be recorded from rectum, vagina and oesophagus.

It is about 0.5 to 1.0 degree C higher than of oral temperature.

4. How much difference in there in oral and axillary temperature?

Ans. Oral temperature is about 0.5 degree C higher than axillary temperature.

5. What is body temperature in hypothermia and hyperpyrexia?

6. What is the average value of body temperature in normal individual?

7. At which temperature patient is labelled as febrile?

8. How long a thermometer is placed for recording the body temperature?

9. What are the factors determine body temperature?

EXPERIMENT 3.7B

To study the response of skin to blunt injury (Triple response)

THEORY

A firm strong stroke across the skin using a pencil point or a key evokes series of responses classified as:

1. Red reaction
2. Flare
3. Wheel

This is called as **Triple response**.

1. Red Reaction

Just at the site of stroke, a red line appears. It is because of histamine and polypeptide released from damaged skin. Which cause capillary vasodilatation.

2. Flare

It is due to dilatation of the arterioles and precapillary sphincter which causes irregular erythematous area which surrounds the site of red line. Skin temperature overlying this area is raised. It is mediated by nerves but does not involve central nervous system (axon reflex).

3. Wheal

If the stroke stimulus has been strong enough, a swelling or oedema develops spreading from the margins of the red line within the flare area. This is because of increase capillary permeability coupled with size in capillary pressure because of vasodilatation.

APPARATUS

A stick/key, spirit and cotton swab.

PROCEDURE

1. Stroke the skin lightly by smooth end of a stick or a key. A white line appears along the line.
2. Stroke the skin firmly. It evokes series of responses as follows:
   (a) Red line outline along the stroke.
   (b) Flare, irregular red area surrounding the red line.
   (c) Wheal, swelling and oedema like appearance spreading from margins of red line with in the flare area.

PRECAUTIONS

1. Clean the area over the skin with spirit swab (to make the skin sterile because there may be scratch during the process of stroke).
2. A stick or key should be washed properly in a antiseptic solution.

QUESTIONS

1. What is triple response?
2. What is axon reflex?
3. What are the causes for red line, flare, and wheal?

EXPERIMENT 3.8

To study the cardiovascular response to exposure of hand to cold

APPARATUS

Thermometer, cold water at 5°C, sphygmomano-meter and stethoscope.

PRINCIPLE

The change in heart rate and of blood pressure (magnitude and duration) in response to a brief exposure of the hand to cold is a measure of vasomotor tone and autonomic activity in man.

RESULT AND DISCUSSION

Tabulate the result as follows:

PROCEDURE

1. The subject is seated or made to lie down on a couch in quiet surroundings.
2. The blood pressure and heart rate (radial pulse) is recorded repeatedly at an interval of 2 minutes till three successive readings are identical.
3. Now one hand of subject is immersed in cold water at 5°C. Stir the water to maintain uniform temperature.
4. After 2 minutes hand is removed from cold water.
5. Record the blood pressure and heart rate immediately after removing the hand from cold water.
6. Recordings are repeated at the interval of one minute till blood pressure and heart rate comes to normal level.

S.No.	Time of readings	Heart rate (Per min)	SBP (mmHg)	DBP (mmHg)
1.	In the beginning			
2	- do -			
3.	- do -			
4.	Immediately (After removing hand from cold water)			
5.	After one min			
6.	After two min			
7.	After three min			
8.	After four min			
9.	After five min			

QUESTIONS AND ANSWERS

1. Why there is increase in blood pressure when hand is immersed in cold water?

Ans. Cold afferents from the hand are going to the sensory cortex and ultimately responsible for increase in sympathetic activity via hypothalamus. Probably this is one the factors responsible for increase in the blood pressure. Other factor is local vasoconstriction which causes hypoxia in hand. It is responsible for pain which also increases the BP.

2. What is the mechanism of pain following immersion of hand in cold water?

Ans. Local vasoconstriction in hand in response to cold causes hypoxia. This hypoxia responsible for pain.

3. What is the local effect of cold exposure to hand?

Ans. It is responsible for vasoconstriction which causes hypoxia and pain in the hand.

4. What is the neural pathway of pain?
5. What is the neural pathway for cold sensation?

EXPERIMENT 3.9

Determination of physical fitness of a subject using Harvard step test

THEORY

To a physiologist "physical fitness" implies the ability to make adequate physiological adjustment to the stresses imposed by a specific task. Research findings have indicated that good cardiorespiratory function (as reflected by the ability to deliver oxygen to the tissues to maintain continuous activity) is perhaps the single most important physiological factors in this respect.

There are number of tests to measure physical fitness of an individual out of which maximum oxygen intake test is considered to be the best single method for measuring the cardiorespiratory response to exercise. Fortunately, pulse rate which is very easy to measure, correlates significantly with oxygen consumption during exercise. The response of heart, reflected in the heart oxygen intake and the maximum heart rate are reached at approximately the same time. This correlation has been employed successfully in a number of fitness tests.

Reasons for Testing Physical Fitness are

1. Determination of ability to perform a specific work task.
2. Providing basis for exercise prescription.
3. Evaluation of cardiac and respiratory function.
4. Screening for coronary heart disease.

In the present experiment heart rate during recovery following a standard exercise will be used as a criterion of fitness of an individual. The test used are:

(a) Harvard step test.
(b) Minute step test.

Because of some obvious advantages, step tests are chosen.

The apparatus is inexpensive and portable, and requires no maintenance, calibration or electricity. It offers much freedom from undesirable features.

PROCEDURE (HARVARD STEP TEST)

This test exposes the subject to a standard exercise that no one can perform in a "steady state" for more than a few minutes. It takes into account two factors: the length of time the exercise can be sustained and deceleration of heart rate after exercise. It consists of measuring the endurance in stepping up and down on a bench of standard height and the pulse response to this exercise.

1. It is desirable to use a subject in good physical condition. Have the subject sit quietly for at least 5 minutes.
2. The subject should be lightly clothed and wear rubber shoes or no shoes at all.
3. The exercise of protocol is similar to one which is used in Harvard step test for physical fitness. In the original test, a 20-inch step is used. This height is generally difficult to apply for Indian standard, people below 17 years of age and also to short people. Therefore, the height of the step has been lowered to 41 cm (16½ inches).
4. The subject steps on to and down from 41 cm platform 30 times per minute. At the signal 'start' the subject places one foot on the platform, steps up, places other foot on the platform, straightens the legs and backbone and again steps down, bring down the same foot that he placed up first. At two seconds interval the signal 'up' is given. The subject should 'lead of' with the same foot each time and not alternate the foot. The observer has to call the rhythm by adjusting the metronome and asking the subject to perform at the above rate. Subject performs this exercise as long as he can, but not more than 5 minutes.
5. After the cessation of exercise, record heart rate for 30 seconds from 1 min to next 30 seconds.

PRECAUTIONS

If the subject is dyspnoeic, feels pain in chest or in legs, or gets exhausted during the exercise period, ask to discontinue the exercise immediately.

RESULT AND OBSERVATION

The subject performs the exercise for five minutes, unless he stops from exhaustion before that. Two things are carefully noted down.

1. *Duration of exercise in minutes*: Begin counting the time when subjects starts exercising, for 5 minutes continuously unless he stops before exhaustion or if he falls behind the normal rate of stepping, stop him after he has been unable to keep up the pace for 20 seconds. Note the duration of effort to the nearest second.

2. *Pulse rate*: It is counted from one to one and half minute after the exercise. The count gives half a minute value. When the subject stops, start counting the time and ask him to sit quietly on a chair. After exactly one minute, count the number of heart beats for exact 30 seconds.

The Score

The score depends up on two values

1. Duration of exercise.
2. Pulse rate after the exercise.

The score is obtained from the formula:

$$\text{Index of fitness} = \frac{\text{Time of stepping in sec.} \times 100}{5.5 \times \text{pulse count}}$$

The interpretation of score is as follows:

Below 50	Poor
50–80	Average
Above 80	Good

Score may be recorded directly from Table 3.9.1.

Table 3.9.1: Scoring table for Harvard Step test

Duration of effort	Heart beats from 1 min to 1 min 30 seconds in recovery effort										
	40 to 44	45 to 49	50 to 54	55 to 59	60 to 64	65 to 69	70 to 74	75 to 79	80 to 84	85 to 89	90 to more
0"–20"	5	5	5	5	5	5	5	5	5	5	5
30"–59"	20	15	15	15	15	10	10	10	10	10	10
1'0"–1'29"	30	30	25	25	20	20	20	20	15	15	15
1'30"–1'59"	45	40	40	36	30	30	25	25	25	20	20
2'0"–2'29"	60	50	45	45	40	35	35	30	30	30	25
2'30"–2'59"	70	65	60	55	50	45	40	40	35	35	35
3'0"–3'29"	85	75	70	60	55	55	50	45	45	40	40
3'30"–3'59"	100	85	80	70	65	60	55	55	50	45	45
4'0"–4'29"	110	100	90	80	75	70	65	59	55	55	50
4'30"–4'59"	125	110	100	90	85	75	70	65	60	60	55
5"	130	115	105	95	90	80	75	70	65	65	60

Below 50 = Poor general physical fitness
50–80 = Average general physical fitness
above 80 = Good general physical fitness

Instructions for Reading the Table

1. Find the appropriate line for duration of effort.
2. Then find the appropriate column for the pulse count.
3. Read off the score where the line and column intersect.
4. Interpret according to the scale give below the table.

Other Method

The other method for physical fitness is a simple 3 minutes step test. In this method subject is asked to do exercise on a step for 3 minutes and pulse is counted for 15 seconds (from 5 to 20 sec after stopping the exercise) and his energy expenditure is calculated with the help of formula or noted from the table. It expressed in term of MET. MET is a unit for measurement of energy expenditure. (One MET is equivalent to the resting oxygen consumption that is approximately 200 to 250 ml per min.)

QUESTIONS AND ANSWER

1. What is the significance of physical fitness test?

Ans. It is used in:
   (i) Determination of ability to perform a specific work task.
   (ii) Providing basis for exercise prescription.
   (iii) Evaluation of cardiac and respiratory function.
   (iv) Screening for coronary heart disease.

2. When does a person should stop the exercise in Harvard step test?

3. What is the standard height of step for Indian population in Harvard step test?

4. What is MET?

EXPERIMENT 3.10

To measure blood flow to the forearm by plethysmography

THEORY

Plethysmography is the technique to measure the blood flow to particular region of the body. There is different types of plethysmography depending upon to measure blood flow of different parts of the body, e.g. forearm plethysmography and digital plethysmography.

Plethysmograph is an airtight chamber in which we place the part of the body and venous flow is occluded, which leads to change in volume in the chamber and this change is recorded on volume recorder (float recorder or polyrite or student physiograph). In this experiment forearm is placed in airtight chamber which is connected to volume recorder (through transducer to polyrite or directly to float recorder) which records the change in volume.

APPARATUS

Plethysmograph, float recorder or polyrite or student's physiograph with volume transducer.

Plethysmograph

It consists of a rigid walled container, so arranged that forearm or hand can be placed in it. On one end there is rubber collar to make it airtight. On the other end, there is a central opening through which it is connected to one end of a 'T' shaped metallic or glass tube. Other end of 'T' tube is connected to transducer through rubber pressure tube. Third end of 'T' tube is used to calibrate the volume recorder (polyrite or physiograph or float recorder).

PROCEDURE

1. Plethysmograph is connected to transducer.
2. Put forearm at the subject in the plethysmograph. (It should not be too loose and too tight at rubber collar.)
3. Keep the physiograph or polyrite ready after adjusting its sensitivity up to required level.
4. Tie the cuff on the arm in the same hand.
5. Calibrate the volume recorder by injected 2 ml, 4 ml, 6 ml, and 8 ml of air through the 'T' tube with the help of hypodermic syringe.
6. Pressure in the sphygmomanometer is raised suddenly to 70 mmHg to occlude superficial as well as deep veins. Blood goes on flowing in the forearm but not drained and rise in the volume is recorded on the polyrite. Speed of polyrite paper should be about 5 mm/sec. Time tracings are also recorded.
7. First there is gradual increase in volume but later it becomes steady.
8. Now pressure in the cuff is reduced to zero. Blood flow to forearm is calculated with the help of graph recorded (Fig 3.10.1).
9. **Effect of Reactive Hyperemia:**

   After recording the graph for resting blood flow to forearm, raise the pressure in the cuff to 180 to 200 mmHg to occlude the arteries and maintain it for 2–3 minutes.

   After 2–3 minute reduced the pressure in the cuff to 70 mmHg and take the record.
10. **Effect of Exercise:**

    After recording the resting blood flow at resting state ask the person to do the exercise to forearm and hand for 3–5 minutes.

    Now again record the blood flow by raising the pressure in the cuff to 70 mmHg.
11. **Effect of Temperature:**

    To study the effect of temperature on blood flow to forearm, plethysmograph is filled with warm water and cold water each time and blood flow is recorded.

Calculations

(For given Fig. 3.10.1)

Blood flow in forearm at rest:

Volume change in 3.58 sec = 25 mm.

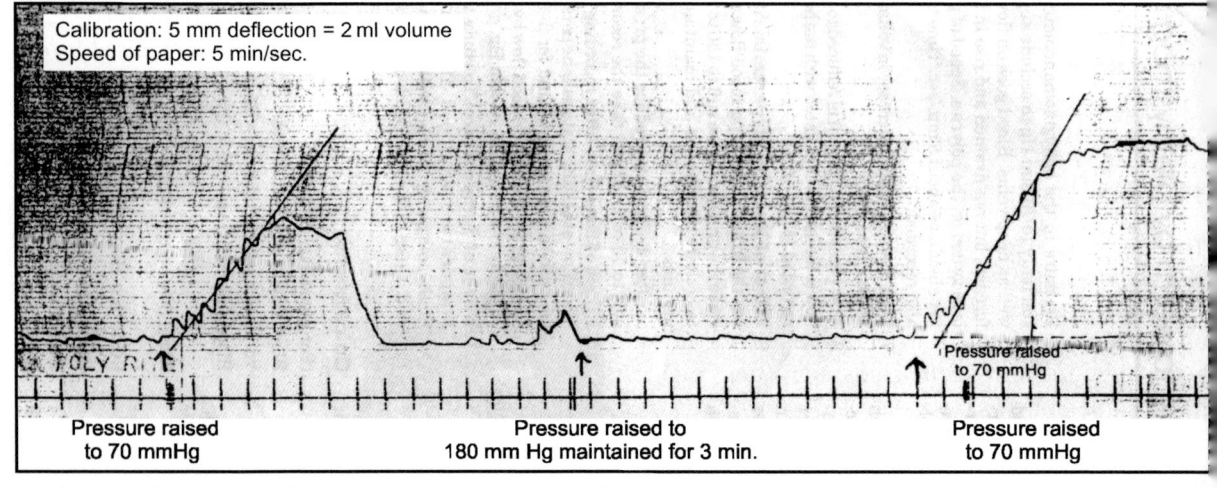

Calibration: 5 mm deflection = 2 ml volume
Speed of paper: 5 min/sec.

POLY R...

| Pressure raised to 70 mmHg | Pressure raised to 180 mm Hg maintained for 3 min. | Pressure raised to 70 mmHg |

Fig. 3.10.1: Blood flow in forearm by plethysmography (First tracing normal blood flow and second tracing reactive hyperemia) using polyrite.

Blood flow in 3.5 sec = $25 \times 2/5$

$= 10$ ml.

(2 ml = 5 mm deflection)

Blood flow = $10 \times 60/3.5 = 171.4$ ml/min.

Reactive Hyperemia

Change in volume in 3 sec. = 31 mm

Blood flow in 3 sec = $31 \times 2/5 = 12.4$ ml.

Blood flow per min = $12.4 \times 60/3 = 248$ ml/min

QUESTIONS AND ANSWERS

1. Why pressure in the cuff is raised to 70 mm Hg to measure blood flow by plethysmography?

2. What is reactive hyperemia?

Ans. When artery is occluded for 2 to 3 min it leads to hypoxia. This hypoxia responsible for marked increase in blood flow because of vasodilatation when pressure in the cuff is reduced to 70 mmHg. This sudden increase in blood flow in response to hypoxia is called reactive hypoxia.

3. What is the effect of exercise on blood flow to forearm?

Ans. There is increase in blood flow in the forearm during exercise. It is because of increase in production of metabolites (CO_2 and H^+) and hypoxia.

4. What is the effect of change in temperature on blood flow to forearm?

Ans. Increase in temperature causes increase in blood flow to forearm and decrease in blood flow decreases the blood flow.

EXPERIMENT 3.11

Recording of human electrocardiogram

THEORY

Electrocardiogram (ECG) is an electrical activity of the heart recorded by electrodes from the body surface.

ECG gives information about :

1. Disturbances of rate rhythm and conduction.
2. Anatomical orientation of heart.
3. The relative size of its chambers.
4. The extent, location and progress of ischaemic damage to myocardium.
5. Effects of altered electrolyte concentrations.

APPARATUS

ECG Machine

1. It is a very sensitive galvanometer.
2. It works on domestic electricity (220 volt AC) and on battery also.
3. Potential picked up by the electrode is amplified before feeding to galvanometer.
4. It has main switch for 'off' and 'on'.
5. 50 Hz filter is fitted to cuts off unwanted interference.
6. Calibration - commonly used sensitivity is 10 mm deflection = 1 mv potential on ECG paper.
7. Centering knob is provided to control base line.
8. Lead selector switch is present to record various leads.
9. Various leads with electrodes.
10. ECG paper:
    - (i) It is a waxed paper.
    - (ii) Speed of paper is 25 mm/sec.
    - (iii) Horizontal scale 25 mm = 1 sec.
    - (iv) Vertical scale 1 mv = 10 mm.

Lead

It is a circuit by which electrical activity of the heart is recorded. The original electrographic lead system was devised by William Einthoven (1860–1927). Leads are of different types.

    A. Standard bipolar limb leads: Lead I, Lead II, and Lead III.

    B. Augmented unipolar limb leads: aVR, aVL and aVF.

    C. Unipolar chest leads: From V1 to V6.

A. Standard Limb Leads

The standard limb leads are shown in Fig. 3.11.1.

Lead I: Left arm is connected with the positive terminal of galvanometer and right arm is connected with negative terminal of galvanometer.

Lead II: Right arm is connected to negative terminal and left leg is connected to positive terminal of galvanometer.

Lead III: Left arm is connected to negative terminal and left leg to positive terminal of galvanometer.

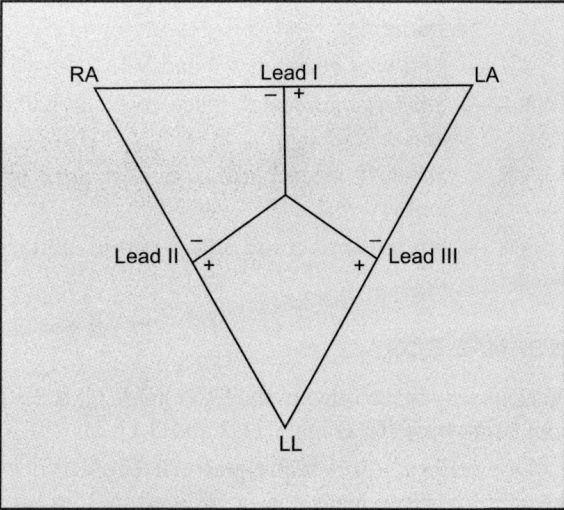

Fig. 3.11.1: Einthoven triangle showing standard limb leads (RA right arm, LA left arm, and LL left leg).

B. Augmented Unipolar Limb Leads

There is recording of potential difference between one limb and other two limbs.

aVL: Between left arm and right arm + left leg.

aVR: Between right arm and left arm + left leg.

aVF: Between left leg and right arm + left arm.

In this lead system two limbs are connected to high resistance (5000 ohms) and then to the galvanometer and other end of galvanometer is connected to 3rd limb. There is increase in size of potential by 50% without any change in the configuration from the nonaugmented bipolar limb lead record because each augmented limb lead is equal to 3/2 of bipolar limb lead.

C. Unipolar Chest Leads

In this lead system all the three limbs (right arm, left arm and left leg) are connected to very high resistance (5000 ohms) to make zero potential. The exploring electrode is placed in the various parts of precordial region to record various chest leads.

Location of various chest-leads is as follows:

V1 — 4th intercostal space just right to the sternum.

V2 — 4th intercostal space just left to the sternum.

V3 — Mid way between V2 and V4.

V4 — 5th left intercostal space mid clavicular line.

V5 — 5th left intercostal space at anterior axillary line.

V6 — 5th left intercostal space at mid axillary line.

NORMAL ECG

Various waves recorded in the ECG are P, Q, R, S, T and some time 'U' (Figs 3.11.2 and 3.11.3).

Depending upon wave pattern (positive or negative) various leads can be divided in 3 groups.

1. Left sided lead: I, aVL, V4, V5, V6. All waves are positive except Q & S.

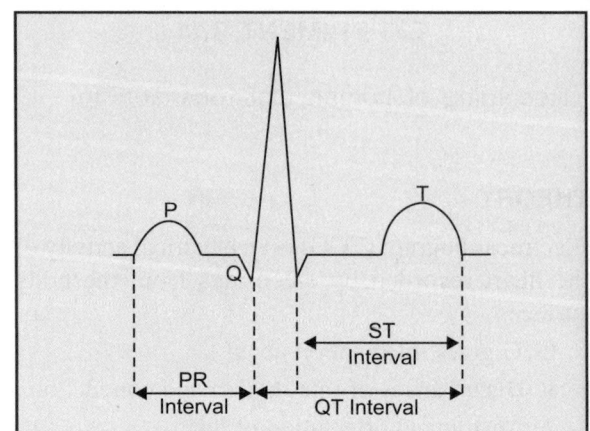

Fig. 3.11.2: Normal cardiogram showing various waves.

2. Right sided leads: II, aVR, V1, V2. All waves are negative except Q & S.

3. Inferiors or diaphragmatic leads: III, aVF, V3. Show biphasic pattern.

PROCEDURE

1. Ask the subject to lie supine on the bed comfortably.

2. Check that ECG machine should be earthed properly.

3. Apply saline gelly on the various body parts where electrodes are applied.

4. Tie the various electrodes and connect the various leads.

5. Adjust the speed of paper to 25 mm/sec. Adjust and record the calibration that 1 mv shows the deflection of 10 mm on the paper.

6. Adjust the lead select in the specific sequence and record ECG (I, II, III, aVR, aVL, aVF, V1, V2, V3, V4, V5 and V6).

CALCULATIONS

Calculation of Heart Rate

Speed of ECG paper = 25 mm/sec.

ECG paper moves in one min = 1500 mm.

RR interval in mm = One cardiac cycle.

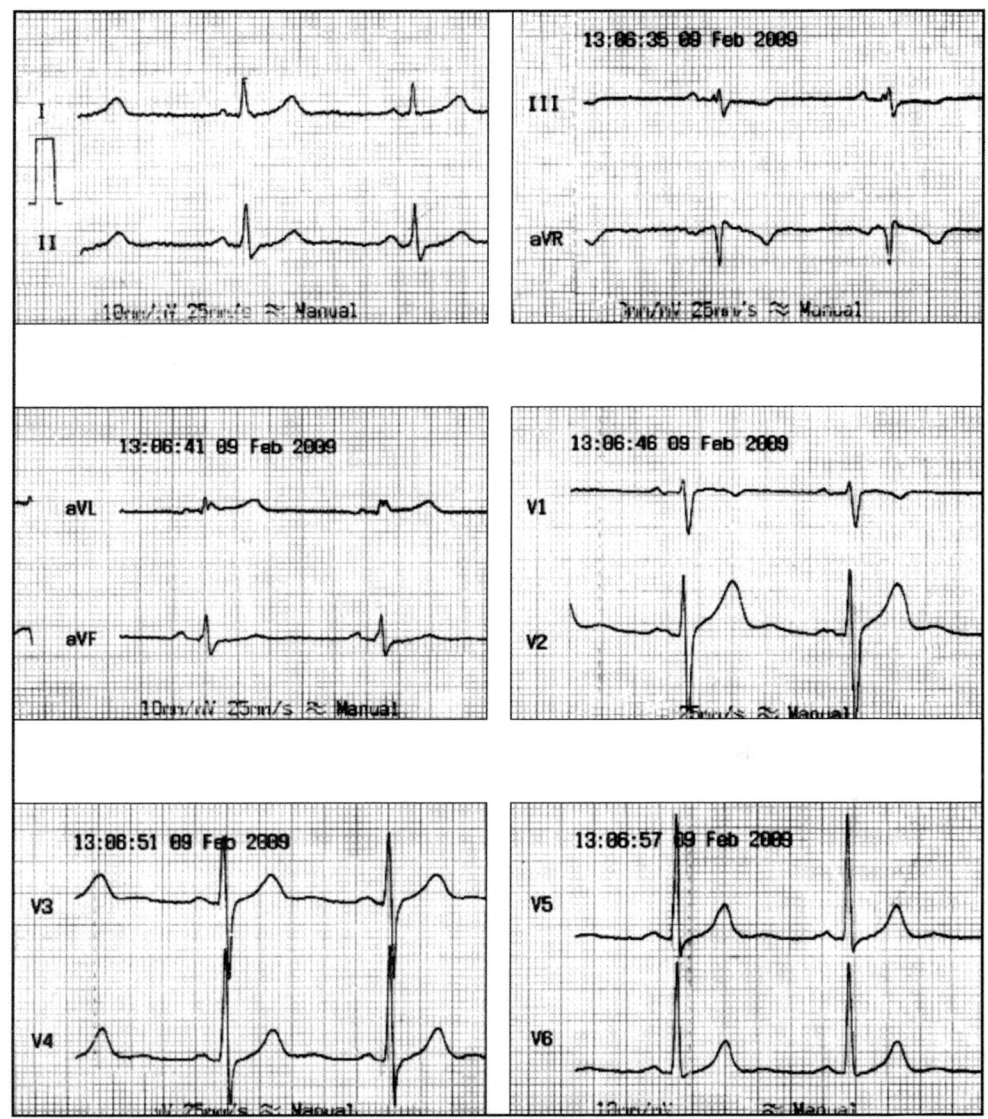

Fig. 3.11.3: ECG in various leads.

$$\text{Heart rate} = \frac{1500}{\text{RR interval in mm}} \text{ per min}$$

Calculation of Cardiac (Vector) Axis

Since the standard limb leads I, II, and III are records of the potential difference between two points, therefore, deflection in each lead at any moment indicates the magnitude and direction in the axis of the electromotive force generated in the heart. This is called as cardiac axis or cardiac vector.

Cardiac axis at any given moment can be calculated from any two standard limb leads. The electrical axis of heart is plotted by using the average QRS deflection (in man) in any two standard limb leads. This is called mean QRS vector. Average QRS deflection means height of R wave minus the height of the largest negative deflection in the QRS complex (Fig. 3.11.4).

For example Average deflection in standard limb lead-I is 18 mm and in lead-II 20 mm (Average deflection is sum of positive and negative deflection, if positive deflection is 21 mm and negative deflection 3 mm it mean average deflection will be 21–3 = 18). Raise a perpendicular on lead-I at 18 mm distance from the centre at 'A'. Another perpendicular is raised at a distance of 20 mm from the centre point at 'C'. These two perpendiculars are intersecting at point 'D'. Draw a line from the centre to the point 'D'. The angle ABD will be the cardiac axis (Fig. 3.11.4).

Normal cardiac axis:

From –30° to +110°

> –30° = Left axis deviation.

> +110° = Right axis deviation.

Analysis and Interpretation

1. Calculate heart rate.
2. Measure and write down the various characteristic features of ECG as shown in Table 3.11.1.
3. Calculate cardiac axis.

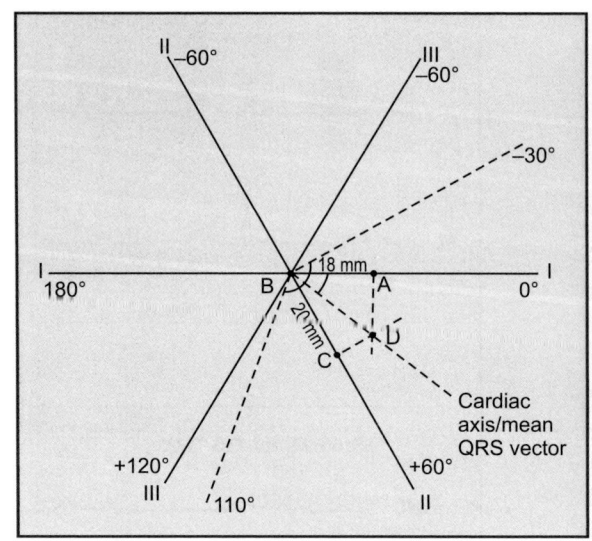

Fig. 3.11.4: Calculation of cardiac axis.

Precautions

1. Ensure that ECG machine should be properly earthed.
2. Subject should not wear any magnetic and metallic article which might interfere with the low voltage electrical signals.
3. Must record calibration before recording ECG.

S.No.	ECG component	Cause	Duration (sec)	Amplitude (mv)
		Table 3.11.1: Characteristic features of normal ECG		
1.	P wave	Atrial depolarisation	0.08–0.1	0.2–0.5
2.	QRS complex	Ventricular depolarisation	0.08–0.12	1.5–2.0
3.	T wave	Ventricular repolarisation	0.27	0.2–0.5
4.	PR interval	Atrial depolarisation and conduction in bundle of His	0.13–0.16	—
5.	QT interval	Ventricular depolarisation and Ventricular repolarisation	0.4–0.43	—
6.	ST interval	Ventricular repolarisation	0.32	—

EXPERIMENT 3.12

To study respiratory movements by stethograph

APPARATUS

Stethograph, Marey's tambour, stop watch, kymograph with drum and time marker.

Stethograph

Stethograph is a corrugated rubber tube, closed at one end and other end is connected to Marey's tambour with the help of pressure rubber tube. Recording of respiratory movements by stethograph is called stethography.

Marey's Tambour

The tambour is a flat saucer-shaped metallic apparatus membrane. To the bottom is fixed a metal tube which is connected with stethograph through a pressure rubber tube.

Working of Stethograph

Stethograph is tied around the chest with the help of a hook and metallic chain. With expension of chest during inspiration, corrugated tube stretches and its length increases which leads to increase and volume and finally there is fall in pressure in stethograph. It is further responsible for down movement of diaphragm (membrane) of Marey's tambour and lever moves downwards. The opposite sequence occurs during expiration and lever moves up.

PROCEDURE

1. The subject sits quietly and comfortably on a stool with his back towards the recording apparatus and stethograph is tied around the chest at the level of nipples or at lower half of the chest.

2. The corrugated tube is left partially stretched so that the respiratory movements can produce pressure changes in it.

3. The connected tube is joined to the Marey's tambour which is mounted on a stand. On the same stand, the time marker is also be fixed.

4. Speed of the kymograph is adjusted to 2.5 mm per second.

5. Respiratory movements are recorded as follows:

   I. **Normal Respiration:** At slow speed quiet breathing movements are recorded. Normal respiratory is calculated from the record.

   II. **Breath Holding:** After normal tracing, breath holding is recorded after holding the breath at the

      (i) end of the quiet expiration.

      (ii) end of maximum expiration.

      (iii) end of quiet inspiration.

      (iv) end of maximum inspiration.

      (v) end of voluntary hyperventilation for 15 to 30 seconds.

   Calculate the breath holding time in the different situation of holding of breath. Breaking point is the point at which breathing can no longer be voluntarily inhibited. Generally young healthy subjects can hold the breath for about 45 seconds.

   3–5 minutes gap should be given after each breath holding

   III. **Effect of Voluntary Hyperventilation:** Record normal respiratory movement and stop the drum. Ask the subject to breath deep and fast to his maximum for one minute. Start the drum and record the breathing movements till it comes back to normal.

   IV. **Effect of Swallowing:** Record normal respiratory movements and ask the subjects to drink water 3 to 4 times in such a way that sometime he will drink it during inspiratory phase and sometime in expiratory phase.

   V. **Effect of Talking, Sneezing and Coughing:** Record normal breathing movements and now ask the subject to read about few sentences from the book to study the effect of talking.

Again record normal movements and record the effect of sneezing and coughing.

VI. **Effect of Exercise:** Disconnect the pressure tube from stethograph ask the subject to do moderate grade exercise (jogging on the same spot) for 2 minutes. Now connect the stethograph to Marey's tambour by pressure tube and take the record till breathing comes to normal.

VII. **Effect of Asphyxia:** Record normal breathing movements. Ask the subject to breath in polythene bag having capacity 5–6 litres for few breathing and take the record, but discontinue to breath in the bag if there is much discomfort.

RESULT AND DISCUSSION

Express your result as follows.

1. Normal respiratory rate.
2. Breath holding time in seconds:

   (i) End of expiration
   (ii) Maximum expiration
   (iii) End of inspiration
   (iv) Maximum inspiration
   (v) After voluntary hyperventilation

3. Effect of voluntary hyperventilation.
4. Effect of swallowing.
5. Effect of taking, sneezing and coughing.
6. Effect of exercise.
7. Effect of asphyxia.

Precautions

1. Stop the subject to hyperventilate if he feels any discomfort or fainting.
2. Stethograph tied around the chest should not be too loose or too tight.
3. Must ask to stop breathing in a polythene bag if subject feels any discomfort.

QUESTIONS AND ANSWERS

1. What is breaking point and what are the causes of it?

Ans. The breaking point is the point when the subject is not able to hold the breath further. It is because of increase in carbon dioxide and hydrogen ions in blood and hypoxia.

2. How much is normal breath holding time?

3. How can we prolong breath holding time?

Ans. It can be done by holding the breath –

   (i) After deep inspiration.
   (ii) After voluntary hyperventilation.
   (iii) After taking deep breath in pure oxygen.

4. What is the effect of voluntary hyperventilation on breathing?

Ans. It is followed by apnoea and periodic breathing.

5. What is periodic/cheyne stoke's breathing?

Ans. Repeated sequence of apnoea followed by breathing till the normal breathing is restored called as periodic breathing. When it is because of certain disease state (heart failure or uremia) it is called cheyne stoke's breathing. It is because of wash out of CO_2 during voluntary hyperventilation which causes apnoea after this CO_2 level rises and further responsible for brief period of increased ventilation. This again responsible for wash of CO_2 and inhibit respiration leading to small phase of apnoea. This cycle is repeated till normal breathing is restored.

6. What is deglutition apnoea and what is its physiological significance.

Ans. During swallowing respiration gets inhibited in what ever the phase the breathing is. This is called as deglutition apnoea. The afferent impulses travel in glossopharyngeal nerve which inhibites the respiratory centre. The reflex is protective in nature and prevents aspiration of food particles into respiratory passage.

7. What is the effect sneezing and coughing on respiration?

Ans. Both sneezing and coughing begin with a deep inspiration followed by forceful expiration.

8. In which phase of respiration person speaks?

Ans. Person speaks in expiratory phase. Before speaking one has to inspire and depth of inspiration depends on length of the sentence a person going to speak.

9. What is asphyxia?

Ans. Occlusion of airway is called asphyxia. In this condition there is hypercapnia and hypoxia both are present.

10. What is hypoxia?

Ans. Deficiency of oxygen at tissue level is called hypoxia.

11. What is hypercapnia?

Ans. Accumulation of carbon dioxide in the body is called hypercapnia.

12. What is hypocapnia?

Ans. Wash out of carbon dioxide from the body is called hypocapnia ($^-PCO_2$ in blood).

13. Which phase in the record is inspiration and which one is expiration and why?

Ans. In the record downward movement is inspiration and upward movement is expiration. During inspiration there is stretching of stethograph tube which causes increase in volume and decrease in pressure in the tube. This fall in the pressure in the tube is responsible for downward movement in the diaphragm of Marey's tambour leading to down movement of writing lever. During expiration recoiling of stethograph tube responsible for up movement of writing lever.

14. Amplitude of tracing is a lung volume or some thing else, explain.

Ans. The tracings on kymograph are not lung volumes. These are the respiratory movements only. Movements during inspiration or expiration are responsible for stretching or recoiling of the stethograph tube.

EXPERIMENT 3.13

To study the effect of posture on vital capacity by vitalograph

APPARATUS

Vitalograph, mouthpiece, nose lip, couch and antiseptic solution.

Vitalograph

1. It is an instrument used to measure vital capacity.
2. It is a double walled metallic cylindrical chamber containing water between two cylinders. Water in the apparatus makes it air-tight (Fig. 3.13.1).
3. Lower cylinder having a metallic tube which passes through centre of its base and projects about 1/2 an inch above the upper edge of outer cylinder.
4. Lower end of the tube is connected to a mouth piece through a corrugated rubber tube.
5. Upper inverted cylinder called as 'Bell' which is made up of copper or aluminium.
6. At the top of the bell a hook is fixed, which is connected to the balancing weight with the help of a metallic chain through a moving disc.
7. Movable disc is having graduations for vital capacity from 0 to 6 litres.
8. Displacement of bell is recorded with the help of a pointer located at disc.

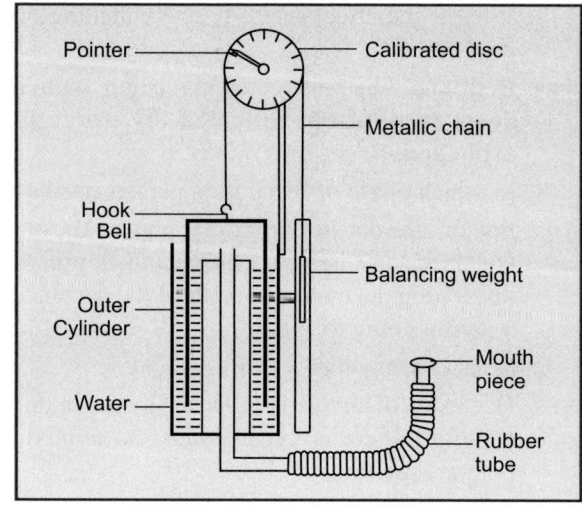

Fig. 3.13.1: Vitalograph.

9. Total capacity of vitalograph is 6 litres.
10. Water level in the vitalograph is kept about 1–2 inches below the upper edge of outer cylinder.

PROCEDURE

1. Mouth piece should be properly washed in 1% solution of savalon and then with tap water.
2. Set the pointer over the movable disc to zero by holding the bell at lowest position.
3. Ask the subject lie supine comfortably on the couch.
4. Give proper instruction to the subject regarding the apparatus.

RESULT AND DISCUSSION

Tabulate your result as follows:

Posture	First reading (L)	Second reading (L)	Third reading (L)
1. Lying			
2. Sitting			
3. Standing			

5. Insert the mouthpiece between lips and teeth.
6. Ask him to breathe through the mouth to his maximum.
7. Close his nostrils with the help of nose clip by his own thumb and fingers.
8. Ask him to blow in the apparatus with maximum effort and to the maximum. Note down the value of vital capacity from movable disc.
9. Wait for 2–3 minutes and take another reading in lying posture. Take third reading after 2–3 minutes of gap in same posture.
10. Now take 3 readings in each sitting and standing posture.

PRECAUTIONS

1. Mouthpiece should be properly cleaned with antiseptic solution.
2. There must not be water in the corrugated rubber tube.
3. Water level in the vitalograph should be about 1–2 inches below upper edge of outer cylinder.

Normal Value

Adult male = 4.8 litres

Adult female = 3.2 litres

Effect of Posture or Vital Capacity

Vital capacity is highest in standing, less in sitting and least in lying posture. Possible cause of more vital capacity in sitting and standing posture is as follows:

1. Decrease in venous return, decrease in pulmonary blood flow in sitting and standing posture causes less blood volume in thoracic cavity.

2. Because of gravity abdominal viscera shift downwards leading to lowering of abdominal diaphragm. This provide more space in thoracic cavity.

Above factors show maximal effect in standing posture as compared to sitting.

Other Factors Affecting Vital Capacity

1. *Sex*: Vital capacity is more in male as compared to female.
2. *Height*: With increase in the height of the individual there is increase in vital capacity.
3. *Body surface area*: Vital capacity increases with increase in body surface area.
4. *Age*: Vital capacity is less in children maximum in adult and in old age it decreases because of loss of elasticity of chest.
5. *Pregnancy*: In first and second trimester of pregnancy there is decrease in vital capacity and in third trimester it becomes normal.
6. *Pathological causes*: Vital capacity decreases in diseases of respiratory system, e.g. pulmonary fibrosis, emphysema, pleural effusion and pulmonary oedema.

Accumulation of fluid in abdominal cavity (ascitis) causes decreases in vital capacity.

QUESTIONS AND ANSWER

1. Define vital capacity.
Ans. This is the volume of the air which can be expired with maximum effort after the maximum inspiration.
2. What is the normal value of vital capacity?
3. What is the effect of posture on vital capacity?
4. What are the other factors effecting vital capacity.

EXPERIMENT 3.14

Determination of various lung volumes and capacities by spirometry

APPARATUS

Simple spirometer/Expirograph, mouth piece, nose clip and antiseptic solution.

Simple Spirometer

1. Simple spirometer is double walled cylindrical chamber containing water between the two cylinders. An inverted cylinder which is very light in weight carries a hook by which is attached to balancing weight and to writing pen through a pulley. This inverted cylinder is called as Bell. Water makes the spirometer airtight. Pen moves up and down when volume of air in the bell decreases or increases during inspiration and expiration.

2. The paper on the kymograph is calibrated for volume as well as time. There are two speeds of kymograph slow (60 mm/min or 1 mm/sec) and fast (1200 mm/min or 20 mm/sec). 10 mm tracing on spirometer paper which is because of movement of bell is equal to 300 ml of change in volume in the bell. (1 mm = 30 ml*).

3. Spirometer is connected to the metallic tube with the help of two corrugated/plain rubber tubes. A mouthpiece is connected to third end of the metallic tube (Fig 3.14.1).

4. Kymograph of spirometer works on 220 volt AC.

THEORY

A convenient way of measuring the lung volumes and capacities is by using a spirometer, and the procedure of recording is called as spirometry. Various lung volumes and capacities are as follows:

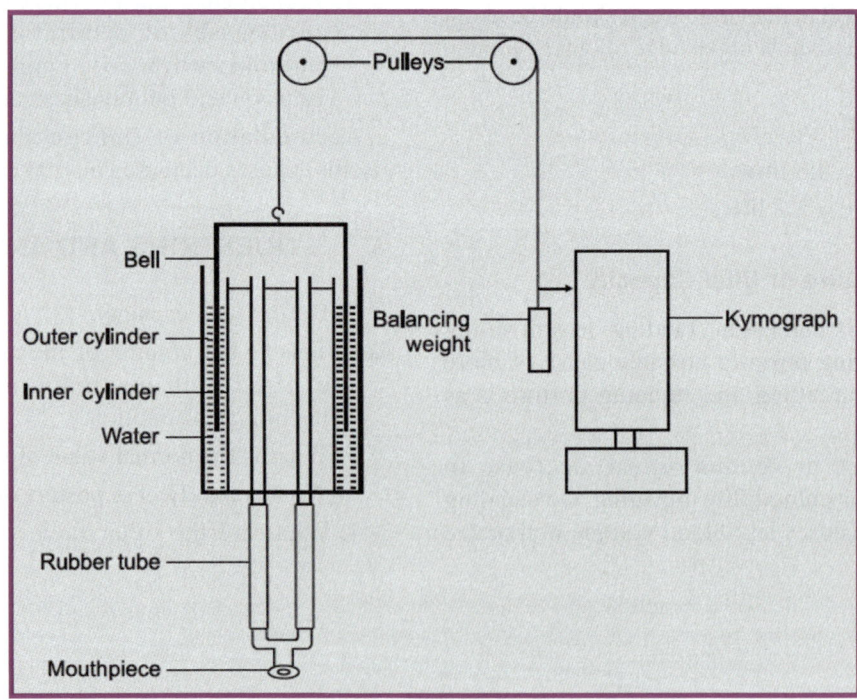

Fig. 3.14.1: Basic diagram of simple spirometer.

1. *Tidal volume* (TV): The volume of the air breathes in or out in one breath is called as tidal volume.

   Normal: 500 ml.

2. *Inspiratory reserve volume* (IRV): It is the maximum volume of the air which can be inspired after completing a normal tidal inspiration.

   Normal: 2000 to 3200 ml.

3. *Expiratory reserve volume* (ERV): It is the maximum volume of air which can be expired after a normal tidal expiration.

   Normal: 750–1000 ml.

4. *Residual volume* (RV): It is the volume of the air which remains in lungs after a maximal expirations.

   Normal: 1200 ml.

5. *Inspiratory capacity* (IC): It is the maximal volume of the air which can be inspired after completing the tidal expiration.

   Normal: 2500–3700 ml.

6. *Vital capacity* (VC): This is the volume of the air which can be expired with a maximum expiratory effort after a maximum inspiration.

7. *Function residual capacity* (FRC) or *function residual volume* (FRV): This is the volume of the air which remains in the lungs at the end of tidal expiration.

   Normal: 2500 ml.

8. *Total lung capacity* (TLC): It is the total volume of the air present in the lung at the end of maximal inspiration.

   Normal: 6 litres.

9. *Timed vital capacity*:

   FEV1: Volume of vital capacity expired in one second. FEV1% percentage of vital capacity expired in one second.

   Normal: 75%

   FEV2: Volume of vital capacity expired in two seconds. FEV2% percentage of vital capacity expired in two seconds.

   Normal: 85%

   FEV3: Volume of vital capacity expired in three seconds.

   Normal FEV3%: 95–100%

10. *Minute ventilation* (MV): It is the volume of the air inspired or expired in one minute.

    MV = TV × RR (RR: *respiratory rate*)

    Normal = 500 × 12 = 6000 L/min

11. *Maximum voluntary ventilation* (MVV)/ *Maximum ventilation volume*: This the volume of the air which is breathed in or out with maximal breathing effort (Deep and fast breathing) in one min.

    Normal: 90–170 L/min.

12. *Pulmonary reserve* or *Breathing reserve*:

$$= MVV - MV$$

$$\text{Dyspnoeic Index (DI)} = \frac{MVV - MV}{MVV} \times 100$$

Normal: 90%

< 60% usually associated with dyspnoea.

PROCEDURE

1. Fill the distilled water in the spirometer up to 1–2 inches below the upper edge of outer cylinder.

2. Clean the mouth piece first with antiseptic solution (1% Savalon) and then with water.

3. Ask the subject to sit on a stool facing towards the spirometer.

4. Give instructions to the subject regarding the experiment so that he will not hesitate at the time of recording.

5. Keep the pen of spirometer ready after filling it with ink.

6. Fill the spirometer with fresh air by moving its bell up.

7. Ask the subjects to insert the mouth piece between lips and teeth. Close the nose with the help of nose clip.

8. Subject is asked to breathe through the mouth piece in the spirometer quietly. In case of expirograph three way valve is there and with

the help of it subject breaths from the atmosphere for 1/2 to 1 min. Now connect the subject to spirometer with the help of three way valve.

9. Start the kymograph, adjust it to move at slow speed (1 mm/sec) and take the record for 15 seconds. This graph is used to measure tidal volume and minute ventilation.

10. After taking the record for tidal volume subject is asked to take deep breath in with maximum effort and slow speed of kymograph is changed to fast (20 mm/sec) and then he is asked to blow out in the spirometer with maximum force and to the maximal expira-tion. Vital capacity and timed vital capacities are calculated from this spirogram. Vital capacity calculated from this spirogram (Fig. 3.14.2) is also called as *forced vital capacity* (FVC).

11. Same procedure is repeated three times after filling the spirometer with fresh air each time.

12. For measuring MVV spirometer is filled with fresh air and subject is asked to breath in it deep and fast with maximum effort for 15–20 seconds. This record is taken with fast speed (20 mm/sec) of kymograph.

CALCULATIONS

1. **Tidal Volume:** Draw two lines in such a way that one line should touch maximum number of upper end of tracings and other line should touch maximum number of lower end of tracings. Measure the vertical distances between two lines.

TV = Distance between two lines (mm) × 30
= in ml.
(10 mm vertical distance = 300 ml).

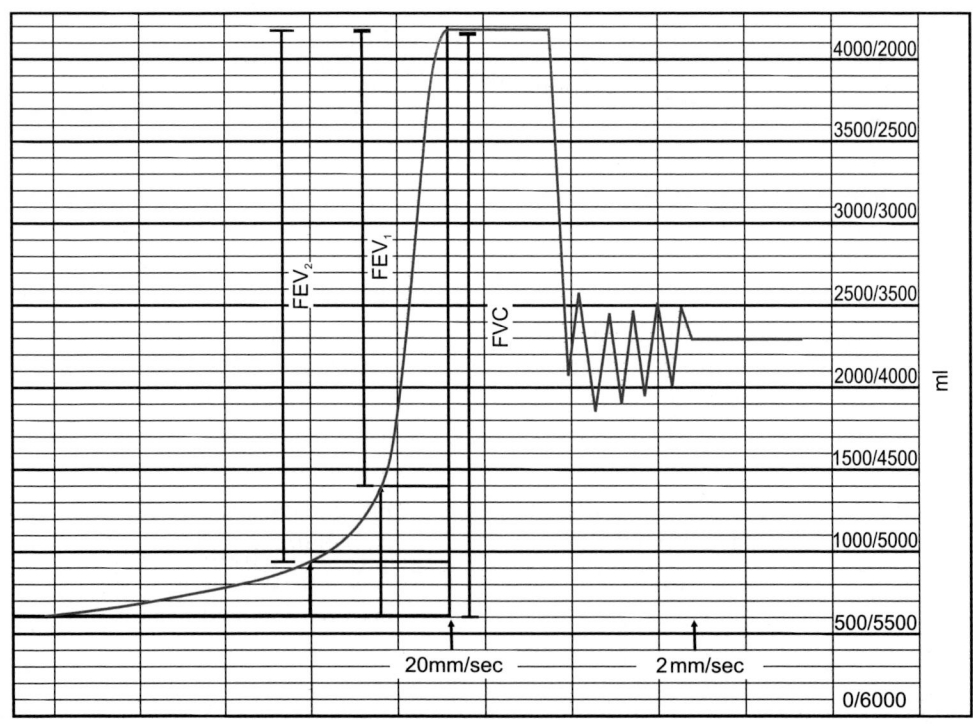

Fig. 3.14.2: Spirogram.

2. Lung Volumes and Capacities: Other lung volumes and capacities are calculated from the forced vital capacity graph by multiplying the various vertical distances (mm) to 30 ml*. (Figs 3.14.2 and 3.14.3).

3. FEV1%: Volume expired in one second of expiration is calculated by considering the zero time from the beginning of expiration. (Horizontal 20 mm distance indicates one second.)

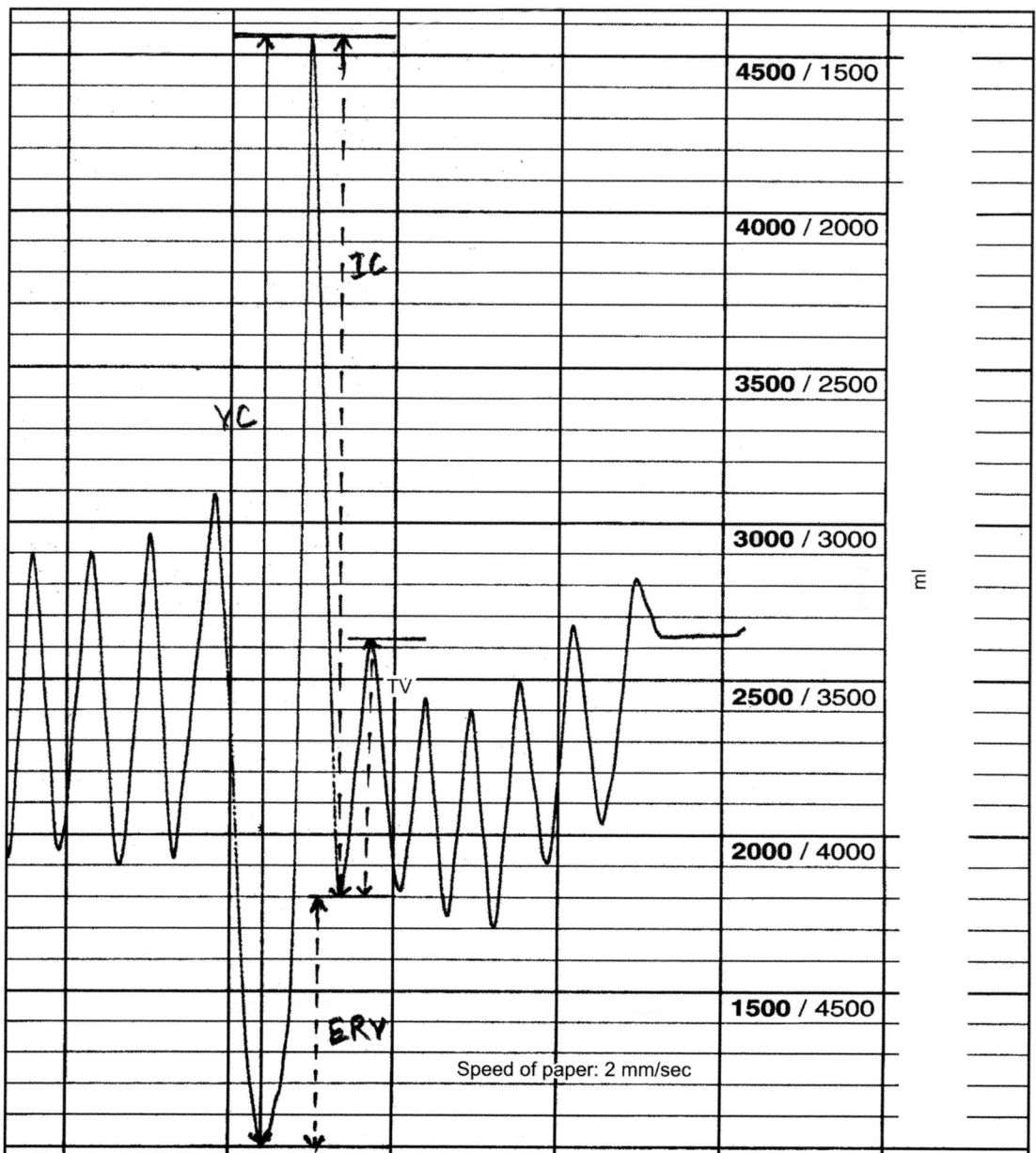

Speed of paper: 2 mm/sec

Fig. 3.14.3: Spirogram.

$$FEV1\% = \frac{FEV_1}{FVC\ (VC)} \times 100$$

4. **Minute Ventilation (MV):** Count inspiratory or expiratory tops for 15 seconds (N) from tidal volume recording.

$MV = TV \times N \times 4 = L/min.$

5. **MVV:** Measure the height of all the inspiratory or expiratory tracings for 15 seconds. Add the height of all the tracings (cm).

MVV = Total height (cm) × 300 (ml) × 4
$= L/min.$

Dyspneic index is also calculated as discussed in the theory part of practical.

* It may vary with spirometer supplied by different companies. This is why the spirogram given in this chapter has different volume calibration.

PRECAUTIONS

1. Must clean the mouth piece with antiseptic solution.
2. Make sure that there should be no water in the rubber tube connecting mouth piece to spirometer.

RESULT AND DISCUSSION

Tabulate your result as follows:

3. Fill the spirometer with fresh air each time after recording one spirogram.

Clinical Significance of Timed Vital Capacity

1. FEV1% is decreased in obstructive lung diseases, e.g. bronchial asthma, but force vital capacity remains normal.
2. FEV1% remains normal in case of restrictive lung diseases, e.g. pulmonary fibrosis, but FVC decreases.
3. In combined lesion (restrictive + obstructive) FEV1% and FVC both decrease.

QUESTIONS AND ANSWER

1. Calculate the various lung volumes and capacities from spirogram.
2. What is FEV1% and what is its significance?

Ans. This is the percentage of the vital capacity which is expired in first second of expiration. In case of obstructive lung disease its value decreases. In case of restrictive lung disease it remains normal.

3. What is breathing reserve?
4. What is dyspneic index and what is its significance?

S. No.	Parameters	Observed	Normal	Remarks
1.	TV			
2.	IRV			
3.	ERV			
4.	IC			
5.	VC (FVC)			
6.	FEV$_1$%			
7.	MV			
8.	MVV			
9.	DI			

EXPERIMENT 3.15

To determine total respiratory compliance

THEORY

Compliance is a change in volume per unit change in pressure.

Total respiratory compliance is 0.13 l/cm of water to 0.21 l/cm of water.

Lung compliance is 0.22 l/cm of water.

APPARATUS

Simple spirometer with water manometer or expirograph with water manometer, oxygen cylinder mouthpiece, nose clip, and antiseptic solution.

PRINCIPLE

Pressure is applied at end expiratory state and change in volume is recorded on spirometer paper on slow moving kymograph. The pressure is changed by applying weight on floating drum (bell) of spirometer. A graph is plotted between change in pressure and change in volume. Value of compliance is found out from the graph.

PROCEDURE

1. Fill the spirometer with pure (100%) oxygen and close the outlet (knob) and now connect it to water manometer.
2. Ask the subject to sit on a stool facing spirometer.
3. Mouthpiece is inserted between lips and teeth. Nose is closed with nose clip.
4. Subject is asked to breath quietly and respiratory tracing are recorded on slow moving (1 mm/sec) kymograph.
5. Add 1/2 kg weight on the bell at the end of expiration (end expiratory state is a static condition). Change in pressure is noted from the water manometer.
6. Now remove 1/2 kg load and add 1 kg weight at end expiratory state on spirometer bell and note change in pressure from manometer.
7. Similarly change in volume and pressure is recorded with 1.5 kg, 2 kg and 2.5 kg of weights.
8. A graph is plotted between change in volume and change in pressure. Value of total respiratory compliance is found out from the graph.

Plot a graph by making pressure change on X axis and volume change on Y axis. Change in volume with 1 cm H_2O pressure is found out. It is expressed in L/cm H_2O. Lung compliance can also be determined by measuring the oesophagial pressure which is equivalent to the pulmonary pressure.

PRECAUTION

1. Same as in recording of lung volumes and capacity.
2. Weight should be added on the bell at end expiratory state and quietly.

Clinical Importance of the Experiment

Distensibility (compliance) is decreased in

1. Smoking
2. Thoracic cage disease: kyphosis and scoliosis.
3. Fibrotic lesions of lungs: Pulmonary tuberculosis and pneumonia.
4. Emphysema.

RESULT AND OBSERVATION

Tabulate your result as follows:

S. No.	Weight applied (kg)	Pressure change (cm H_2O)	Change in volume (ml)
1	0.5		
2	1.0		
3	1.5		
4	2.0		
5	2.5		

EXPERIMENT 3.16

Determination of basal metabolic rate (BMR)

APPARATUS

Expirograph or Benedict's Roth apparatus, soda lime crystals, mouthpiece, nose clip, 1% savalon solution, oxygen cylinder, weighing machine, barometer, Dubois normogram for calculation of body surface area and normal BMR table (Tables 'A' and 'B').

Expirograph (Fig. 3.16.1)

1. It is a spirometer having double-walled cylinder and an inverted light weight cylinder (Bell).
2. Plastic bottle containing sodalime crystals fixed in the spirometer.
3. Two metallic tubes are connected to mouth-piece through two one way valves.
4. Another two way valve is present near the mouth piece to connect the respiratory system of the subject to atmosphere or spirometer.
5. There are two speeds of expirograph at which spirometer paper moves (slow speed: 1 mm/sec, fast speed: 20 mm/sec).
6. 10 mm vertical scale of spirometer paper is equal to 300 ml of volume.
7. There are two metallic knobs at the base of spirometer, one for filling the oxygen in the spirometer and other to drain the water from spirometer at the end of the experiment.
8. Antiseptic solution (1% savalon) is used to clean the mouthpiece.

THEORY

Basal metabolic rate: Energy expenditure of the body for minimal level of activity (basal condition) is called as Basal Metabolic Rate. Basal conditions are complete physical and mental rest, 12–16 hours after the last meal and comfortable environmental temperature (20–25°C).

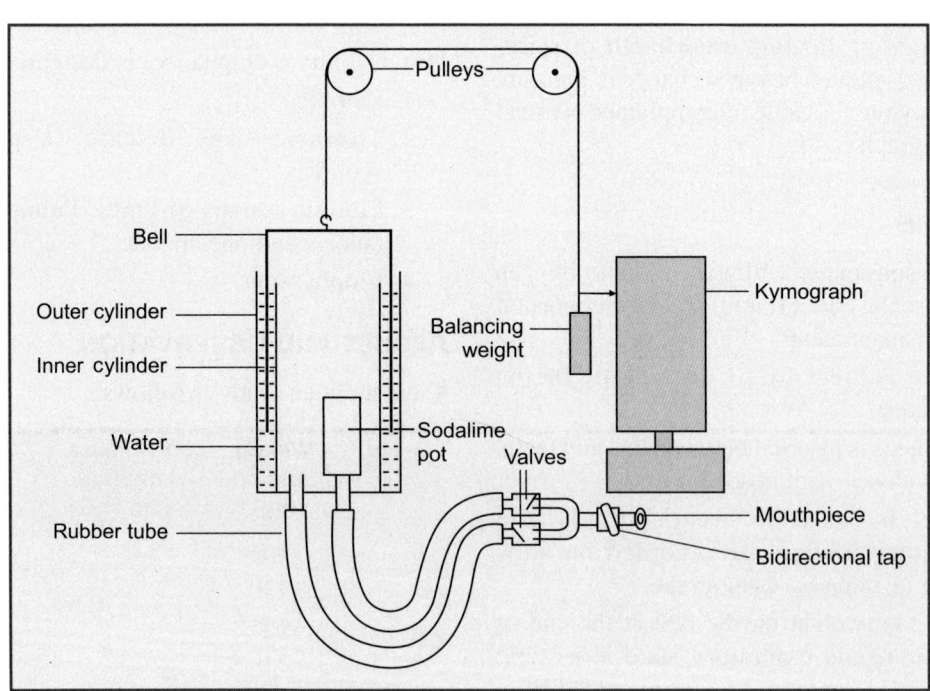

Fig. 3.16.1: Basic diagram of expirograph.

BMR can be estimated with sufficient accuracy merely by measuring the oxygen consumption of the subject for six minutes period under basal conditions. If BMR is not estimated in basal conditions then it is called as resting metabolic rate.

PROCEDURE

1. Subject is advised not to eat any thing after evening meal and to sleep early.
2. He is asked to come to the laboratory in fasting condition on the next day in the morning.
3. He is to take rest for about half an hour before the investigation.
4. Note down age height and weight of the subject.
5. Note down room temperature and atmospheric pressure.

6. Fill the expirograph/spirometer with pure oxygen to its 2/3 volume.
7. Subject is asked to sit on a stool in front of expirograph.
8. He is asked to breath in the expirograph through mouthpiece after applying the nose clip for 6 minutes.
9. Spirogram is recorded during this period at 1.0 mm/sec speed (Fig. 3.16.2).

CALCULATIONS

1. Draw a horizontal (base) line from the lower end of the first tracing to the total distance of spirometer paper moves in six minutes.
2. Draw a straight line passing through the maximum number of lower ends of tracing.

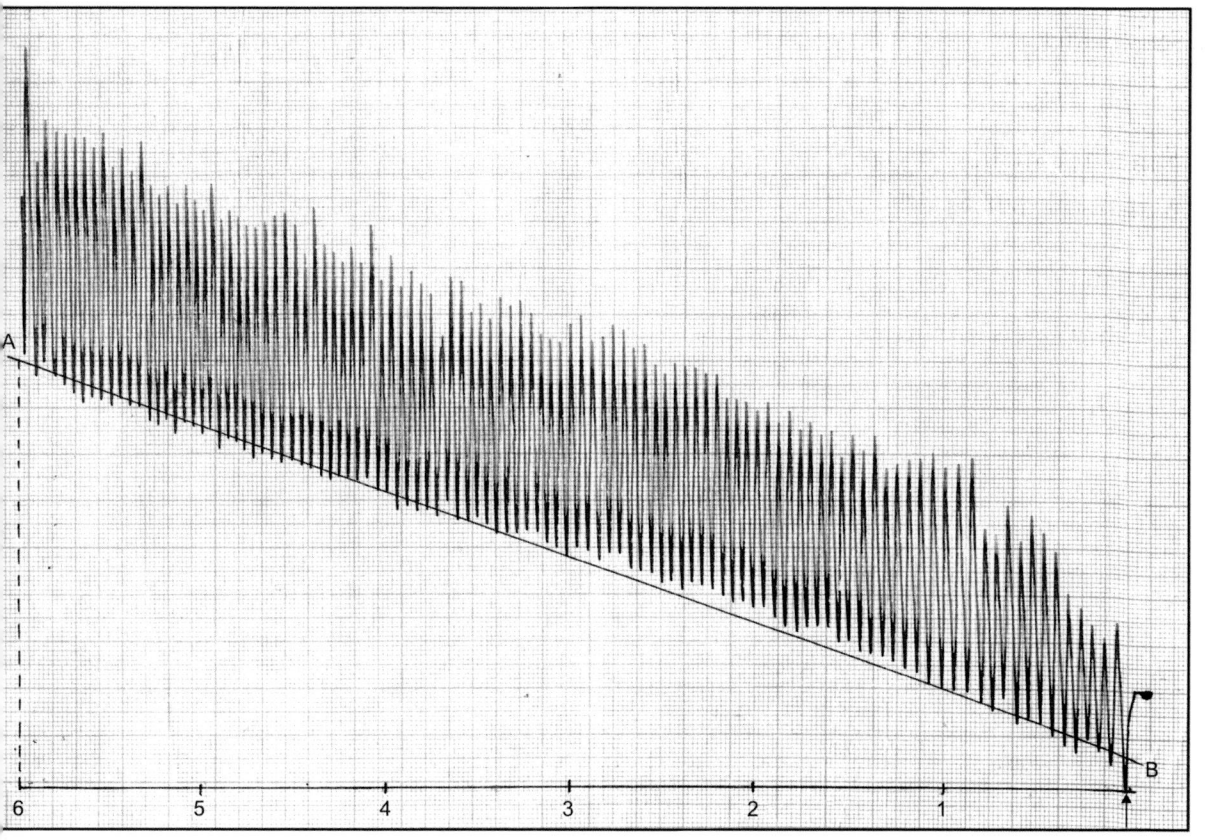

Fig. 3.16.2: Spirogram recorded for six minutes to find out oxygen consumption.

3. Measure the total vertical displacement from the baseline after 6 minutes of time distance on the graph.

4. Multiply vertical distance (cm) to 300 (1 cm = 300 ml) to find out oxygen consumed in 6 minutes.

5. Calculate per hour oxygen consumption by multiplying it by 10.

6. Convert the volume of oxygen to Standard Temperature (0°C) and pressure (760 mmHg) by multiplying it by specific factor (Table 'C').

7. Calculate energy produced by this corrected volume of oxygen.

   Energy produced = Corrected volume of oxygen × 4.875 kcal

   (Energy produced at STDP by one litre of O_2 is 4.875 kcal at RQ of 0.8)

8. With the help of body surface area (from Dubois normogram, Table 'A') of the subject energy produce per square meter of surface area is calculated. BMR is expressed kcal/m²/hour.

9. It can be further compared from the Table 'B'. BMR may be expressed as percentage from expected value at particular age. BMR value from –15 to +20% is considered as normal.

FACTORS AFFECTING BMR

1. *Age*: In children BMR is more as compared to adult.

2. *Sex*: BMR is slightly higher in male as compared to female.

3. *Body surface area*: It increases with increase in body surface area.

4. *Body temperature*: With increase in body temperature there is increase in BMR (0.5°C rise in temperature causes 7% rise in BMR).

5. *Environmental temperature*: Increase in environmental temperature decreases BMR and decrease in temperature increases BMR.

6. *Atmospheric pressure*: At high altitude BMR increases because of decrease in arterial PO_2.

7. *Food intake*: BMR increases after meals.

8. *Exercise*: BMR increases during exercise.

9. *Pregnancy*: It increase during pregnancy.

10. *Endocrinal influence*:

    (i) *Thyroxine level:* BMR increases in hyperthyroidism and decreases in hypothyroidism.

    (ii) *Blood catecholamine level:* Increase level of epinephrine and norepinephrine in blood causes rise in BMR.

QUESTIONS

1. What is BMR?

2. What is resting metabolic rate?

3. What are the various physiological factors effecting BMR?

4. What are the pathological factors affecting BMR?

5. What is the normal value for BMR?

TABLE 'A'

Dubois Body Surface Chart
(As prepared by Boothby and Sandiford of the Mayo Clinic)

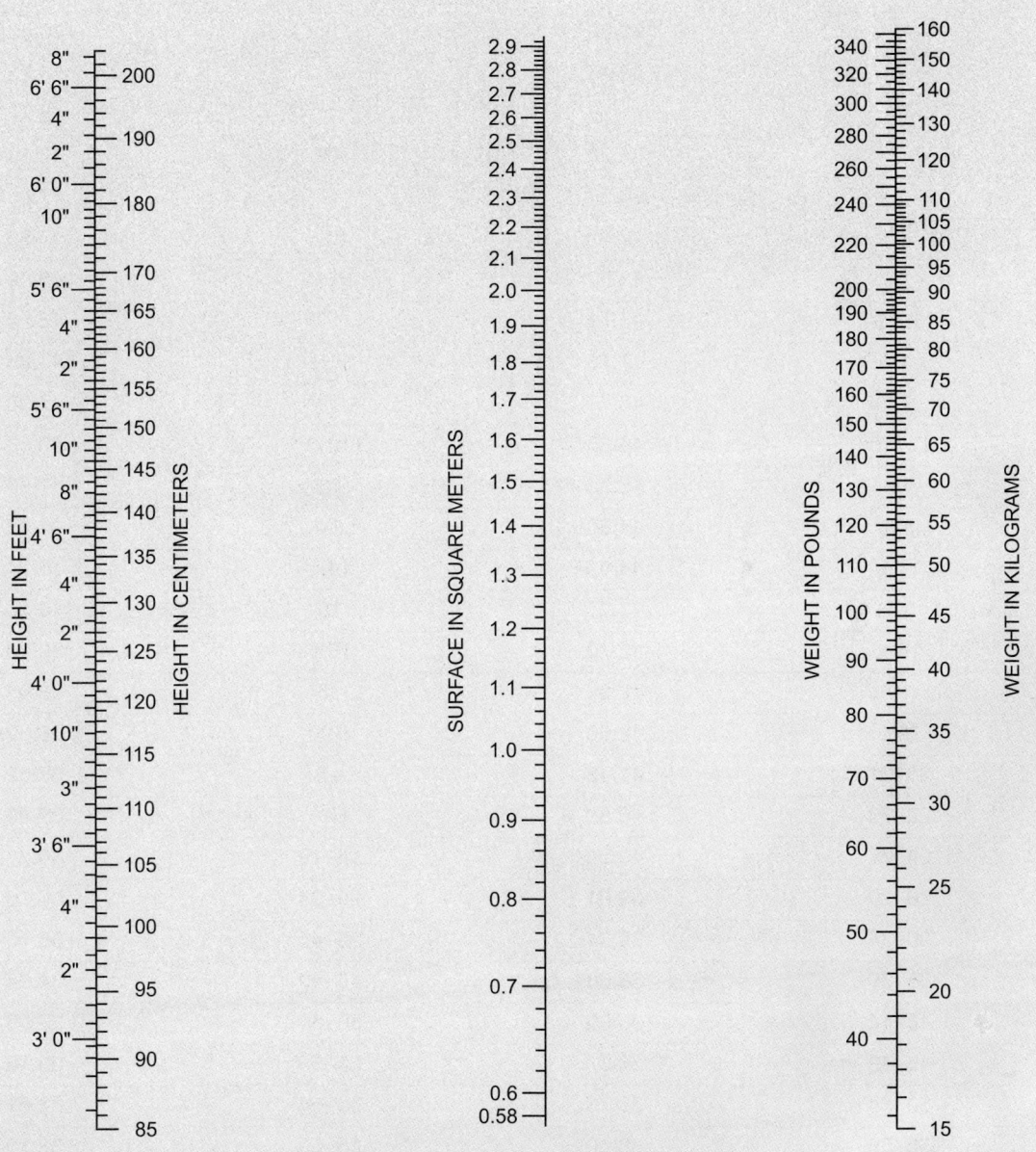

TABLE 'B'
THE MAYO FOUNDATION NORMAL STANDARDS
(American Journal of Physiology, July 1936) Calories per square meter per hour)

Age at Last Birthday	Mean	Age at last birthday	Mean
6	53.00	6	50.62
7	52.45	6½	50.23
8	51.78	7	49.12
8 ½	51.20	7½	47.00
9	50.54	8	47.00
9½	49.42	8½	46.50
10	48.50	9.10	45.90
10½	47.71	11	45.26
11	47.18	11½	44.80
12	46.75	12	44.28
13–15	46.35	12½	43.58
16	45.72	13	42.90
17	44.80	14	41.45
17½	44.03	14½	40.74
18	43.25	15	40.10
18½	42.70	15½	39.40
19	42.32	16	38.85
19½	42.00	16½	38.30
20–21	41.43	17	37.82
22–23	40.82	17½	37.40
24–27	40.24	18–19	36.74
28–29	39.81	20–24	36.18
30–34	39.34	25–44	35.70
35–39	38.68	45–49	34.94
40–44	38.00	50–54	33.96
45–49	37.37	55–59	33.18
50–54	36.73	60–64	32.61
55–59	36.10	65–69	32.30
60–64	35.48	*	
65–69	34.80		

TABLE 'C'
CORRECTION FOR TEMPERATURE AND PRESSURE

Temperature in Degree Centigrade

mm	15	16	17	18	19	20	21	22	23	24	25	26	27	28	29	30	31	32	33	34	35
600	0.735	0.732	0.728	0.725	0.721	0.718	0.715	0.712	0.708	0.704	0.701	0.697	0.693	0.689	0.685	0.681	0.677	0.673	0.669	0.665	0.661
605	0.742	0.739	0.735	0.731	0.727	0.724	0.721	0.718	0.714	0.710	0.707	0.703	0.699	0.695	0.691	0.687	0.683	0.679	0.675	0.671	0.667
610	0.746	0.745	0.741	0.737	0.733	0.730	0.727	0.726	0.720	0.716	0.713	0.709	0.705	0.701	0.697	0.693	0.689	0.685	0.680	0.675	0.672
615	0.754	0.751	0.747	0.744	0.740	0.737	0.734	0.730	0.726	0.722	0.719	0.715	0.711	0.707	0.703	0.699	0.695	0.691	0.686	0.682	0.678
620	0.760	0.757	0.753	0.750	0.744	0.743	0.740	0.737	0.733	0.729	0.725	0.721	0.717	0.713	0.709	0.705	0.701	0.696	0.692	0.688	0.684
625	0.767	0.764	0.760	0.756	0.752	0.749	0.746	0.742	0.739	0.735	0.731	0.727	0.723	0.719	0.715	0.711	0.707	0.702	0.698	0.694	0.690
630	0.773	0.770	0.766	0.762	0.758	0.755	0.752	0.749	0.745	0.741	0.737	0.733	0.729	0.725	0.721	0.717	0.713	0.708	0.704	0.700	0.696
635	0.779	0.776	0.772	0.768	0.764	0.761	0.758	0.755	0.751	0.747	0.743	0.739	0.735	0.731	0.727	0.723	0.719	0.714	0.710	0.706	0.702
640	0.785	0.782	0.778	0.774	0.770	0.767	0.764	0.761	0.757	0.753	0.749	0.745	0.741	0.737	0.733	0.729	0.725	0.720	0.716	0.711	0.707
645	0.792	0.788	0.784	0.781	0.777	0.773	0.770	0.767	0.763	0.759	0.755	0.751	0.741	0.737	0.733	0.729	0.725	0.720	0.716	0.711	0.707
650	0.798	0.794	0.791	0.787	0.784	0.760	0.777	0.773	0.769	0.765	0.761	0.757	0.752	0.748	0.744	0.740	0.736	0.732	0.727	0.723	0.719
655	0.804	0.800	0.797	0.793	0.790	0.786	0.783	0.779	0.775	0.771	0.767	0.763	0.758	0.754	0.750	0.746	0.742	0.738	0.733	0.729	0.724
660	0.810	0.806	0.803	0.799	0.796	0.792	0.789	0.785	0.781	0.777	0.773	0.769	0.764	0.760	0.756	0.753	0.748	0.744	0.739	0.735	0.730
665	0.816	0.812	0.809	0.805	0.802	0.798	0.795	0.791	0.787	0.783	0.779	0.775	0.770	0.766	0.762	0.758	0.754	0.749	0.745	0.741	0.736
670	0.822	0.819	0.816	0.812	0.809	0.805	0.801	0.797	0.793	0.789	0.785	0.781	0.776	0.772	0.768	0.764	0.760	0.755	0.751	0.746	0.742
675	0.828	0.825	0.821	0.818	0.815	0.811	0.807	0.803	0.799	0.795	0.791	0.787	0.782	0.778	0.774	0.770	0.766	0.761	0.757	0.752	0.748
680	0.834	0.831	0.827	0.824	0.821	0.817	0.813	0.809	0.803	0.801	0.797	0.793	0.789	0.784	0.780	0.778	0.771	0.767	0.763	0.758	0.754
685	0.841	0.837	0.833	0.830	0.827	0.823	0.819	0.815	0.811	0.807	0.803	0.799	0.794	0.790	0.786	0.782	0.777	0.773	0.769	0.764	0.760
690	0.848	0.844	0.841	0.837	0.833	0.829	0.825	0.821	0.817	0.813	0.809	0.805	0.800	0.786	0.792	0.788	0.783	0.779	0.775	0.770	0.765
695	0.854	0.850	0.847	0.843	0.839	0.835	0.831	0.827	0.823	0.819	0.815	0.811	0.806	0.802	0.798	0.794	0.789	0.785	0.780	0.776	0.771
700	0.860	0.856	0.853	0.849	0.845	0.841	0.837	0.833	0.829	0.825	0.821	0.817	0.812	0.808	0.804	0.800	0.795	0.791	0.786	0.781	0.777
705	0.866	0.862	0.859	0.855	0.871	0.847	0.843	0.839	0.835	0.831	0.827	0.823	0.818	0.814	0.810	0.806	0.801	0.796	0.792	0.787	0.783
710	0.872	0.868	0.865	0.861	0.857	0.853	0.849	0.845	0.841	0.837	0.833	0.829	0.824	0.820	0.816	0.812	0.807	0.802	0.798	0.793	0.788
715	0.878	0.874	0.871	0.867	0.863	0.859	0.855	0.851	0.847	0.843	0.839	0.835	0.830	0.826	0.822	0.818	0.813	0.808	0.804	Q.799	0.794
720	0.885	0.881	0.877	0.873	0.869	0.865	0.861	0.857	0.853	0.849	0.845	0.841	0.836	0.832	0.828	0.824	0.819	0.814	0.810	0.805	0.800
725	0.891	0.887	0.883	0.978	0.876	0.872	0.867	0.863	0.959	0.855	0.851	0.847	0.842	0.838	0.834	0.830	0.825	0.820	0.816	0.811	0.806
730	0.897	0.894	0.890	0.886	0.882	0.878	0.874	0.869	0.865	0.861	0.857	0.853	0.848	0.844	0.840	0.836	0.831	0.826	0.822	0.817	0.812
735	0.904	0.900	0.896	0.892	0.888	0.884	0.880	0.875	0.871	0.867	0.863	0.859	0.854	0.850	0.846	0.842	0.37	0.832	0.827	0.822	0.817
740	0.910	0.905	0.902	0.898	0.894	0.890	0.886	0.881	0.877	0.873	0.869	0.865	0.860	0.856	0.852	0.848	0.843	0.838	0.833	0.828	0.823
745	0.916	0.912	0.908	0.904	0.900	0.896	0.892	0.887	0.883	0.879	0.875	0.871	0.866	0.862	0.857	0.853	0.848	0.844	0.839	0.834	0.829
750	0.922	0.918	0.914	0.910	0.907	0.902	0.898	0.893	0.889	0.885	0.881	0.877	0.872	0.868	0.863	0.859	0.854	0.849	0.845	0.840	0.835
755	0.928	0.924	0.920	0.916	0.912	0.908	0.904	0.899	0.895	0.891	0.887	0.883	0.878	0.874	0.869	0.865	0.860	0.855	0.851	0.846	0.841
760	0.934	0.930	0.926	0.922	0.918	0.914	0.910	0.905	0.901	0.897	0.893	0.889	0.884	0.880	0.875	0.871	0.866	0.861	0.857	0.852	0.847
765	0.941	0.936	0.932	0.928	0.924	0.920	0.916	0.911	0.907	0.903	0.899	0.895	0.890	0.886	0.881	0.877	0.872	0.867	0.863	0.857	0.852
770	0.947	0.943	0.939	0.935	0.930	0.926	0.922	0.917	0.913	0.909	0.905	0.901	0.896	0.892	0.887	0.883	0.878	0.873	0.869	0.863	0.858
775	0.954	0.949	0.945	0.941	0.936	0.932	0.928	0.923	0.919	0.916	0.911	0.907	0.902	0.898	0.893	0.889	0.884	0.879	0.875	0.869	0.864
780	0.960	0.956	0.952	0.948	0.943	0.939	0.935	0.930	0.926	0.921	0.917	0.913	0.908	0.904	0.899	0.895	0.890	0.885	0.880	0.875	0.870

EXPERIMENT 3.17

To determine energy cost of work and mechanical efficiency by using bicycle ergometer

APPARATUS

Bicycle ergometer (Fig. 3.17.1), expirograph or Benedict's Ruth apparatus, nose clip, mouthpiece, 1% Savalon solution, oxygen cylinder, stethoscope, measuring tape, stopwatch and sphygmomanometer.

THEORY

1. Energy is constantly used by the body and the rate of utilisation is determined by:
   (i) BMR.
   (ii) Physical activity.
   (iii) Specific dynamic action of food.

   The extra amount of oxygen consumed during performance of a work of moderate severity is a measure of energy cost of work.

2. To assess the energy utilised during a specific activity, it is necessary to know the energy utilised for basal metabolism and subtract this from the total energy utilised. The energy utilised is calculated from the spirometric record of oxygen consumption obtained after the steady state has been reached during exercise.

3. Metabolic requirement of the body at rest or during exercise are met with by supplying oxygen to the tissues and by removing carbon dioxide from them. This primarily governed by the CVS and respiratory system.

4. In order to load these mechanisms maximally, large muscle groups must be engaged during exercise. For this reason, treadmill and bicycle ergometer are most commonly used which enable a known power output to be used.

5. Steady state or constant power output: In this test, a power output is maintained constant for long enough for most variables to reach relatively constant steady state values. Rapid increase in oxygen consumption and carbon dioxide output occurs in the first 2–4 minutes at a given work load, but changes thereafter are small. Thus, after 4–5 minutes of exercise at constant work rate, a steady state is assumed to have been reached for measurement of cardiorespiratory responses.

PROCEDURE

1. Note down age, height, weight, temperature, pulse rate and blood pressure of the subject.
2. Note down room temperature and barometric pressure.

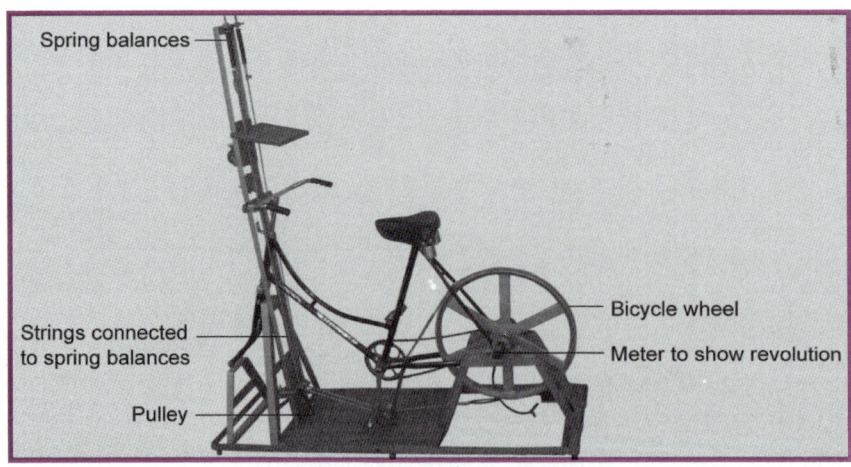

Fig. 3.17.1: Bicycle ergometer.

3. Fill expirograph (spirometer) with 100% oxygen up to 2/3 of its volume.

4. Measure resting oxygen consumption of the subject on expirograph after recording the spirogram for 6 minutes.

5. After a short rest subject is asked to sit on a bicycle ergometer; adjust metronome and he is instructed to pedal the bicycle at a rate of 50 times per minute against the load of 1.0 kg. He is asked to breath from the mouthpiece of expirograph which is connected to the room environment. For first 5–6 minutes, pedalling rate is kept constant and note the heart rate, respiratory rate and blood pressure.

6. When three readings are constant, the subject has reached a steady state and is connected to spirometer filled with oxygen and a one minute of record should be taken.

7. Disconnect the subject from expirograph and allow him to recover.

8. Calculate oxygen consumption per minute from the spirogram.

CALCULATIONS

1. Energy Cost of Work

Oxygen utilised at rest = 'a' litre

1 Liter of oxygen gives = 4.86 cal. (with mix diet)

Energy utilised per minute at rest (Eo)

= 'a' × 4.86 cal

Oxygen utilised during moderate exercise

= 'b' liters

Energy utilised during exercise (Ex)

= 'b' × 4.86 cal

Energy utilised during steady state moderate grade exercise (E) = Ex – Eo

2. Calculation of Work

Circumference of bicycle wheel = 'c' meters

Load (Tension) on the wheel = 1 kg

Rate of revolution of wheel during steady state exercise = n per min

Work done = W = Distance (c × n) × load (1 kg)

3. Calculation of Mechanical Efficiency

$$\text{Mechanical efficiency} = \frac{\text{Output}}{\text{Input}} \times 100$$

Output = Work done per min

$$= \text{W (kg m/min)} = \frac{\text{W (kg m/min)}}{427} \text{Kcal}$$

(427 kgm/min = 1 kcal)

Input E = Ex – Eo kcal

$$\text{Mechanical efficiency} = \frac{\text{W}}{427 \times \text{E}} \times 100$$

RESULT AND DISCUSSION

1. Energy cost of work:
2. Work done during steady state exercise:
3. Mechanical Efficiency:

Relevance to Medical Physiology

1. To assess work capacity of healthy individual.
2. To determine physical fitness of population group.
3. To improve the performance of athletes, sportsmen, and military personals.
4. Pre- and postoperative measurement of cardio-thoracic patients.

PRECAUTIONS

Subject is asked to stop exercise immediately if he feels intolerably breathless, giddiness and pain or constriction or suffocation in chest.

QUESTIONS

1. What is the physiological and clinical significance of the experiment?
2. What are the criteria to stop the exercise during test?
3. Define steady state exercise.
4. Give WHO classifications of exercise.

EXPERIMENT 3.18

To study human diuresis

THEORY

Human kidneys are able to produce diluted or concentrated urine depending upon the osmotic pressure and volume of the body fluids.

When osmotic pressure of body fluids rises more solute is excreted in the urine than water and concentrated urine is passed. When osmotic pressure of body fluids falls more water is excreted in the urine than solute and diluted urine is passed. Urine volume and its specific gravity is measured after drinking of water or normal saline at different time intervals.

APPARATUS

Measuring cylinders and urinometers.

PROCEDURE

The experiment is conducted in a group of 8 volunteers among the students. Students are asked to report to the department at 8.30 a.m. after a light breakfast at 7.00 a.m. omitting coffee or tea. At 8.30 a.m. they are asked to empty the urinary bladder and their BP and weight are recorded.

These students are placed in 4 groups of 2 student in each group.

Group I: Act as control.

Group II: They drink one litre of water.

Group III: They drink one litre of water but undergoes (moderate grade) exercise after 1 hour of drinking of water.

Group IV: They drink one litre of normal saline.

Now urine samples are collected after one hour, 1.5 hour, 2 hour, 2.5 hour, and 3 hours of fluid intake. Volume of each sample measured by measuring cylinder and specific gravity of each sample is measured by urinometer.

OBSERVATIONS

All the data are filled in the table given below.

Urine Samples after	Parameters	Group I control		Group II		Group III		Group IV	
		1	2	1	2	1	2	1	2
1 hour	Urine volume (ml)								
	Specific gravity								
1.5 hour	Urine volume (ml)								
	Specific gravity								
2 hour	Urine volume (ml)								
	Specific gravity								
2.5 hour	Urine volume (ml)								
	Specific gravity								
3.0 hour	Urine volume (ml)								
	Specific gravity								

QUESTIONS AND ANSWERS

1. What is the normal urinary volume in adult human in one day.

Ans. It is about 1500 ml per day.

2. What is the normal specific gravity of the urine in human?

Ans. Normal specific gravity of urine is 1.001 to 1.040.

3. What happens to urinary output and to specific gravity of urine when person drinks water or saline?

Ans. There is increase in urine volume in both the situations. With in take of water specific gravity of urine is less as compared to the saline.

4. What is the effect of exercise on urinary output and why?

Ans. There is decrease in urinary output during exercise. This is because of more loss of water from the body surface and lungs during exercise.

5. What is anuria?

Ans. When urine formation ceases, it is called as anuria.

6. What is oliguria?

Ans. When urinary output is less than 500 ml per day it is called oliguria.

7. What is polyuria?

Ans. When urinary volume is more than 2500 ml per day it is called polyuria.

EXPERIMENT 3.19A

To map the peripheral field of vision with perimeter (Perimetry)

THEORY

Field of vision can be defined as many ways. It is an extent of an area in the space that can be seen at particular moment with an eye fixed at one point. When we fix the eye upon an object, we not only see the object but also a number of objects in the neighbourhood more or less distinctly.

Perimetry means measurement of boundaries and in this case the boundaries of visible area. It is the method of recording field of vision by perimeter.

Normal extent of field of vision with 5 mm of object in good illumination are :

1. Upward   – 60°
2. Outward (temporal) – 90° or more
3. Downward   – 70°
4. Inward (nasal) – 60°

Field of vision can be measured at bed site to detect any gross changes in the field by confrontation method.

Physiological Blind Spot: It is because of absence of photoreceptors in optic disc area. It is located in temporal field from 10° to 15° isoptor and 86° to 93° meridian.

APPARATUS

Perimeter, perimeter chart, test objects of different sizes and colours.

Perimeter (Fig. 3.19a.1)

It consists of vertical stand on which a metallic arc is pivoted. Arc can be rotated in any direction and can also be fixed at any position with the help of a screw. Arc is graduated from 0° to 90°. A test object of specific size and colour can be moved along the length of the arc. The centre of the arc (pivot) is occupied by 5 mm of white circular spot known as fixation point.

A chin-rest and levelling bar is present at base to bring the eye of subject at the level of fixation point.

A scale and a chart frame are present on a wooden disc behind the metallic arc. A movable pin-punch pointer is also present to mark the extent of field of vision in particular meridian.

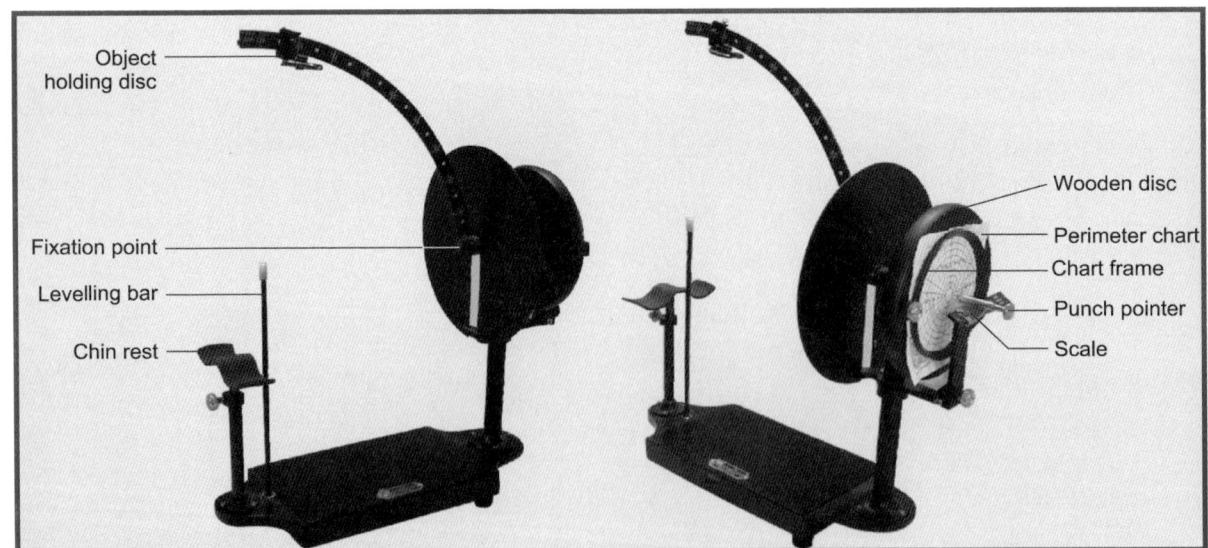

Fig. 3.19a.1: Perimeter (views from front and back).

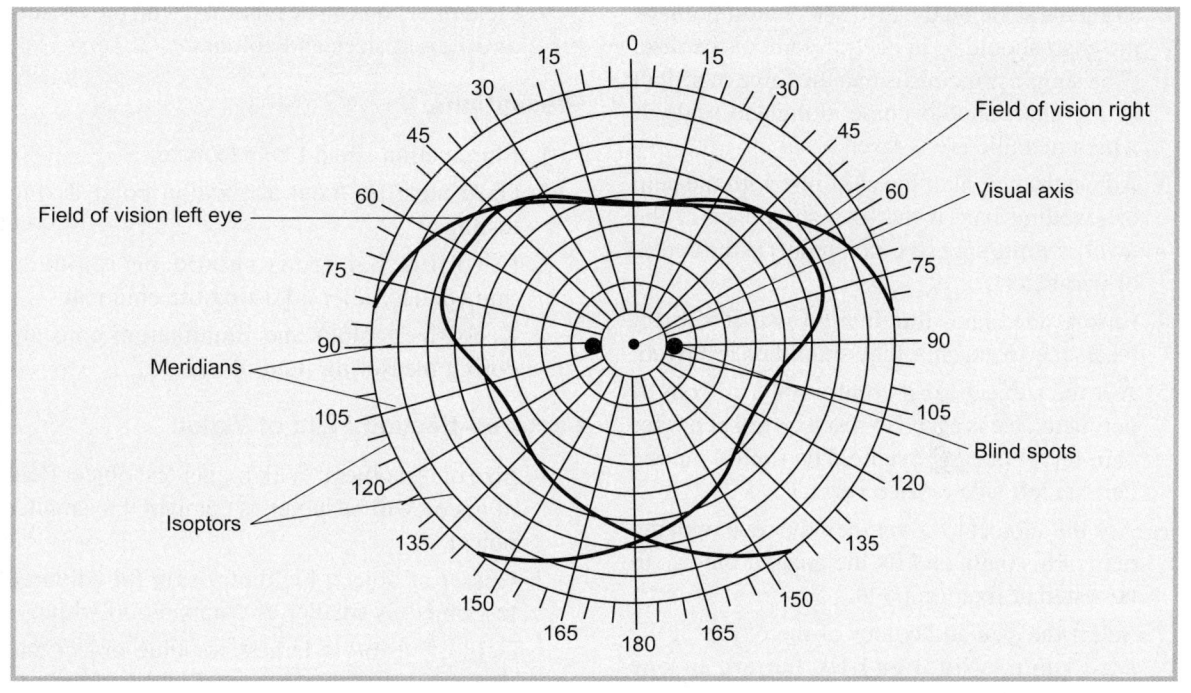

Fig. 3.19a.2: Perimeter chart.

Perimeter Chart

It is a graduated paper used to record field of vision. Central point of chart corresponds with visual axis.

The concentric circles drawn at an interval of 10° are called as isoptors (Fig. 3.19a.2). Particular isoptor denotes the visual angle at nodal point of the eye. The radii of the circles are marked as 15° intervals, which denote the various meridians. Perimeter chart is fixed at wooden disc with the help of chart frame.

PROCEDURE

(I) Confrontation Method

1. Here the patient field of vision is compared with that of observer having a normal field of vision. This method gives rough idea of visual field.
2. The examiner sits facing the patient at a distance of one meter.
3. The patient covers his left eye and fixes his vision of right eye on examiners left eye.
4. The examiner closes his right eye and moves his hand in from the periphery halfway between him and patient.
5. When he sees it himself, the patient ought to say that he also sees it.
6. The movements of the hands are repeated in various parts of field—above, below, to left and to right.

(II) Perimetry

1. *Recognition of Perimeter Chart:* Place the chart in front of your eyes in such a way that temporal field is on outer side.
2. *Fixation of Chart:* Fix the metallic arc at 90° on right side or left side of the subject with respect to specific eye. Fix the chart on wooden disc behind the perimeter in such a way that the same meridian of the chart should come

along the scale on the disc and central point of the chart should be at central point of the disc. (The simple principle is that the same meridian of the chart should come along the scale at which metallic arc is fixed.)

3. Adjust the height of the chin-rest with the help of levelling bar so that eye should be at the level of white spot (fixation point) at the centre of perimeter.

4. Ensure adequate illumination and if subject wears the spectacles, they should be removed.

5. Ask the subject to sit comfortably in front of perimeter. He is asked to rest his chin at proper chin-rest (For right eye field he should put the chin on left side or vice versa.).

6. Ask the subject to cover the other eye with the help of his palm and fix the gaze of the eye to be tested at fixation point.

7. Select the size and colour of the object at the arc (5 mm, white) and fix the arc in one particular meridian. Bring the object at peripheral end of the arc and move it from periphery to centre with the help of a rod.

   Note down the angle at which object is first seen by the subject. Mark the point on the perimeter chart with the help of the pointer on the same isoptor.

8. The above process is repeated in 12 meridians. All the points are joined together to plot the field of vision on the chart.

9. Field of vision can be recorded with the objects of different sizes and colours.

Precautions

1. Illumination should be adequate.
2. Gaze must be fixed at fixation point during testing.
3. Levelling bar (rod) should be removed immediately after adjusting the chin rest
4. Keep size, colour and illumination constant during measuring field of vision.

Factors Affecting Field of Vision

1. Size of test object: With bigger test object field of vision will be larger as compared to smaller object.
2. Colour of object: Field of vision for coloured test object is smaller as compared to white.

   Field of vision is largest for blue object and then yellow, red, and green. Field for blue and yellow is roughly 10° less in each direction than that for white and for red and green is further 10° less.

3. Contrast of the test object with background.
4. State of object: For moving object it is more as compared with stationary objects.
5. Illumination of object.
6. Nature of object: Constant or flickering.
7. Features of face of the subject.

QUESTIONS AND ANSWERS

1. Define the field of vision.
2. What is the extent of normal field of vision?
3. What is anopia?

Ans. The anopia is complete blindness.

4. What is homonymous hemianopia?

Ans. When half of the visual field of same side of both the eyes is gone it is called as homonymous hemianopia.

5. What is heteronymous hemianopia?

Ans. When half of the visual field of the different side of the eyes is gone it is called as heteronymous hemianopia.

6. Enumerate the factors affecting the field of vision.
7. What is the cause of physiological scotoma (blind spot)?

Ans. It is because of the area of the optic disc, there are no photoreceptors in this region.

8. What is the location of physiological blind spot?

Ans. It is present at 12° to 18° isoptor and just below 180° meridian (in temporal field).

9. Can you measure the blind spot with the help of perimeter or not? If yes then how?

Ans. Yes. Bring the object of the perimeter from periphery towards centre at 180° meridian and note the isoptor where object starts to disappear and starts to reappear again. Now change the position of the arc at about 185° meridian and find out its location. Adjust the position of the arc at 190° meridian and find out its location. This method is a rough method so practically it is not used to measure physiological blind spot.

10. What happens to the field of vision in optic atrophy?

Ans. The field of vision constricts and it is called tubular field of vision.

11. Why the spectacles are removed during perimetry?

Ans. Because, they produce obstruction in the field of vision.

EXPERIMENT 3.19B

Mapping of physiological blind spot and calculation of optic disc size

APPARATUS

Long black stiff wire and white circular paper of 2 mm diameter.

PROCEDURE

1. Fix the circular paper of 2 mm diameter on the tip of a black stiff wire about 1 meter long.
2. Ask the subject to stand in front of black board at one meter distance.
3. Draw a white mark (small circle) on the black board at the level of the eye to be tested, this is a fixation point.
4. Ask the subject to cover his other eye and fix his gaze on the white mark on the blackboard.
5. Move the white paper mounted on black wire inward from temporal side along the several adjacent radii.

6. Mark the points at which it disappears from the subject's view and reappears. It will be the limits of blind spot.

OBSERVATION

Vertical diameter of mapped blind spot (VD) = ...
Horizontal diameter of mapped blind spot (HD) = ...
Mean diameter of mapped blind spot

$$= \frac{VD + HD}{2} = \times mm$$

Distance between mapped blind spot and eye
= 1000 mm
Distance between the nodal point and retina
= 17 mm (assumed)

CALCULATION

Diameter of optic disc

$$= \frac{\text{Mean diameter of mapped blind spot (mm)}}{\text{Distance between the mapped blind spot and eye}} \times 17$$

EXPERIMENT 3.20A

To test visual acuity

Acuity of vision is the preciseness or the level of accuracy to which one can see the shape form, outline and contour of objects and distinguish them. It is the ability of the eye to resolve two points separately, when situated close to each other. It can be expressed in terms of visual angle. We can resolve two points or parallel lines and recognise them as two only, when visual angle is of one minute (1° = 60 min). This is tested for near vision and distant vision.

PRINCIPLE

Letters used to find out the acuity of vision are made in such a way that when they are read from the distance specified in the chart at the specific line, each letter subtends an angle of five minute and each part of the letter (necessary to identity it) subtends an angle of one minute at nodal point of the eye (Fig. 3.20a.1).

Near Vision

Ask the subject to read Jaeger's chart (N Printer series) (Fig. 3.20a.2) after holding it at 25–30 cm away from the eye. The card (chart) is well illuminated. Smallest letter in the chart is N6. Individuals with normal activity are able to read letters of N series.

Distant Vision

This is tested with the help of Snellen's chart by the ability of the subject to recognise test letters illuminated suitably.

(a) The test 'block' letters/pictures which are black on a white background are of different sizes. Each line of letters has a figures of 60, 36, 24, 18, 12, 9, 6, and 5 meters noted beside it (Fig. 3.20a.3).

(b) The chart is so designed that each letter a normal individuals can read at a required distance, subtends a visual angle of 5 minutes and each part of the letter subtends an angle of one minute.

PROCEDURE

1. Subject is asked to stand at a 6 meter distance from the chart.
2. He is asked to read the letters with one eye after covering the other eye.
3. Note down which line he is able to read. Repeat the same procedure with other eye after covering the first one.
4. If he is not able to read even the top line marked 60, ask him to come 1 meter closure to the chart, if he is not able to see the top letter even at 1 meter distance, do finger counting. If not then do hand movements. If hand movements are also not perceived then projection and perception of light is checked with the help of torch light.

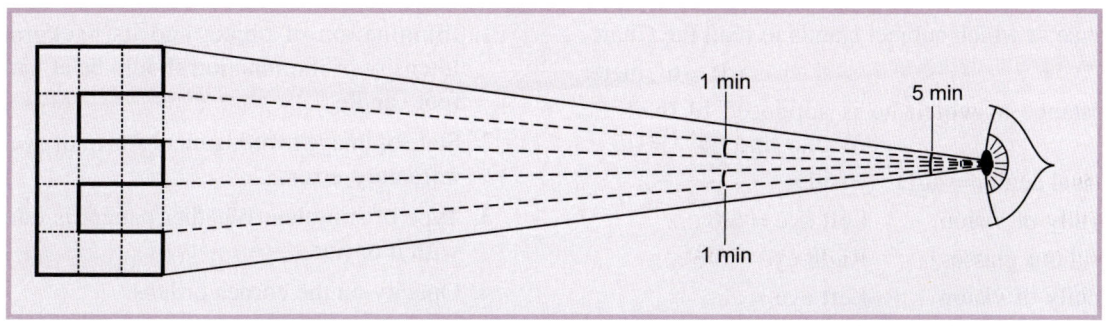

Fig. 3.20a.1: Basis of designing test letters of Snellen's chart and Jaeger's chart.

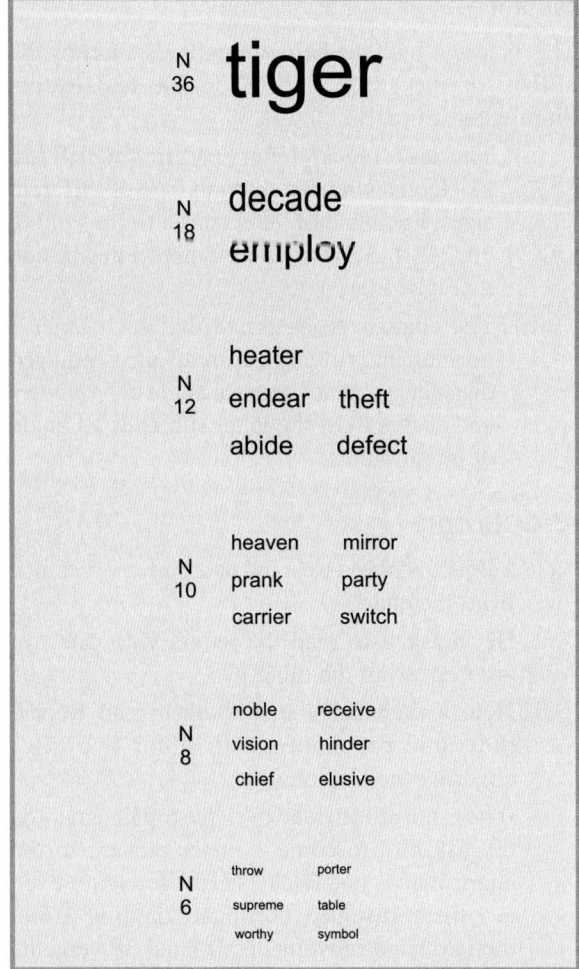

Fig. 3.20a.2: Jaeger's chart (N Printer series).

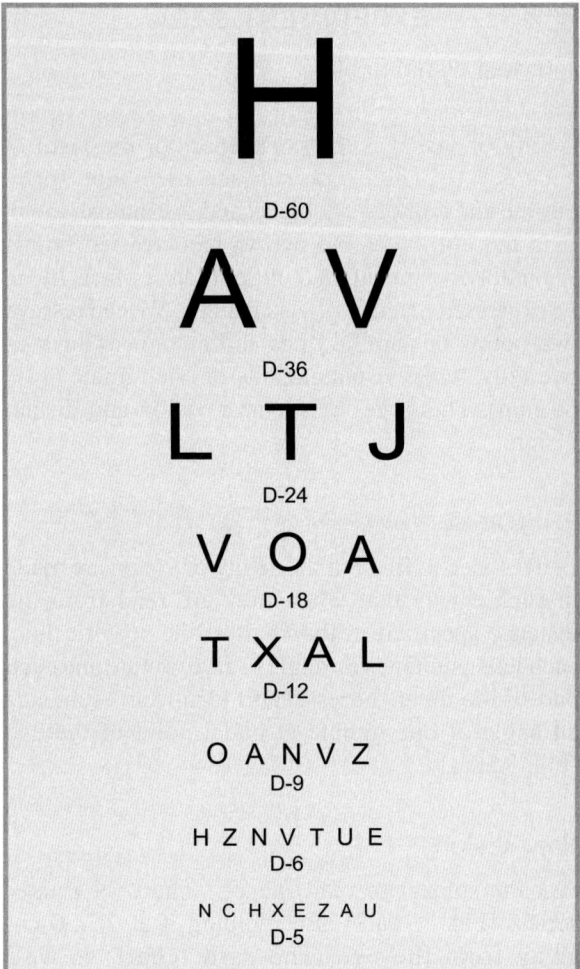

Fig. 3.20a.3: Snellen's chart.

OBSERVATION AND RESULT

Distance at which subject stands to read the Chart

$$(d) = 6 \quad \text{meter}$$

Distance at which he is supposed to read the

particular line 'D' = ...

Visual acuity = d/D = 6/D

Acuity of vision   Left eye = 6/6 ......

(without glasses)   Right eye = 6/6 .....

Acuity of vision   Left eye = ...

(with glasses) Right eye = ...

Factors Affecting Visual Acuity

1. Illumination of object and its background. Intensity of illumination should be at least 20 foot candle.

2. State of image forming mechanism of eye. e.g. refractory errors.

3. Type of stimulus: Whether patient is familiar with it or not.

4. Opacity on the cornea or lens.

5. Foreign body in the eye.

QUESTIONS

1. Define the acuity of vision.
2. What are the factors effecting acuity of vision?
3. What is the visual angle?
4. What is the base of designing of Snellen's chart?

5. At what distance from the eyes Jaeger's chart is held for testing acuity of near vision?
6. If the subject is not able to see even the top letter of Snellen's chart what will you do?

EXPERIMENT 3.20B

To test colour vision

Appreciation of colour is a function of cones. Inability on the part of an individual to recognise the colours is called colour blindness. Following tests are used in the laboratory for testing colour vision.

COLOUR VISION TESTS

1. Ishihara Charts (Ishihara's Isochromatic Colour Plates)

These plates have figures outline in lots of primary colours, painted on background of dots of confusion colours (Fig. 3.20b.1). A normal person sees all the figures at a glance, the colour blind person is unable to do so.

2. Holmgren's Wool Test

The subject is asked to match a piece of wool from the collection of skeins (bundle of yarn) of various colours.

3. The Edridge Green Lantern

This device used to find out blindness as a pre-employment test for pilots, and drivers. The lantern exhibits several standard colours different shades of red, yellow, green, blue, and purple. Three rotating discs make various combinations possible. The size

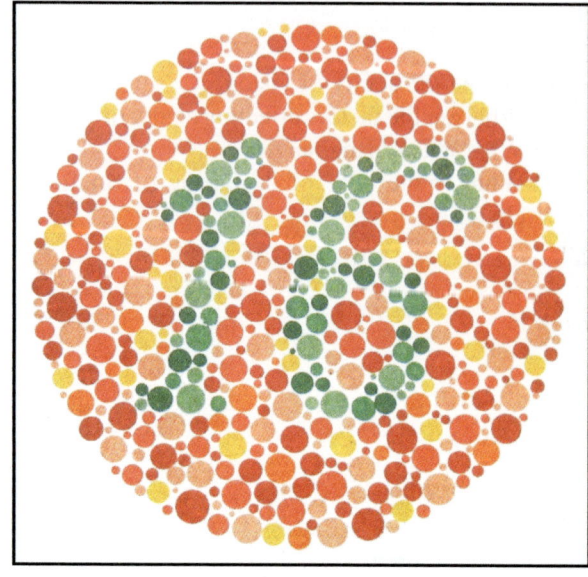

Fig. 3.20b.1: Ishihara chart

of the light can be varied by a diaphragm. The patient is seated in a dimly lighted room about six metres away from the lantern and he is asked to name the colour of the light produced by the coloured glasses either alone or in combinations.

Significance of Colour Vision Testing

It is used to find out colour weakness or colour blindness in the individual like pilots and drivers as a fitness test.

QUESTIONS

1. What are the primary and the secondary colours?
2. Who are trichromate, dichromate, and mono-chromate?
3. What is colour anomaly?
4. What is anopia?
5. What are the different types of cones present in human eye?
6. What is the significance of testing colour vision?

EXPERIMENT 3.21

Cardiopulmonary resuscitation: To demonstrate the technique of artificial respiration and
cardiac resuscitation

Cardiorespiratory arrest is defined as the abrupt
failure of the heart or respiration or both to maintain
an adequate cerebral circulation. Cardiopulmonary
resuscitation is an emergency life-saving procedure.

Causes of Cardiorespiratory Arrest

Acute Conditions

1. Drowning
2. Anaphylactic shock
3. Coronary thrombosis
4. Inhalation of poisonous gases like CO.
5. Head injury
6. Electrocution
7. Cardiac surgery
8. Overdose of anaesthesia

Chronic Conditions

1. Chronic lung disease.
2. Congestive heart failure.
3. Progressive obstruction in the air flow.

Signs and Symptoms of Cardiorespiratory Arrest

1. Person becomes unconscious with cold, moist
   and pale skin.
2. Presence of weak or no pulse.
3. Blood pressure not recordable.

First aid Measures before Resuscitation

1. Ensure that the airway passage is clean. To
   remove mucus or other secretions from the air
   passage.
2. Extend the neck so that tongue should not fall
   back and block the airway.

3. All tight clothing such as tight collar should
   be loosened.
4. In case of drowning, turn the patient upside
   down by holding his ankles so as to remove
   water, also apply strong pressure on the
   abdomen.

Pulmonary Resuscitation (Artificial Respiration)

Time is an important factor in resuscitation so should
be started as quickly as possible.

Methods

Manual methods and mechanical methods.
  A. *Manual methods:*
     1. Mouth-to-mouth breathing
     2. Holger–Nielsen method
     3. Sylvester–Brosche method
  B. *Mechanical methods:*
     1. Drinker's method
     2. Paul–Bunnell method
     3. See Saw or Rocking method

A. Manual Methods

Mouth-to-Mouth Breathing
Procedure
  (i) Ensure the first aid measures before artificial
      respiration
  (ii) Extend the neck close the nostrils and open
       the mouth of the subject (patient) (Fig. 3.21.1).
  (iii) Take a deep inspiration yourself.
  (iv) Apply your mouth to subject's mouth.
  (v) Look at the chest for expansion.
  (vi) Maintain a rate of 10–12 breaths per minute.
  Advantages of this method:
  (i) Simple procedure.
  (ii) No instrument is needed.
  Disadvantage of this method:
  (i) Unpleasantness
  (ii) Cannot be performed for long

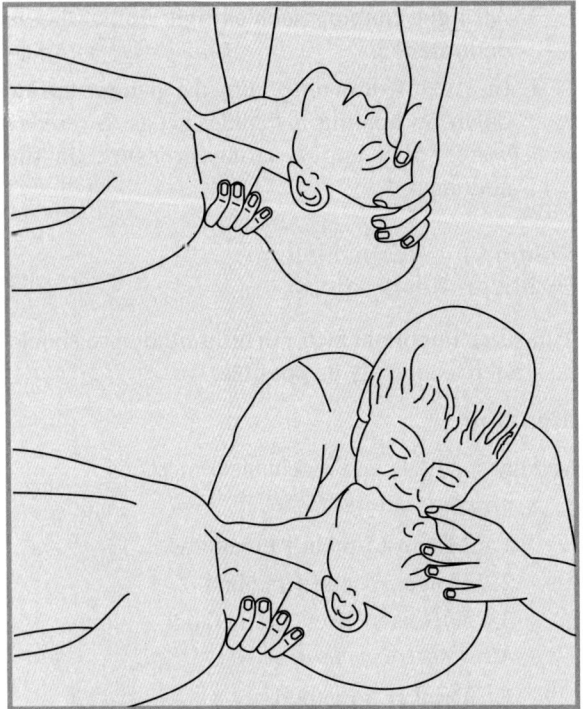

Fig. 3.21.1: Mouth-to-mouth breathing.

(iii) Risk of spread of infection from one to other.

(iv) Rise in intrapulmonary pressure hinders venous return.

(v) Tongue of the subject keeps falling back obstructing airway.

Holger–Nielsen method (back pressure arm lift method)

Procedure

(i) The subject is made to lie prone. The arm are abducted at the shoulders and elbows flexed, the head is turned to one side resting on the hands.

(ii) The operator kneels down with one knee near subject's head. The subject's arms are held just above the elbow and operator gently straightens himself, while raising the subject's arm until resistance is felt. During this manoeuvre the thorax expands and intrathoracic pressure drops and inspiration takes place.

(iii) The subject's arms are then gently dropped.

(iv) The operator's hands and fingers spread apart are placed on the back of the subject immediately below the scapulae; the operator moves forward till his elbows are extended vertically above the patient. This procedure produces active expiration (Fig. 3.21.2).

(v) The whole cycle is repeated 12 times per minute.

Advantages

Both inspiration and expiration are actively brought about. Method is simple and no instrument is required.

Sylvester–Brosche Method

Procedure

(i) The subject is made to lie in prone position.

(ii) The operator kneel behind the subject and support his head behind operator's knees.

(iii) The subject's forearms are held at the wrist and place them across the lower part of the chest.

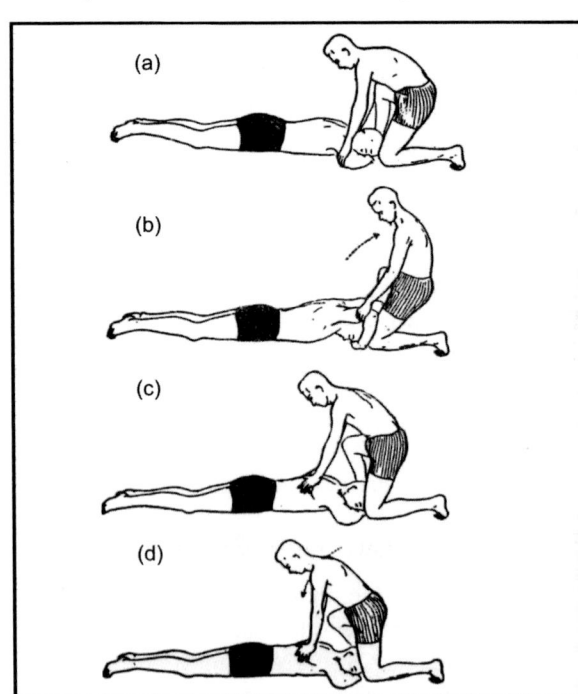

Fig. 3.21.2: Holger–Nielsen method.

(iv) The operator slowly rock forwards on straight elbows until his arms are nearly vertical; keeping the arms straight press down on the lower part of the subject's chest wall for 2 seconds. This procedure produces active expiration.

(v) The operator then draws the subject's arms upwards, outwards, and backwards in a sweeping movement as far as they can go. This produces inspiration.

(vi) The whole cycle is repeated 12 times per minute.

B. Mechanical Methods

Drinkers Method

In this method patient is kept inside the iron respirator cabinet, his head remains outside. Pressure in the cabinet is raised or lowered rhythmically to produce expiration and inspiration respectively.

Other mechanical methods are Paul–Bunnell method and Rocking method.

CARDIAC RESUSCITATION

In cardiac arrest the heart stops either in systole or ventricular fibrillation. A systole is revived by external cardiac message and ventricular fibrillation either by internal (open) cardiac massage or by using an electric shock defibrillator.

1. External Cardiac Massage

The heart is compressed between the sternum and the vertebral column, and then released so that circulation is established and maintained.

Procedure

(i) Place the heel of the hand over the site of compression (at the junction of upper two-thirds and lower one-third of sternum).

(ii) Place the heel of the second hand over the first parallel to it.

(iii) Finger should not touch the body.

(iv) The elbows should be straight.

(v) Force should be vertically downwards.

(vi) The movements should be at the shoulders so that the body weight of resuscitator is transmitted through the hands to the sternum so that it should be compressed by 1.5 to 2.0 inches.

(vii) It should be maintained at the rate of 70/min.

In infants

(i) Place the thumb over middle of the sternum and fingers supporting the back.

(ii) The fingers of the hand pressing over the sternum can also be used.

(iii) It is maintained at 100–120/min.

(iv) Compress the chest by 1 inch.

If resuscitator is one person, ratio of chest compression and breath should be 15:2. If the resuscitation is carried out by two persons, the ratio should be 5:1.

2. Internal Cardiac Massage

This method should be used only in a hospital in operation theatre. It is done either during operation or in postoperative stages of cardiac arrest.

3. Electronic Shock Defibrillator

This is a method of choice in abolishing ventricular fibrillation via electrodes placed across the chest cavity or directly to the heart in open cardiac preparations.

QUESTIONS

1. What are the advantages and disadvantages of mouth-to-mouth breathing?

2. What are the signs and symptoms of cardio-respiratory arrest?

3. What are the causes of cardiorespiratory arrest?

4. What are the first-aid measures, which are required before cardiorespiratory resuscitation?

5. What are the methods of artificial respiration?

EXPERIMENT 3.22

General physical examination

Examination of general state of the patient before any systematic examination is the minimum necessary requirement. Following conditions should be fulfilled before the start of any clinical examination:

1. Day light is better than artificial light because latter may mask the changes in skin colours.
2. Every attempt should be made to reassure and relax the subject.
3. Ideally, a relative or a female attendant should be present when a male doctor is examining a female patient.
4. For a thorough examination, the subject should be asked to take off all his clothes.
5. Always stand on right side of the patient (in case of the right-handed doctor).

The following points should be observed in General Physical Examination

1. **General Appearance:**
   (i) Does patient look healthy, unwell, or ill.
   (ii) Gait should be observed whether the subject is able to walk or not.

2. **Mental and Emotional State:** An over-anxious person may be restless, with wide palpebral fissures and sweating palms.

3. **Physique and Build:** It tells about nutritional status. Fluid retention (oedema) may cause an increase in the weight.

4. **Facial Expression and Speech:** Expression and particularly eyes, may indicate feelings better than do words. Patient is able to speak at all or he is silent.

5. **Eyes:** See for exophthalmos or ptosis, see the conjunctiva for anaemia (pallor), jaundice (yellowness) or inflammation (redness). In pupils see for size, equality, regularity, reaction to light and accommodation, look for nystagmus.

6. **Skin:** See for – pallor, yellowness, pigmentation, cyanosis (blue colouration), cutaneous eruptions, texture, and oedema.

7. **Hands:** Observe strength of grip as he shakes hand and see for character of nails and clubbing of fingers.

8. **Feet:** See for oedema (pitting or non pitting), ulceration and any growth.

9. **Neck:** Look for enlargement of thyroid gland, lymph nodes, distension of veins, pulsations of carotid vessels, position of trachea and jugular venous pressure.

10. **Temperature:** When taking the temperature, remember the following points:
    (i) In conscious adult temperature is taken in the mouth. In young children it should be taken from axillae or groin folds. Temperature of mouth is 0.5°C higher than axillae or groin.
    (ii) Thermometer should be kept for 1–2 minutes for temperature recording.

11. **Pulse:** Count the radial pulse for a full minute and observe rate, rhythm, character, volume and condition of vessel wall. Observe presence or absence of delay of femoral pulse compared with radial.

12. **Blood Pressure:** Record the blood pressure of the patient.

13. **Respiration:** Rate of respiration and type of respiration.

14. **Thorax:** Look for dilated vessels, apex beat, retraction of one nipple, discharge from nipple of breast, discharged from nipple, any lump (palpate it).

15. **Abdomen:** Any distension, its symmetry, scars, dilated vessels, visible pulsations, inguinal glands, impulse on coughing and any redness.

EXPERIMENT 3.23

Clinical examination of cardiovascular system (CVS)

EXAMINATION OF CARDIOVASCULAR SYSTEM

This includes the following:
   I. Examination of arterial pulse.
   II. Recording of blood pressure.
   III. Venous pulse in neck.
   IV. Examination of precordium.

I. Examination of Arterial Pulse

Arterial pulse can be examined (palpated) in main peripheral arteries—the radial, brachial, carotid, femoral, popliteal, posterior tibial and dorsalis pedis.

Radial pulse examination is preferred as it can be easily felt. It is best felt with the tips of the three fingers, slightly compressing the vessel against the underlying bone. Patient's forearm should be pronated and wrist slightly flexed.

Observations

Following observations should be made during the examination of pulse.
   1. Rate
   2. Rhythm
   3. Character
   4. Volume
   5. Condition of vessel wall
   6. Presence or absence of delay in femoral and radial pulse.
   7. Compared the pulse with other side.

1. Rate

Radial pulse is expressed in terms of beats per minute. Beats are counted for full one minute.

Causes of increase in pulse rate: Anxiety, excitement, exercise, fever, thyrotoxicosis.

Causes of decrease in pulse rate: Athletes, hypothyroidism and complete heart block.

2. Rhythm

Normally the pulse beat at regular interval so decide whether it is regular or irregular. If it is irregular decide if it is completely irregular, whether the irregularity has a recurring pattern, or whether an otherwise regular rhythm is occasionally interrupted by some slight irregularity. The pulse of arterial fibrillation is completely irregular.

3. Character

By feeling of radial pulse character of pulse cannot be appreciated. It is felt by palpation of carotid pulse. Normal pulse having P, t, n, and d waves, which are identified in sphygmograph (Fig. 3.23.1).

Abnormal Characters

   (i) *Anacrotic pulse:* This occurs in aortic stenosis. There is slow rise in p wave and small volume. This known as an anacrotic pulse.

   (ii) *Collapsing or Water hammer pulse:* It is characterised by a rapid upstroke and descent of the pulse wave. It occurs most often in aortic regurgitation. Collapsing character is due to regurgitation of blood from aorta back in to the left ventricle or due to abnormal leak from arterial system.

   (iii) *Biferiens pulse:* It is a combination of the slow rising and collapsing pulses occurring when aortic stenosis and incompetence are present.

   (iv) *Pulses alternans:* When ventricle beats strongly then weakly in successive beats of normal rhythm, alternation is present. It happens in case of severe left ventricular damage.

4. Volume

This refers to the amplitude of movement of the vessel wall during passage of pulse wave. This gives rough guide to pulse pressure which depends on the stroke volume and the compliance of the arteries.

Causes of abnormal volume of pulse are:
   (i) In shock pulse is weak and thready.

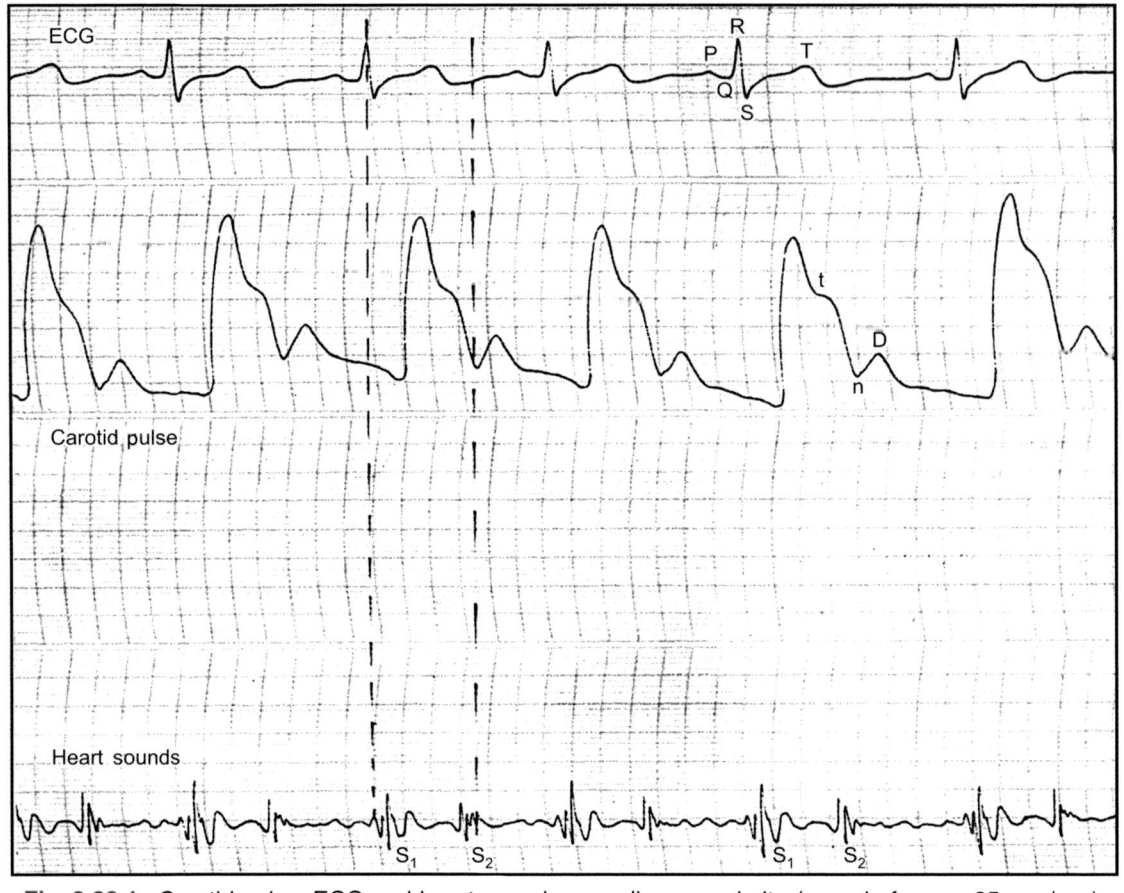

Fig. 3.23.1: Carotid pulse, ECG and heart sounds recording on polyrite (speed of paper 25 mm/sec).

(ii) Pulse is strong and high volume during exercise and old age.

5. Condition of Vessel Wall

To assess this sufficient pressure should be exerted on radial pulse and it should be rolled beneath the fingers against underlying bone.

(i) Arterial wall cannot be felt or it is soft in youngers.

(ii) It is easily palpable and felt like whip cord due to arteriosclerosis in old people.

6. Delay of the Femoral Pulse

As compared with right radial pulse, it is found in coarctation of aorta.

7. Compare the Right Radial Pulse with the Left Side

This is done to find any delay or to check synchronicity.

How to Describe the Pulse

72 per min, regular, good in volume, equal on both the sides, normal character and synchronous on opposite side. No delay of femoral pulse as compared to right radial pulse.

II Recording of Blood Pressure

It is an important part of clinical examination of cardiovascular system.

III Venous Pulse in Neck

The external jugular veins can be seen on the surface in the posterior triangle of neck. They communicate directly with the right atrium, therefore level of the pressure in these veins can be regarded as an increase of right arterial pressure (central venous pressure). In health, in whatever position the subject may be (reclining at angle of about 45° sitting or standing), the external jugular veins get filled up to the level of manubriumsterni only. If veins are filled up to higher than this, it indicates the presence of increased central venous pressure. Neck veins are examined with the patient in a good light and reclining at an angle of about 45° (Fig. 3.23.2). The neck should be supported so that the neck muscles, especially the sternomastoid, are relaxed. The veins normally show slight pulsation, and three small waves (the a, c, and v waves) can be distinguished in each cardiac cycle (Fig. 3.23.3).

Raised jugular venous pressure (JVP) is seen in:
 (i) Right heart failure
 (ii) Obstruction to superior vena cava.
 (iii) Slight rise in JVP is seen in pregnancy because of increase in circulatory blood volume.

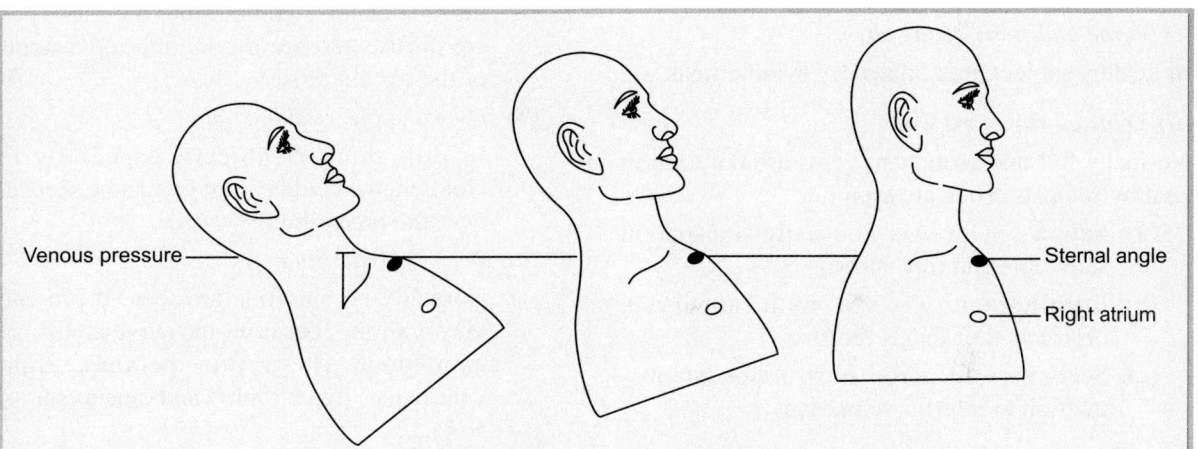

Fig. 3.23.2: Examination of neck veins and Jugular venous pressure (In normal individual peaks of right atrial pressure waves are just visible in the internal jugular vein at the angle of 45°).

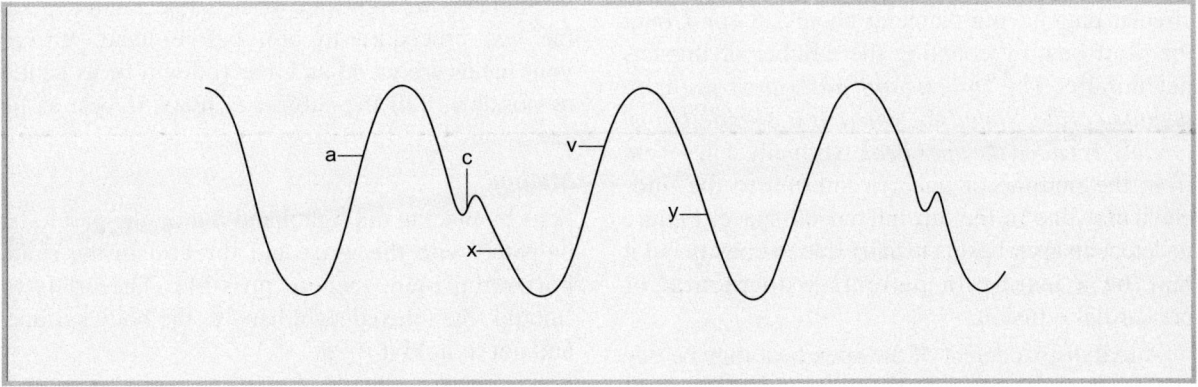

Fig. 3.23.3: Normal jugular venous pulse.

IV Examination of Precordium

Precordium is the portion of the anterior aspect of the chest wall which overlies the heart. Its examination is carried out under following headings:

1. Inspection
2. Palpation
3. Percussion
4. Auscultation

1. Inspection

Clothing of the patient should be removed up to waist. Look for:

(i) Shape and form of the chest

In healthy subject, it is bilaterally symmetrical.

(ii) Veins on the chest wall

Normally full and prominent veins are not seen in healthy subjects. They are seen in

(a) Subjects with skin unusually transparent show thin and tiny veins.

(b) Intrathoracic growth with aneurysm obstructs the venous return.

(c) Secondary to portal obstruction or obstruction to inferior vena cava.

(iii) Cardiac impulse

It refers to the movements occurring due to the impact of the heart against the chest wall during systole. The area over which the impact is seen is a circular area having diameter about 2.5 cm. Count the heart beat by counting the number of impacts per minute. *The lowest and outermost point of definite cardiac impulses, where it is seen/felt most forcibly, is called the apex beat.* Normally it lies 9 cm from the midline or one cm internal to the mid-clavicular line in the 5th intercostal space. Failure to detect an apex beat is usually due to obesity but it may be a feature in patients with pleural or pericardial effusion.

A real displacement of the apex beat may be due to disease of the surrendering viscera, which 'push' or 'pull' it from its usual site. Instances of 'pushing'

are found in pleural effusion and pneumothorax, and 'pulling' in pulmonary fibrosis and collapse of the lung.

The left ventricular hypertrophy, the beat becomes more forceful and may extend outwards towards the axilla.

Apex beat becomes prominent due to anxiety, nervousness and exercise.

(iv) Other pulsations

(a) *In the neck*:

Carotid artery pulsations are visible on either side in the anterior triangle of the neck by the side of the sternomastoid muscle. They are diffuse and are transmitted movements of the carotid pulse.

(b) *Over the precordium*:

In thin slender subjects, especially in children, the cardiac impulse can be seen all over the precordium.

(c) *In the epigastrium*:

Normally no pulsation are seen. If present, they can be because of nervousness or excitement (in a thin person), right ventricular hypertrophy and aneurysm of aorta.

2. Palpation

It means examination by fingers and palm.

Stand on the right side of the subject and explain the test procedure to him before hand. Ensure your hands are warm and that you will be as gentle as possible. Tell the subject to relax as best as he can.

Method

Start by placing the right hand flat on the part to be palpated with the wrist and forearm in the same horizontal plane, where possible. The art is to 'mould' the relaxed right hand to the body surface, and not to hold it rigid.

(i) *Feel for* temperature and texture of skin of chest.

(ii) *Feel for cardiac impulse:*

Confirm the findings obtained by inspection with respect to the location, extent, repetition rate and rhythm.

(iii) *Feel the pulsations in neck:*

Carotid artery pulsations are to be felt and venous pulsation are best visible than palpation. Check the direction of blood flow in neck veins.

(iv) *Feel for a thrill:*

Any sound or murmur which is loud an low pitched will be palpable like a worm moving under the hand. These palpable vibration are called a thrill.

3. Percussion

Method

Place the middle finger (pleximeter finger) of left hand firmly on the part to be purcussed, other fingers should be well separated apart and should not touch the surface.

The back of middle phalanx of pleximeter finger is then struck with tip of the middle finger (plexor finger) of right hand in a perpendicular direction. Sound produced after percussion may be tympanic (from hollow viscera containing gas), resonant (as from lungs) and dull (from solid viscera).

(i) By percussing the fourth intercostal space from the left lung towards the heart, it is possible to defined the left border more or less precisely. It is about 1.5 cm internal to mid-clavicular line.

(ii) The right border of the heart is just to the right of the sternum at the level of fourth rib. It is difficult to define since the sternum acts as a sounding board.

(iii) The upper border of the heart cannot be defined accurately as the dullness of the heart tissue continuous with the dullness of the big vessels.

(iv) Similarly, the lower border of the heart can not be defined as it lies in relation with the diaphragm and the left lobe of the liver below it.

Area of pericardial dullness increases due to large pericardial effusion and aortic aneurysm. Area of pericardial dullness decreases or absent in emphysema.

4. Auscultation

Stethoscope is used to listen the heart sounds. The heart sounds produced by closure of hearts valves can be heard all over the precordium but are heard best over four cardiac areas on the chest wall. These areas are customarily called by the name of the valve from which sounds and murmurs arise.

(i) The mitral area, which corresponds to the apex beat.

(ii) The tricuspid area, which lies just to the left of the lower end of the sternum.

(iii) The aortic area, which is to the right of the sternum in the second intercostal space.

(iv) The pulmonary area, which is to the left of the sternum in the second intercostal space.

Usually two heart sounds are heart (S1 and S2) 'lub' and 'dub'. First heart sound (S1) is because of closure of the mitral and tricuspid valves, it is low pitched loud round at the onset of ventricular systole. Second heart sound (S2) is because of closure of pulmonary and aortic valves, it is high pitched sharp sound at the onset of ventricular diastole. Splitting of first heart sound is difficult to detect because mitral and tricuspid valves close almost at the same time.

Splitting of second heart sound can be detected because pulmonary valves close after the aortic valve. Splitting is widest during inspiration and narrowest during expiration called as physiological splitting.

Third (S3) and fourth (S4) heart sounds usually not audible with stethoscope.

Murmurs are abnormal sounds which are produced due to turbulence in the blood flow at or near a valve or an abnormal communication within the heart. Murmurs may be systolic, diastolic or continuous throughout systole and diastole.

QUESTIONS AND ANSWERS

1. How will you assess for raised jugular venous pressure (JVP) is an individual?
2. How will you differentiate between arterial and venous pulsation?
3. How will you count the intercostal spaces and ribs?

Ans. They are best counted downwards from the second costal cartilage which articulates with the sternum at the extremities of the angle of Louis (transverse bony ridge at the junction of the body and the manubrium) which is easily felt beneath the skin.

4. How will you describe radial pulse?

5. What is pulse deficit? Give its causes.

Ans. The difference between the hear rate and pulse rate is called pulse deficit. It is seen in atrial and ventricular fibrillations.

6. What are the causes for first and second heart sounds?
7. What are the differences between first and second heart sounds?
8. How will you define the apex beat?
9. Name the condition in which apex beat can not be visualised.
10. What is murmur?
11. Define thrill.

EXPERIMENT 3.24

Clinical examination of respiratory system

IMPORTANT POINTS TO BE TAKEN CARE OF, DURING CLINICAL EXAMINATION

1. Patient should be examined preferably in good daylight. Artificial light tends to cast shadow and also induces errors in appreciation of colours.
2. Patient should be asked to loosen all the garments so that any part to be examined could be exposed easily without loss of time. The physical signs cannot be elicited through clothings. Clothes reduce the sensitivity and acuteness of observation. The patient should be provided with a light covering sheet so that no part of the body remains unnecessarily exposed.
3. The male doctor is advised to carryout the examination of a female patient in the presence of another female person, whose presence is not objected by the patient.
4. Customarily the right-handed examiner stands on the right side of the bed and carries out the examination.
5. Be careful and be thorough in the examination. If you are not careful, harm may be done to the patient by the disease. If you are not thorough correct diagnosis may not be reached. Examination, therefore, should be done in routine fashion. Observe correctly; make sure that you are correct before you record any finding. Use accurate terms during recording.
6. Always compare your observation to the other side of the body in the respective area.
7. Before proceeding to the systemic examination, valuable information regarding the function of that system can be obtained from general physical examination of the patient (Exp. 3.22).

Examination of Respiratory System

It is conducted under the four headings.

    I. Inspection   II. Palpation

    III. Percussion   IV. Auscultation

I. Inspection

The subject should be stripped to waist and examined on a bed lying or sitting comfortably. Look at the chest from the front, then from the side, and then from the back and finally over the shoulders from behind and front. Following observations should be made:

1. Shape of the Chest

    (i) The normal chest is bilaterally symmetrical. It may become asymmetrical by diseases of lungs or of body cage.

    (ii) Any bony prominence, deformities of sternum, ribs and vertebral column (scoliosis, kyphosis and pigeon chest).

2. Movements of the Chest

Observe whether movements are similar on both the sides of the chest or different.

    (i) Count respiratory rate by observing breathing movements of abdominal wall for complete one minute. The normal breathing rate in adult is 12 to 16 breaths per minute. Increase in respiratory rate (tachypnoea) may be because of nervousness, exercise, fever and hypoxia. Decrease in respiratory rate may be because of brain damage.

    (ii) Rhythm of respiration—to look whether breathing is regular or irregular.

    (iii) Type of breathing—see whether thoracic or abdominal breathing. Normally it is abdomino-tharacic, in pregnancy it becomes thoracic.

II. Palpation

To check for tenderness on the chest. Other points noted during palpation are:

1. Position of Trachea

Feel the position of trachea at the suprasternal notch in the neck. It is done by placing the index finger and ring finger on lateral bony prominent points of the suprasternal notch and middle finger is used to feel the position of trachea by feeling the space between trachea and lower end of sternomastoid muscle, on both the sides.

(i) Normally it is central or slightly deviated towards right side.

(ii) Trachea may be pushed away from the affected side by pleural effusion.

(iii) Trachea may be pulled towards affected side by fibrosis or collapse of the lung.

2. Position of Apex Beat

Feel the apex beat of heart as described in clinical examination of cardiovascular system. It may be displaced in shifting of mediastinum lung in different lung disease.

3. Expansion of Chest

Asymmetrical expansion of chest is observed during inspection may further be confirmed by palpation. This is done by fixing the fingers of either hand at the sides of patient's chest and making the tips of the thumbs, just meet (not fixed) in the middle line in front of chest. As the patient takes deep breath, the increasing distance between the thumbs indicates the degree of expansion.

4. Vocal Fremitis

Vocal means pertaining to voice and fremitis a vibrating sensation perceived by palpation. It is done with palm of hand placed flat on the chest. The patient is asked to repeat "one, one, one" in a clear normal voice.

(i) Vibrations in the corresponding areas on two sides of chest are approximately equal in intensity.

(ii) Vocal fremitis decreased when the corresponding bronchi are obstructed and in pleural effusion.

(iii) Vocal fremitis increased when the lung consolidates or contains a large cavity near the surface.

III. Percussion

The middle finger (pleximeter) of left hand is placed firmly on the part which is to be percussed and is adapted to any inequality of surface, so that no air is interposed between it and the skin. The back of its middle phalanx is then struck with the tip of the middle finger (plexor) of the right hand. The stroke should be delivered from the wrist and finger joints and the percussing finger should be so bent that when the blow is delivered its terminal phalanx is at right angle to the metacarpal bones and strikes the pleximeter finger perpendicular. The character of the sound produced depends on the body part percussed, accordingly it varies quantitatively and qualitatively. They are of three types.

1. Tympanic

Hollow viscera containing gas gives this type of sound. It is of musical character.

2. Resonant

A viscous like lungs in which air is trapped gives this type of sound. It is of low pitch and clear in character.

3. Dull

Solid viscera containing no air give dull sound. It is of high pitch and a short duration.

Percussion is done in order to ascertain the following points:

(i) Limit of the lung resonance.

(ii) Area of cardiac dullness.

(iii) Area of the liver dullness.

Beginning in front, the examiner should tap lightly and directly (that means without pleximeter finger) on the most prominent part of each clavical at the corresponding points. There after the other corresponding areas on both the sides, should be carefully percussed. Then find out the area of cardiac dullness.

The back and axillary regions should be examined in the same manner.

The lower limits of lung resonance should be examined from above downwards. The lower border of right lung lies over the liver and is thin; therefore, its exact situation is made out by light percussion. Posteriorly the muffling is due to thick muscles and fat of the back, which makes it necessary to percuss more firmly. In quite respiration, the lower border is found to lie in the mammary line at the sixth rib, in mid axillary line at the eighth rib. On the left side, the lower border overlaps the stomach, so the change is not from the lung resonance to dullness, but to the tympanic stomach resonance. Posteriorly there is splenic dullness and because of other solid structures, the condition resembles that of the right side. The position of lower border corresponds closely with that of right side.

IV. Auscultation

This is done with the help of stethoscope.

Stethoscope

It consists of two ear pieces which are joined together with the help of a metallic tube to a Y-shaped rubber tube. The other end of rubber is connected to the chest piece of stethoscope. It has two sides, a bell and a diaphragm. The ear knobs of ear piece are put in the ears in such a way that they will come along the direction of external auditory canal (medially and forwards). Diaphragm and bell are used for auscultation by rotating them to either side.

During auscultation subject is asked to breath with his mouth open, regularly, slightly deeper and faster than normal. The following observation should be made.

1. Character of Breath Sounds

There are two types of breath sounds.

(i) Vesicular

These are produced by the passage of air in and out of normal lung tissue. Vesicular breathing is heard all over the healthy chest and, most typically in the axillary region and infrascapular region. Through out inspiration the sound is fairly intense and of low pitch, with a characteristic rustle. There is no distinct pause before the expiratory sound, which is heard only in the early part of expiration. Normally the inspiratory sound is heard for at least twice as long, as the expiratory sound.

(ii) Bronchial

These sounds are produced by the passage of air through the trachea and large bronchi. Bronchial breathing is heard normally over the trachea, where it is very intense. The bronchial breathing heard over a disease lung is far less intense but of the same quality. The inspiratory sound of bronchial breathing is harsh and aspirate, becoming audible shortly before the end of inspiration. The expiratory sound has the same character but is more intense and of higher pitch than the inspiratory; the sound lasts through most of expiration. Bronchial breathing is recognized best by the quality of expiratory sound and the silent gap between inspiration and expiration.

2. Intensity of Breath Sounds

Intensity of breath sound is reduced in extensive damage in lungs or pleural effusion or pleural thickening. It is increased in very thin subjects and children.

3. Vocal Resonance

When the subject is asked to repeat the words "one, one, one" or "nine, nine, nine" the ears perceive, not the distinct syllables but a resonant sound. The intensity of the sound depends on the conductivity of his lungs; the nearer the stethoscope is to a large bronchus, the more intense the sound is.

Normal intensity of vocal resonance conveys the impression that is being produced at the chest piece of stethoscope.

Increase intensity conveys the impression that it is being produced near the ear piece of stethoscope and it is described as bronchophony.

When the vocal resonance is markedly increased it conveys the impression that it seems to be spoken in auscultator's ear, it is called as whispering pectoriloquy.

4. Added Sounds

(i) Ronchi or wheeze

Prolonged uninterrupted noises, arise in the bronchi and are due to partial obstruction of their lumen as in bronchial asthma.

(ii) Crepitations

These are discontinuous crackling or bubbling sounds.

QUESTIONS

1. How will you palpate the trachea?
2. What are the different steps of clinical examination of respiratory system?
3. How will you count the intercostal spaces?
4. What is vocal fremitis?
5. How will you percuss the chest during clinical examination of respiratory system?
6. What are the normal breath sounds heard during auscultation?
7. What are the added breathe sounds?

EXPERIMENT 3.25

Clinical examination of the abdomen

CLINICAL EXAMINATION

Clinical examination of abdomen of a subject is carried out in a standard sequence of examination.

    I. Inspection

    II. Palpation

    III. Percussion

    IV. Auscultation

It is helpful for recording in notes or when communicating information to colleagues to think of the abdomen as divided in to regions (Fig. 3.25.1).

The two lateral vertical planes (CC', DD') pass from the femoral artery blow to cross the costal margin close to the tip of the 9th costal cartilage.

The horizontal planes (AA', BB'), the subcostal and inter-tubercular, pass across the abdomen to connect the lowest points on the costal margins, and the tubercles of the iliac crests respectively.

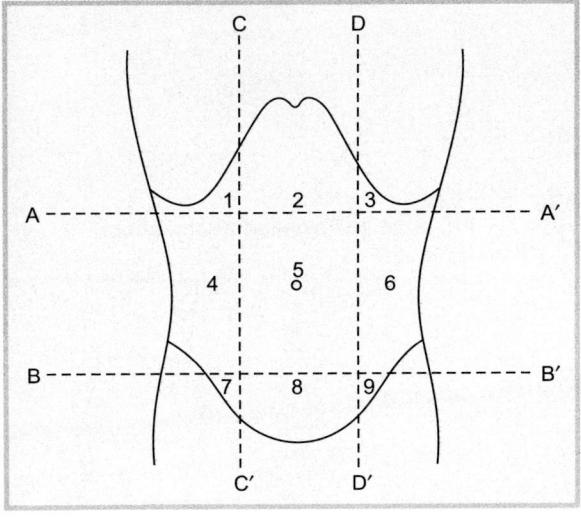

Fig. 3.25.1: Regions of abdomen. 1 and 3: Right and left hypochondria; 2: Epigastrium; 4 and 6: Right and left lumber; 5: Umbilical; 7 and 9: Right and left iliac; 8: suprapubic.

I. Inspection

The subject should be lying flat on his back, arms by his sides, on a firm couch, the head and neck supported by pillows, to make him comfortable. Make sure there is a good light and the room is warm. Stand on the patient's right side and ensure your hands are warm. The abdomen is fully exposed up to just above the xiphisternum and note the following features:

1. Shape

Look for normal abdominal contour and presence of sunken, fullness or distension.

    (i) A sunken (scaphoid) abdomen is seen in severe malnutrition and starvation.

    (ii) Generalized fullness or distension may be due to fat, fluid, flatus and faeces.

    (iii) Localised distension may be due to gross enlargement of liver, spleen or any other organ.

2. The Umbilicus

Normally the umbilicus is slightly retracted and inverted. If it is everted then an umbilicus hernia may be present.

3. Movements of Abdominal Wall

Normally there is a gentle rise in the abdominal wall during inspiration and a fall during expiration; the movements should be free and equal on both sides. In generalized peritonitis this movement is absent or markedly diminished.

4. Presence of Visible Pulsations

    (i) Visible pulsations of abdominal aorta in the epigastrium is a frequent finding in nervous thin patients.

    (ii) Visible peristalsis of stomach or small intestine may be observed in normal very thin elderly patient with lax abdominal muscles, in patient having obstruction at pylorus and in patient having obstruction in the distal small bowel.

5. Skin and Surface of the Abdomen

    (i) In marked distension the skin is smooth and shiny.

(ii) White or pink wrinkled linear marks on the abdominal skin are produced by gross stretching of the skin in pregnancy, ascites and Cushing's syndrome.

(iii) Pigmentation of the abdominal wall may be seen in the midline below the umbilicus in pregnancy (Linea nigra).

6. Presence of Prominent Veins

Look for any prominent vein on the abdomen in various areas.

Small, thin veins over the subcostal margin in thin individuals is a common finding.

Distended veins around the umbilicus (caput medusae) are seen in portal hypertension.

Distended veins on the abdominal wall and chest wall appear in patient with obstruction to inferior vena cava.

7. Genitalia

Inspect both groins, the penis and scrotum of a male, for any swelling and to ensure that testes are in their normal position.

II. Palpation

Palpation of abdomen should be done in the same posture as described in inspection. Make sure that in the winter your hands and room should be warm.

Palpation should be started in the left iliac region lightly and move anti-clockwise to end in the suprapubic region.

Start by placing the right hand flat on the part to be palpated with the wrist and forearm in the same horizontal plane, where possible. The art is to 'mould' the relaxed right hand to the body surface, and not to hold it rigid. The best movement is gentle but with firm pressure with the finger held almost with slight flexion at metacarpophalangeal joints (Fig. 3.25.2).

1. Palpation of Abdominal Regions

During palpation of different regions, note down any tenderness or rigidity. In the patient having peritonitis palpation leads to rigidity because of reflex contraction of abdominal muscles.

2. Palpation of Kidneys

The right hand is placed anteriorly in the lumber region while the left hand is placed posteriorly in the loin (Fig. 3.25.3). Ask the subject to take a deep breath in, press the left hand forwards, and the right hand upwards and inwards. The kidney is not usually palpable except its lower pole is felt as a smooth, rounded firm swelling between both right and left hand. It can be pushed from one hand to the other and descends on deep inspiration.

3. Palpation of Spleen

Usually, the spleen is not normally palpable. It has to be enlarged two or three times it's usual size before it becomes so and then is felt under the left subcostal margin.

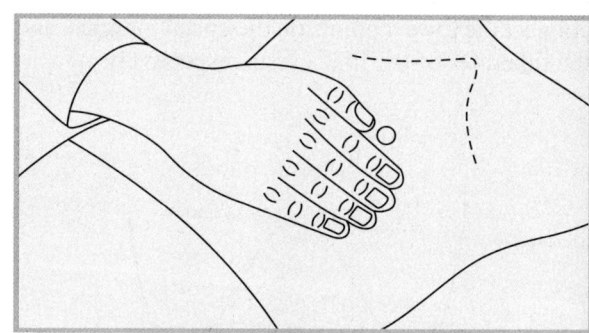

Fig. 3.25.2: Palpation of abdomen.

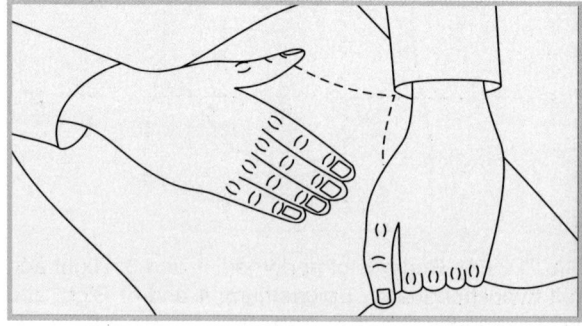

Fig. 3.25.3: Palpation of left kidney.

Place the left hand flat over the lower most rib cage posteriorly, and the right hand beneath the costal margin (Fig.3.25.4). Ask the subject to breathe in deeply, press it deeply with the fingers of the right hand beneath the costal margin, at the same time exerting pressure medially and downwards with the left hand. If enlargement is suspected and it is still not palpable, turn the subject onto his right hand side and repeat the whole procedure.

4. Palpation of Liver

Sit beside the right hand side of the subject, place both hands side by side flat on the abdomen in the right subcostal region, lateral to the rectus with the fingers pointing towards the ribs. If resistance is felt move the hands further down till the resistance disappears. Ask the subject to breathe in deeply and at the height of inspiration press the fingers firmly inwards and upwards.

Normally the liver is not palpable in healthy individuals, if it is enlarged, it is felt as a sharp regular border which slides beneath the fingers.

III. Percussion

In the abdomen only light percussion is necessary — a tympanic note is heard throughout except over the liver, where note is dull.

1. Defining the Boundaries of Abdominal Organs

(i) Liver

The upper and lower borders of the right lobe of the liver can be defined accurately by percussion. Start anteriorly, at the fourth intercostal space, where the note will be resonant over the lungs and move vertically downwards. In the healthy individual the upper border of liver is at about the fifth intercostal space here the note becomes dull. This dullness extends down up to just below right costal margin.

Dullness in the area over the liver is reduced in severe emphysema and large pneumothorax.

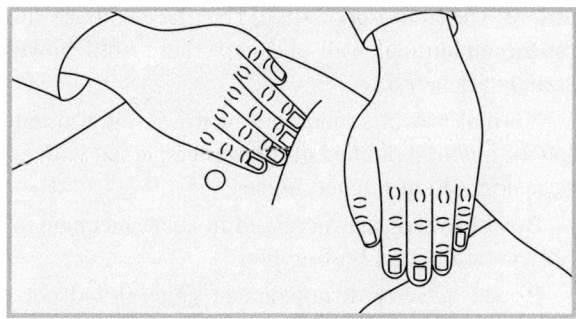

Fig. 3.25.4: Palpation of spleen.

(ii) Spleen

Its dullness extends from the left lower ribs into the left hypochondrium and left lumber region.

2. Confirmation of Pressure of Free Fluid in Peritoneal Cavity (Ascites)

Presence of any one of the two signs: shifting dullness and a fluid thrill, make diagnosis of ascites.

(i) Shifting dullness

Lie the patient supine and, on percussion, note dullness in the flanks and lower abdomen, with a central area of resonance at and above the umbilicus. Now turn the patient on his right side. Allow time for the intestines to float upwards and the free fluid to gravitate down and percuss again.

Now repeat this, turning the patient onto his left side.

(ii) Fluid thrill

To elicit it the patient is again laid on his back. Place one hand flat over the lumber region of one side, get an assistant to put the side of his hand firmly in the midline of the abdomen, and then tap the opposite lumber region. A fluid thrill or wave is felt as a definite and unmistakable impulse by watching hand held flat in the lumber region. As a rule a fluid thrill is felt only when there is a large amount of ascites present which is under tension.

IV. Auscultation

It is a useful way of listening for bowel sounds and deciding whether they are normal, increased or absent. The stethoscope should be placed on one site on the abdominal wall and kept there until bowel sounds are heard.

Normal bowel sounds are heard as intermittent low or medium pitched gurgles interspersed with an occasional high-pitched noise.

Bowel sounds are increased in acute mechanical obstruction called borborygmi.

Bowel activity disappears in generalized peritonitis and abdomen is silent.

QUESTIONS

1. Palpate liver or spleen in the given subject.
2. What is fluid thrill and how is it elicited?
3. What is ascites?
4. How to palpate kidneys?
5. Describe different steps of clinical examination of abdomen.
6. What are the various regions of abdomen used during clinical examination?

EXPERIMENT 3.26

Clinical examination of sensory system

During examination of sensory system test various types of sensations:

1. Tactile sensibility
2. Pain
3. Temperature
4. Sense of position
5. Vibrations
6. Recognition of size, shapes, weight and form of objects (stereognosis).
7. Presence of any abnormal sensation.

Before starting the examination, explain the nature of the test to be performed to the patient to get his full cooperation. *The eyes should then be closed and test different forms of sensations. Always compare corresponding points on both sides of the body.*

1. Tactile Sensibility

(i) Light Touch

Use a wisp of cotton wool or hair aesthesiometer. Tell the patient to say yes every time he feels a touch – comparing corresponding points on both side of the body.

It is not enough to find out that the patient can feel the touch. One should find out whether he can localise it and whether he can discriminate between two points (Two point discrimination). It is done with the help of compass aesthesiometer. Normally 2 mm of separation of points can be appreciated on the palmar surface of the thumb and fingers. This distance depends upon the number of tactile receptors in the area (density of receptors).

(ii) Pressure Touch (Sense)

Repeat the above test with the tip of a finger on any blunt object the temperature of which does not differ much from that of the skin.

Loss of tactile sensation is called anaesthesia, if it is partial loss it is called hypoaesthesia.

2. Pain sensation

(i) Superficial Pain

Use the point of a steel pin or a needle to test superficial pain sensation. The technique is same as that used for touch.

(ii) Pressure Pain

It is tested by squeezing the muscle or the tendo-achilles. It can also be done with the help of Algometer. With help of this instrument, we can measure the threshold pressure, which causes the pressure pain.

Absence of sensibility of pain is termed analgesia, partial loss of pain sensation is called as hypoalgesia, and exaggerated pain, sensibility is known as hyperalgesia.

3. Temperature (Thermal) Sensibility

It is tested using test tubes containing hot and cold water. The part to be tested is touched with each in turn, and the patient says whether each tube feels hot or cold.

4. Sense of Position

(i) Ask the patient to close his eyes, take hold of one of his limbs and move it about in various directions through the air, finally leaving in some definite position say semi-flexed and slightly elevated, ask him to put the corresponding limb in a similar position. If the subject is able to place the other limb in same position – sense of position is intact.

(ii) In case of foot he may be told that the great toe will be placed pointing upwards or downwards and he is asked to tell where it is.

Patient with defective sense of position may not be able to manipulate small objects without visually observing their movements (sensory ataxia).

5. Vibration Sense

A tuning fork (128 Hz) is made to vibrate by striking the prongs gently on a firm object like rubber pad or wooden table. Its foot is then placed on some subcutaneous bone in the region to be tested. The ankle is a commonly tested site. Ascertain if the patient receives the vibrations, and if so, ask him to say once again when he ceases to feel them. The fork is transferred to the same region of the observer for comparison. If the examiner still perceive the vibrations, the patient's perception of vibration is impaired. There is often loss of vibration sense in the feet and legs in old age. Vibration sensibility may be lost in tabes dorsalis, peripheral neuritis and posterior column disorders.

6. Recognition of size, shape, weight and form of objects (stereognosis)

These faculties can be tested most accurately in the hands with the eyes closed.

To test size, place in the patient palm objects of same shape, but of different sizes, for example small rods of different lengths. Ask him to say which is the larger. To test recognition of shape familiar objects such as coins, a pencil, scissors, etc. are placed in the hand, and patient is asked to identify them. Loss of this faculty is known as astereognosis.

It may occur, with patient lesions, when position sense and light touch are normal, although there is usually some defect in these modalities. When astereognosis occurs with posterior column lesions, position sense, vibration sense and light touch are invariably profoundly disturbed.

7. Presence of any Abnormal Sensation

This is termed as paraesthesia and consists of various sensations experienced by the patient in the absence of any outside stimulus. The commonest of these are: feeling of 'pins and needles', of numbness, of heats or chills, of pressure of tightness, of itching sometimes termed pruritus or a feeling as if insects were crawling over the body (formication).

QUESTIONS

1. Demonstrate the testing of touch sensation in the right forearm of the subject.
2. Demonstrate the examination of temperature sensation in right forearm of the subject.
3. What are anaesthesia, hypoaesthesia and hyperaesthesia?
4. What are analgesia, hypoalgesia and hyperaesthesia?
5. How to test sense of position in upper and lower limb of a subject given to you?
6. Give neural pathway of various somatic sensations.

Examination of motor system is done under following headings:

I. Bulk of muscles

II. Tone of muscles

III. Strength (Power) of the muscles

IV. Reflexes

V. Coordination of movements

VI. Gait

VII. Involuntary movements.

I. Bulk of Muscles

This is estimated by inspection and palpation. Measure the circumferences of arm, forearm, thigh and leg at identical level of both sides. The level should be decided in relation to some fixed, subcutaneous bony landmarks. The bony point selected may be the medial epicondyle of the humerus, the anterior superior iliac spine, the medial malleolus, etc. Judgment regarding the presence of muscular wasting or otherwise depends most often on a comparison of the two sides. But occasionally both sides may show wasting. Therefore, common-sense about what should be normal muscle mass for given person should also be employed.

Wasted or atrophic muscles are smaller, softer and more flabby than normal when they are contracted. Muscle wasting associated with fibrosis is called contracture. The muscle feels hard, inelastic and shortened, therefore, it is not possible to stretch them passively to a normal degree.

Muscle atrophy is seen in injury and disease of muscle or joint. Generalised muscular atrophy is seen in cachexia of any cause. Neurological disorder also causes muscle atrophy.

II. Tone of Muscles

Muscular tone is a state of tension or contraction present in the resting healthy muscle. It depends on the integrity of stretch reflex which is under the control of higher centres. Muscle tone is regulated by corticospinal and extrapyramidal pathways. Increase in the tone is called hypertonia and decrease in tone is hypotonia. The degree of tone is estimated by handling the limbs and moving them passively at their various joints.

Hypotonia is seen in damage to reflex arc (lower motor neurone lesion). Tone is also decreased during sleep.

Hypotonia following lesions of the corticospinal system (upper motor neurone lesions) is termed as *spasticity*. It is confined to one group of muscles (flexes or extensor).

Hypertonia resulting from disease of basal ganglia is termed as extrapyramidal rigidity. Both the group of muscles (flexes or extensor) are involved in rigidity.

III. Strength (Power) of the Muscles

The general rule in this investigation is to ask the patient to throw into action the particular muscle or group of muscles which one wishes to test, while the observer offers to that action a greater or lesser degree of passive resistance.

1. Testing the Power of Muscles of Upper Limb

(i) *Abductor pollicis brevis*: The patient is asked to abduct his thumb in a plane at right angle to the palmar aspect of the index finger, against the resistance of the examiner's own thumb. The muscle can be seen and felt to contract.

(ii) *Opponens pollicis*: Ask the patient to touch the tip of his little finger with the point of his thumb. Oppose the movement with your thumb or index finger.

(iii) *Interossei and lumbricals*: Test the patient's ability to flex his metacarpophalangeal joints and to extend the distal interphalangeal joints. The interossei also adduct the fingers.

(iv) *Flexors of fingers*: Ask the patient to squeeze your fingers. Allow him to squeeze only your index and middle fingers – this is sufficient to assess strength of grip without his painfully crushing your fingers.

(v) *Flexors of the wrist*: Ask him to bring the tips of his fingers towards the front of the forearm.

(vi) *Extensors of the wrist*: Ask the patient to make a fist, and try to forcibly flex the wrist against his effort to maintain his posture.

(vii) *Brachioradialis*: Place the arm of the patient midway between the prone and supine position then ask the patient to bend up the forearm, whilst you oppose the movement by grasping his hand.

(viii) *Biceps*: Ask the patient to bend up the forearm against resistance, with the forearm in full supination.

(ix) *Triceps*: Ask the patient to straighten out his forearm against your resistance.

(x) *Supraspinatus and deltoid*: Ask the patient to lift his arm straight out at right angles to his side against resistance. The first 30° of his movement is carried out by the supraspinatus and the remaining 60° is produced by the deltoid.

2. Testing the Power of Muscle of Trunk

(i) *Muscle of abdomen*: Weakness of these muscles is shown by the patient's inability to sit up in the bed from the supine position with out the aid of his arms.

(ii) *Trapezius*: Upper part: Ask the patient to shrug his shoulders against examiner's resistance. Lower part: Ask him to approximate the shoulder blades.

3. Testing the Power of Muscles of Lower Limb

(i) *Dorsiflexion and planter flexion* of the feet and toes are tested by asking the patient to elevate or depress the part against resistance.

(ii) *Extensors of the knees*: Bend up the patient's knee, and then, pressing with your hand on his skin, ask him to try to straighten it out again.

(iii) *Flexors of the knee*: Raise the leg up from the bed, supporting the thigh with your left hand and holding the ankle with your right hand.

Then ask the patient to bend his knee.

(iv) *Flexors of the thigh*: With the leg extended ask the patient to raise his leg off the bed against your resistance.

(v) *Adductors of the thigh*: Abduct the limb and then ask the patient to bring it back to the midline against resistance.

(vi) *Abductors of the thigh*: Place the patient's legs together and ask him to separate them against resistance.

IV. Reflexes

Superficial and deep reflexes are described in Exp. 3.28.

V. Coordination of Movements

Coordination of muscle movement means the cooperative contraction of separate muscle or groups of muscles in order to accomplish a definite act. Absence or imperfection of such cooperation is called incoordination or ataxia.

(a) Test for Coordination in Upper Limbs

1. *Finger nose test*: Ask the patient to touch first his nose with his own index finger and then the examiner's index finger. If he performs these movements without making errors, coordination is normal. He is then asked to perform the same action with his eyes closed, irregularity indicates impairment of position sense in limb.

2. Ask the patient to make a circle in the air with his index finger, first with eyes open and then with eyes closed. All normal persons can draw a circle smoothly and accurately whether the eyes are open or closed.

3. *Diadochokinesia and dysdiadochokinesia*: The patient is asked to flex his elbows to a right angle and then alternatively to supinate and pronate his forearms as rapidly as possible. All normal persons can do this very rapidly. When movements are slow, awkward and incomplete,

and often become impossible after few attempts, it is referred as dysdiadochokinesia.

(b) Test for Coordination in Lower Limb

1. Ask the patient to walk along a straight line. If incoordination is present he will soon deviate to one side or the other.

2. *Heel–knee test*: If he cannot walk, ask him, as he lies in bed, to lift one leg high in the air, to place the heel of this leg on the opposite knee and then to slide the heel down his shin towards the ankle. In cerebella ataxia a characteristic, irregular side to side series of errors in the speed and direction of movement occurs.

3. *Romberg's sign*: The patient is asked to stand with his feet close together, and if he can do this, he is then asked to close his eyes. If Romberg's sign is present, as soon as his eyes are closed he begins to sway about or may even fall. This is present in sensory ataxia (loss of posterior sense). Cerebellar ataxia results due to cerebeller dysfunctions.

VI. Gait

Gait means the manner of walking. It is of major importance in diagnosis. Some common abnormal types of gait recognised are described as under.

(i) *Spastic or hemiplegic gait*: This is a characteristics feature of persons with pyramidal tract lesions. The patient walks on a narrow base, has difficulty in bending his knees and drags his feet as if they are glued to the floor. The foot is raised from the ground by tilting the pelvis, and leg is then put forward so that the foot tends to describe an arc, the toes scraping along the floor.

(ii) *Stamping gait*: Stamping means to strike the ground heavily with the sole of foot. This is a characteristic of a person with sensory ataxia.

(iii) *Drunken or reeling gait*: This is seen in person with cerebella lesions. The person walks in a zigzag line and deviates to the affected side due to hypotonia.

(iv) *Festinant gait*: This is characteristic of Parkinson's disease. The person bend forward, and walks quickly with short steps as if trying to catch up centre of gravity.

(v) *Waddling gait*: Waddling means to walk with short steps like the gait of a duck. This is typically seen in persons with proximal muscular weakness (Myopathies, muscular dystrophies). The feet are planted widely apart and the body sways from side to side as each step is taken. The heel and toes tend to be brought down simultaneously.

VII. Involuntary Movements

Abnormal movements present in the patients are – tremors, athetosis, chorea, tics, and epilepsy.

Tremors

Regular or irregular distal movements having an oscillatory (vibrating) character are referred as tremors. Intentional tremors are seen in cerebellar dysfunction. These are coarse and clearly seen when the part is used in voluntary movements.

Fine and rapid tremors are seen in anxiety and thyrotoxicosis. In Parkinson's disease tremors are present at rest and disappear during activity. Its frequent presence can be seen as pin-rolling movements (rhythmic contraction of thumb over first fingers).

QUESTIONS

1. How will you grade the power of the muscle?
2. How will you test the power of flexors of fingers?
3. How will you test coordination of muscle movements in upper limb and lower limb?
4. What are the differences between intention tremors and Parkinson's disease tremors?
5. What is Romberg's sign? Give its clinical significance.
6. What are the signs of cerebellar lesions?

EXPERIMENT 3.28

To study superficial and deep reflexes

APPARATUS

Patellar hammer and examination couch.

Patellar hammer consists of a long metallic handle, at one end of it a triangular rubber piece is attached. The rubber piece has two ends, one pointed and other broad. This rubber piece is used to give a sharp blow to a tendon, in order to cause sudden stretching of the muscle.

During eliciting the reflex, make sure that subject should be comfortable and relax. Skin overlying the muscle tested should be uncovered to see the contraction (response) of the muscle.

EXAMINATION

I. Superficial Reflexes

These reflexes are of significance in unilateral lesions when healthy side is taken as standard for comparison purposes.

1. Plantar Reflex

Subject is asked to lie on the bed or couch in supine position. Gently scratch the outer edge of the foot with blunt object (key) from the heel toward toe and then medially (Figs 3.28.1a and b). Flexion of the four outer toes takes place, with increase in strength of stimulus all the toes are flexed and ankle becomes dorsiflexed and inverted. This is called flexor plantar response. With still stronger stimuli withdrawal of the limb occurs. In case of upper motor neurone lesions, plantar response becomes extensor plantar response. It is called as *Babinski's sign*. (In the extensor plantar response there is dorsiflexion (extension) of great toe and spreading out and extension of other toes.) It is also positive in children below one year of age. It is because myelination of corticospinal pathway gets completed in 6–12 month. Level of spinal cord involved in the reflex is L_5 and S_1. Elicit the reflex on other limb also for comparison.

2. Abdominal Reflexes

Stroke the abdominal wall gently with key parallel to costal margin and inguinal ligament when subject lying in supine with uncovered abdomen. Normally, this leads to contraction of underlying muscles. It is usually difficult to obtain this reflex in anxious persons, elderly, obese and multipara women. Level of spinal cord involved in the reflex is T_7 to T_{12}.

3. Cremasteric Reflex

Stroke the skin at upper and inner part of thigh, testicles are drawn upward because of contraction of cremasteric muscle. Spinal segments involved in the reflex are L_1 and L_2.

4. Anal Reflex

Stroking or scratching the skin near anus leads to contraction of anal sphincter. Spinal segments involved in the reflex are S3 and S4.

Conjunctival reflex, pupillary reflex and corneal reflex are discussed in cranial nerve examination.

II. Deep (Tendon) Reflexes

If a tendon of a lightly stretched muscle is struck a single, a sharp blow with a soft rubber hammer, the muscle contracts briefly. This is the monosynaptic stretch reflex. It is a test of the integrity of the afferent and efferent pathways, and of the excitability of anterior horn cells in the spinal segment of the stretched muscle.

Make sure that subject is warm and comfortable. He should be completely relaxed with diverted attention. All these reflexes must be elicited on the other limb also for comparison.

Grading of Reflexes:

Grade 0: Absent,

Grade 1: Present (as a normal ankle jerk)

Grade 2: Brisk (as a normal knee jerk)

Grade 3: Very brisk

Grade 4: Clonus – it is a sign of increased reflex activity characterised by repetitive muscular contraction produced by stretch.

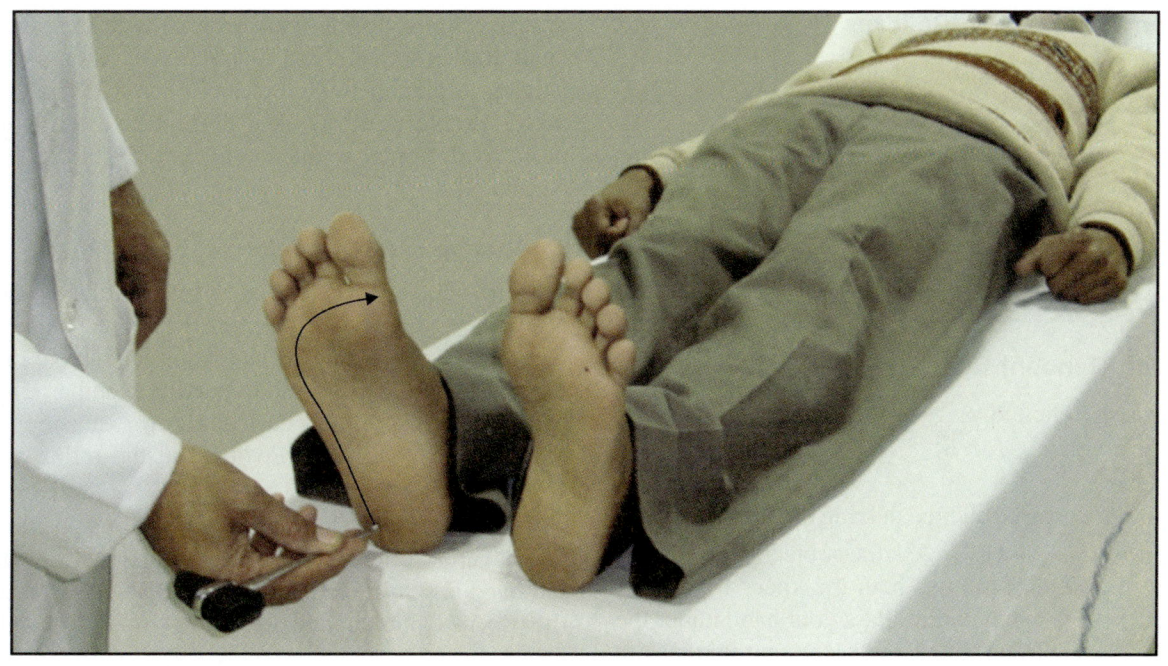

(a) Right

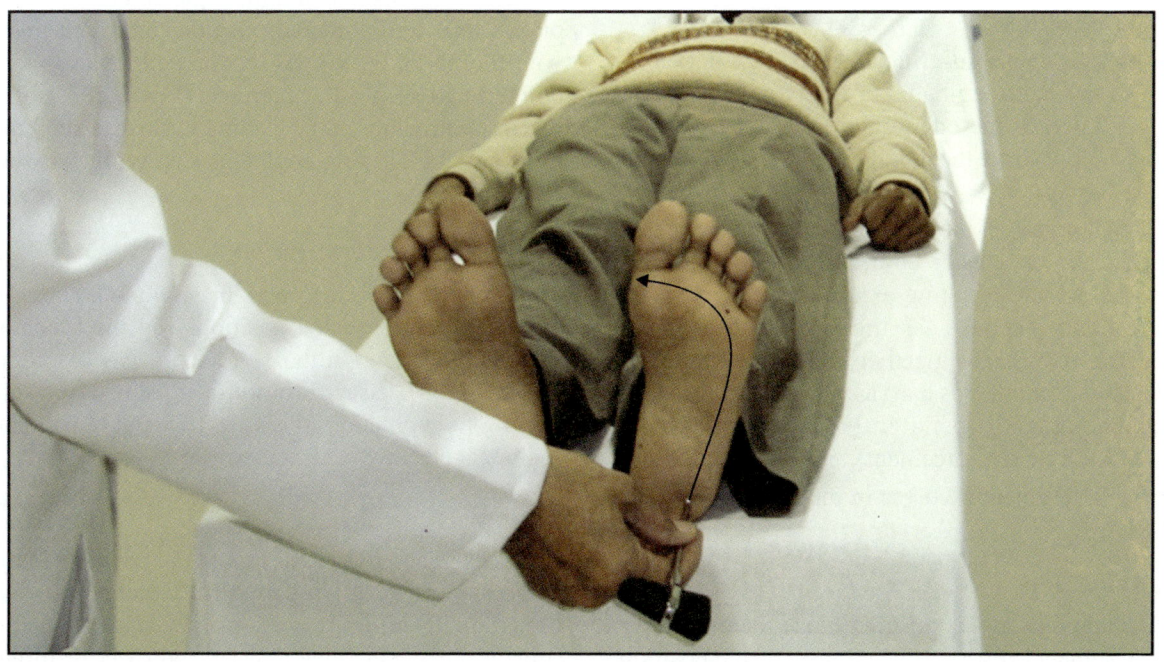

(b) Left

Figs 3.28.1a and b: To elicit plantar reflex.

Abnormal Tendon Reflexes

1. Reflex diminishes or absent
   - During sleep
   - Lower motor neuron lesion
2. Reflex exaggerates:
   - Anxiety or nervousness
   - Upper motor neuron lesion
   - Thyrotoxicosis

Deep (Tendon) Reflexes

These are elicited as

1. Knee Jerk

This reflex can be elicited in lying or sitting position.

(a) *Lying position:* Ask the subject to lie supine. Ask him to raise both the knees by flexing knee and hip joint. Pass your hand under the knee to be tested and place on the opposite knee (Fig. 3.28.2). Now strike the patellar tendon midway between its origin and insertion.

(b) *Sitting posture:* Subject is asked to sit on the bed with leg hanging freely over the other knee or the edge of the bed (Fig. 3.28.3). Now strike the tendon with patellar hammer as above.

Thigh region of the patient should be uncovered. Reflex shows a brief contraction of quadriceps femoris muscle resulting extension of the knee. If there is no response ask the subject to hook the fingers of two hands together and then to pull them against one another as hard as possible or to make a clench fist with ipsilateral hand (Jendrassik's manoeuvre or reinforcement).

Spinal segment involves in the reflex are L_2, L_3, and L_4.

2. Ankle Jerk

It is elicited in supine posture. Place the lower limb of the subject in everted and slightly flexed position, then with one hand, slightly dorsiflex the foot so as to stretch it (Fig. 3.28.4). Strike the tendon of gastrocnemius muscle (calf muscle) with the other hand. Reflex shown sharp contraction of calf muscle leading to planter flexion of ankle joint. If there is no response Jendrassik's manoeuvre may be performed. Spinal segments involved in the reflex S1 and S2.

3. Triceps (Jerk) Reflex

Ask the subject to lie supine. Flex the elbow and allow the forearm to rest across the subject's chest (Fig. 3.28.5). Tap the triceps tendon just above the olecranon with narrow end of patellar hammer. The triceps contracts might be leading to extension at elbow. Spinal segments involved in the reflex are C_6 and C_7.

Other method to elicit the reflex in sitting position is that support the forearm of the subject with your left hand in semiflexed position (Fig. 3.28.6). Strike the triceps tendon above olecranon with right hand.

4. Biceps (Jerk) Reflex

The elbow is flexed to a right angle and the forearm placed in a semipronated position; then you place your thumb on the biceps tendon and strike it with pointed end of patellar hammer (Fig. 3.28.7). The biceps contract might be leading to flexion at elbow joint. C_5 and C_6 spinal segments are involved in this reflex.

5. Supinator (Jerk) Reflex

The elbow is flexed to a right angle and forearm placed in semipronated position. Tap the brachioradialis tendon upon the styloid process of radius (Fig. 3.28.8). Brachioradialis muscle contracts leading to supination of elbow. C-5 and C-6 spinal segments are involved in the reflex.

6. Jaw Jerk

Ask the subject to open his mouth but not too widely. Place one finger of left hand firmly on his chin and then tap it suddenly with finger of right hand (Fig. 3.28.9). Masseter muscle contracts resulting closure of the jaw. Trigeminal nerve (V cranial nerve) is involved in this reflex.

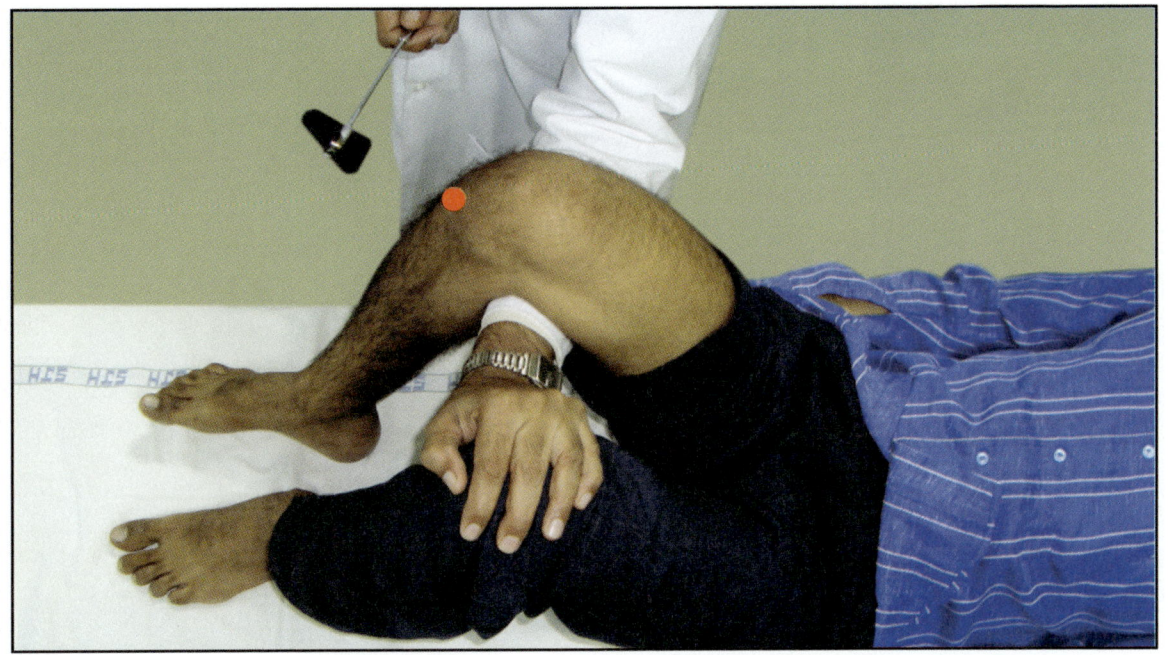

(a) Right

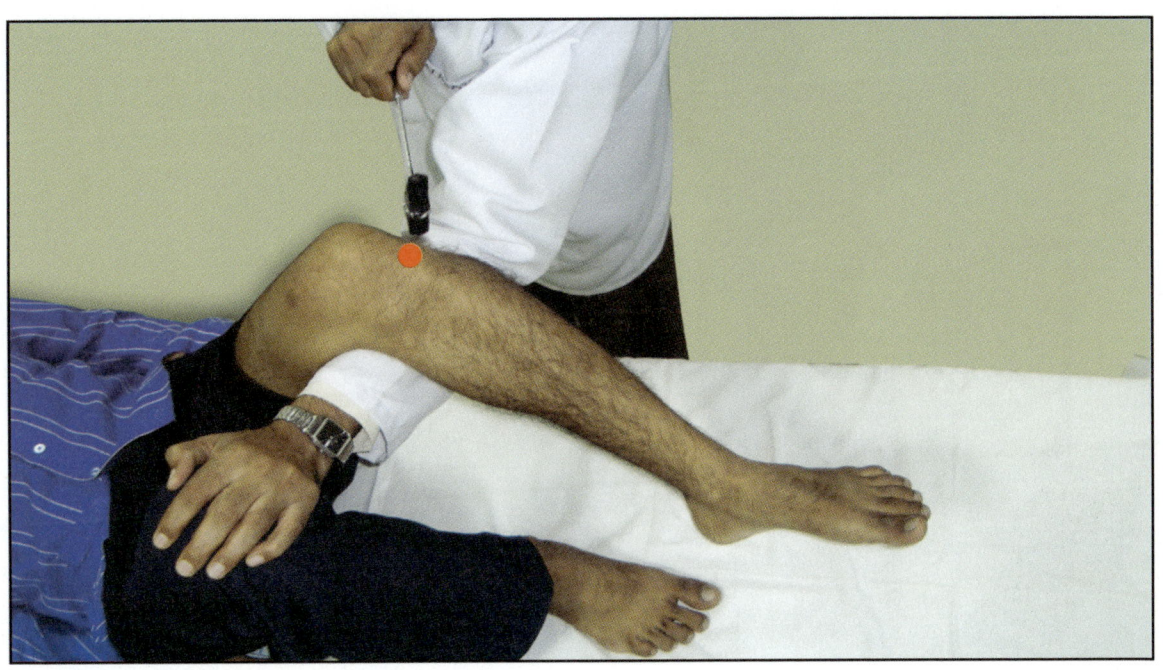

(b) Left

Fig. 3.28.2: To elicit knee-jerk in lying position.

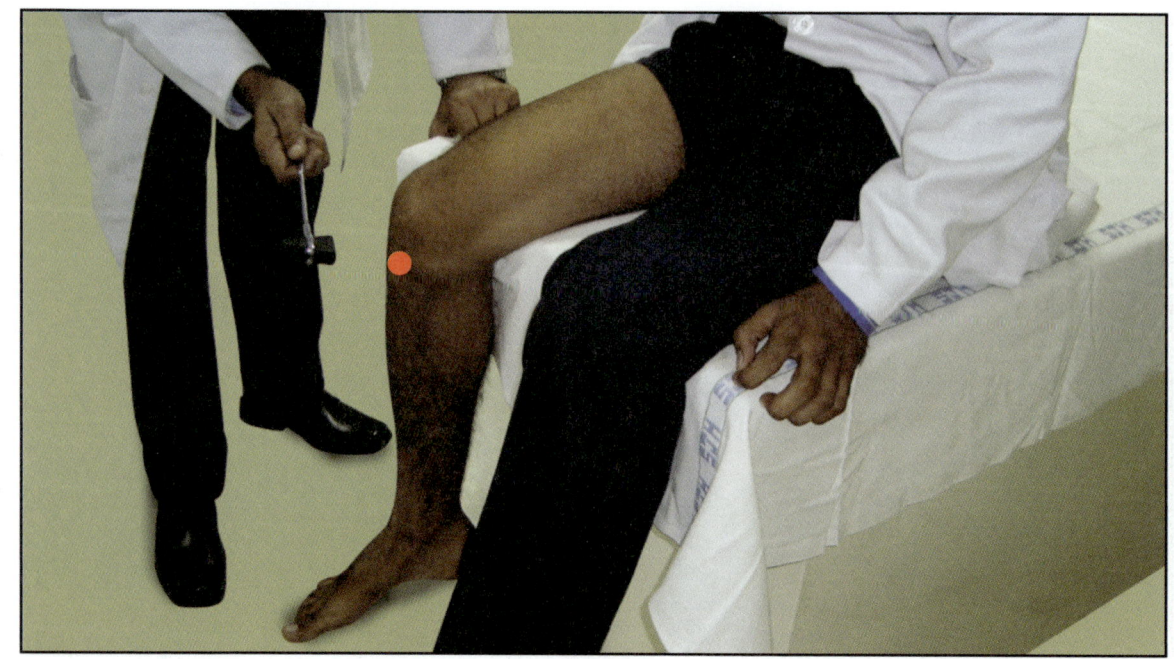

(a) Right

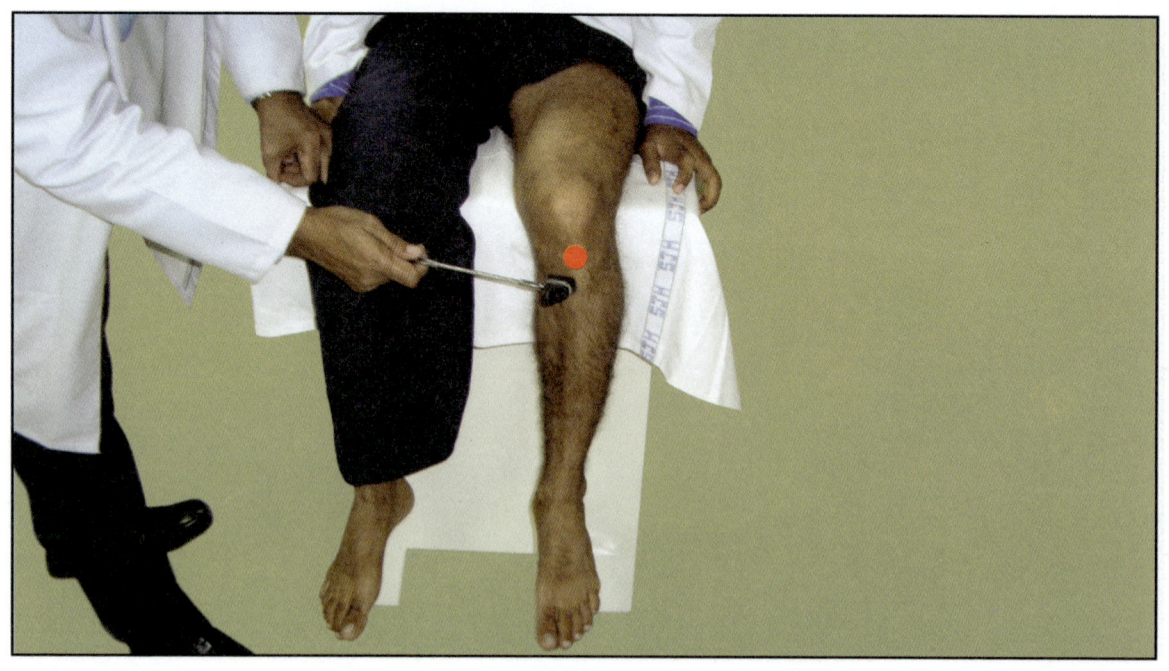

(b) Left

Fig. 3.28.3: To elicit knee-jerk in sitting position.

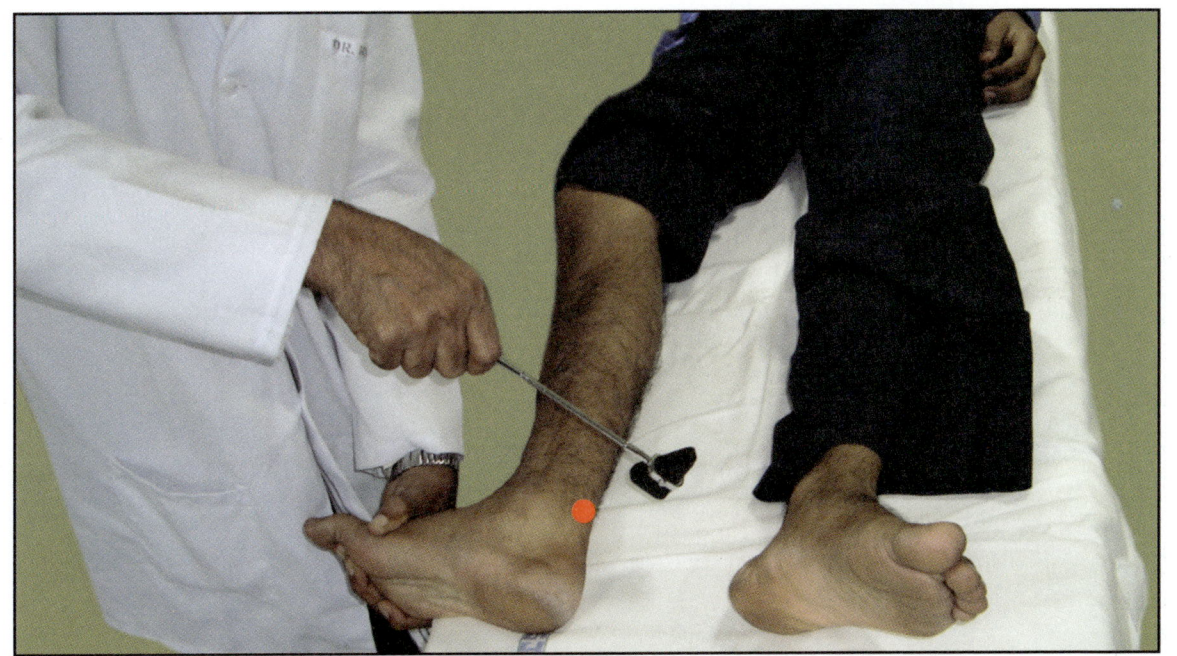

(a) Right

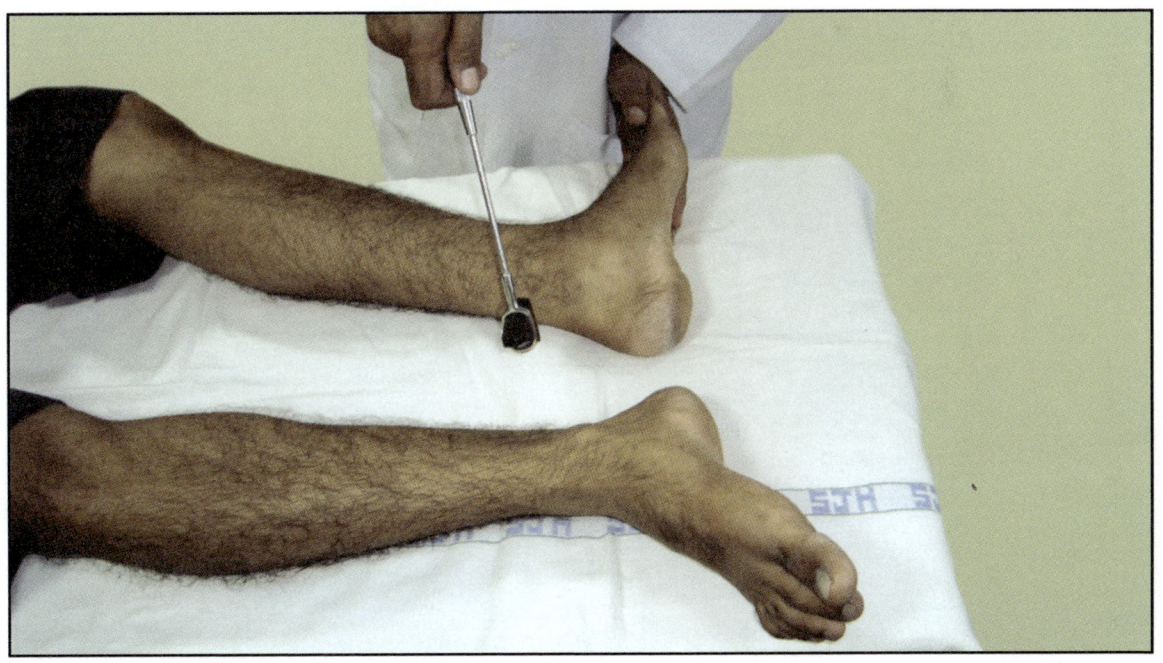

(b) Left

Fig. 3.28.4: To elicit ankle jerk in lying position.

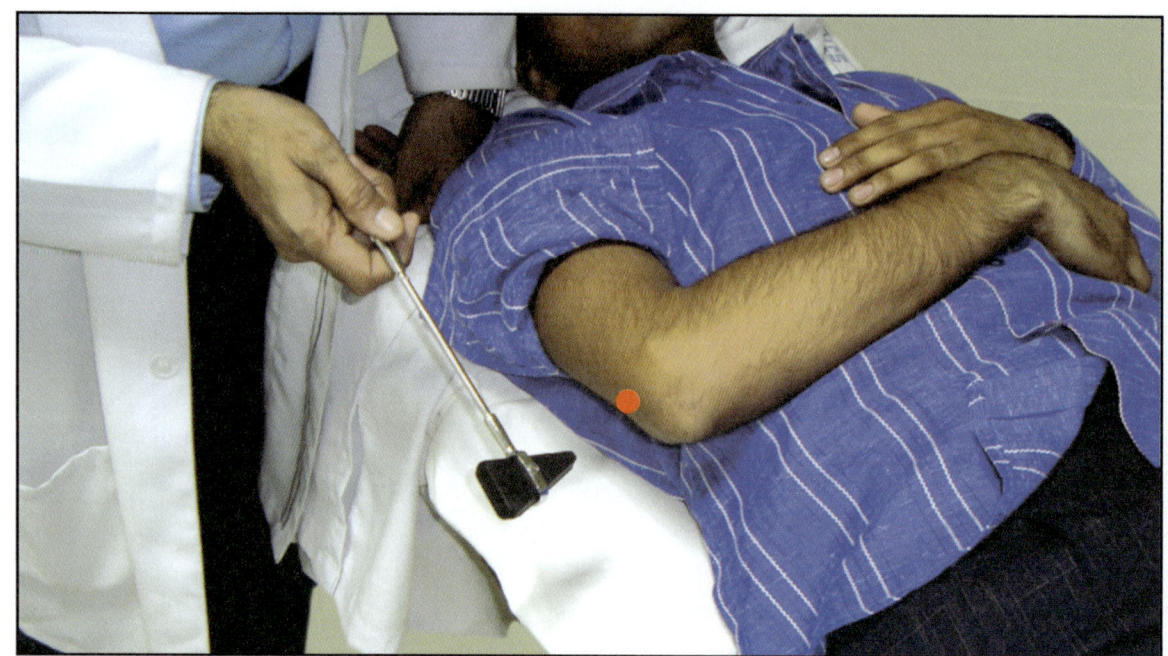

(a) Right

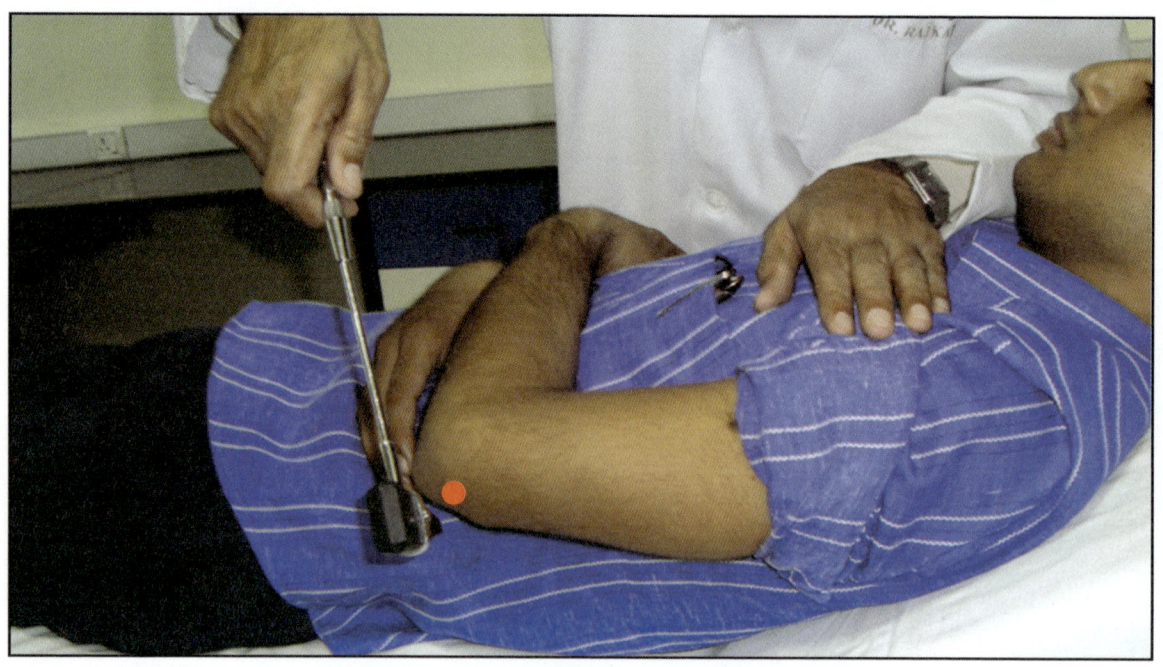

(b) Left

Fig. 3.28.5: To elicit triceps reflex in lying position.

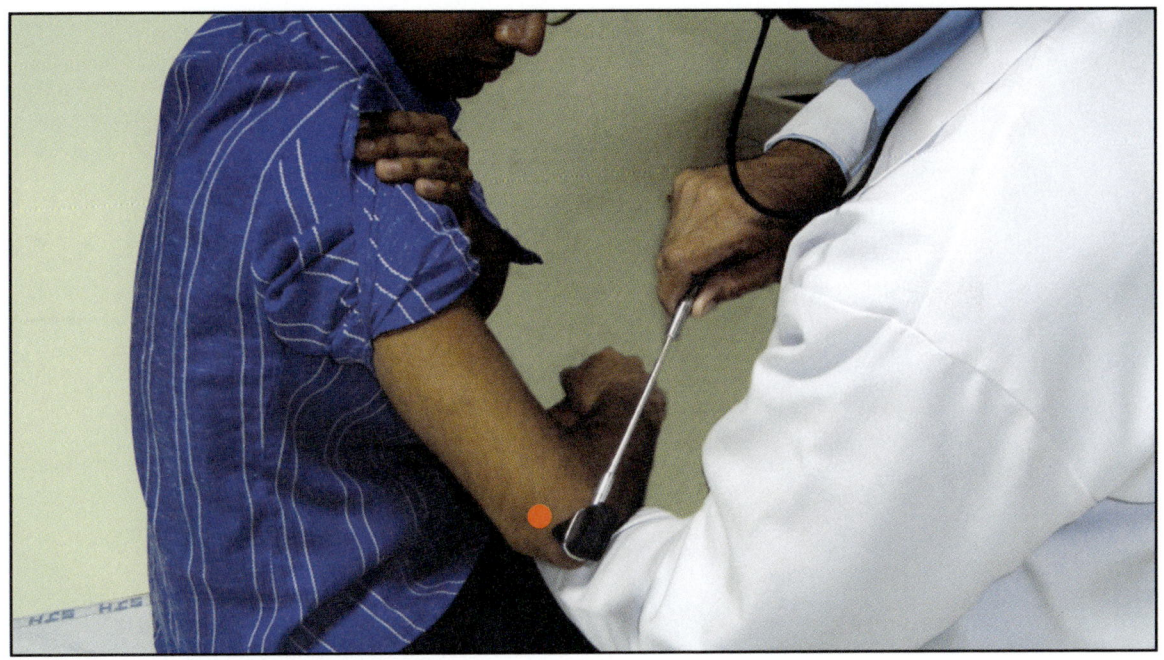

(a) Right

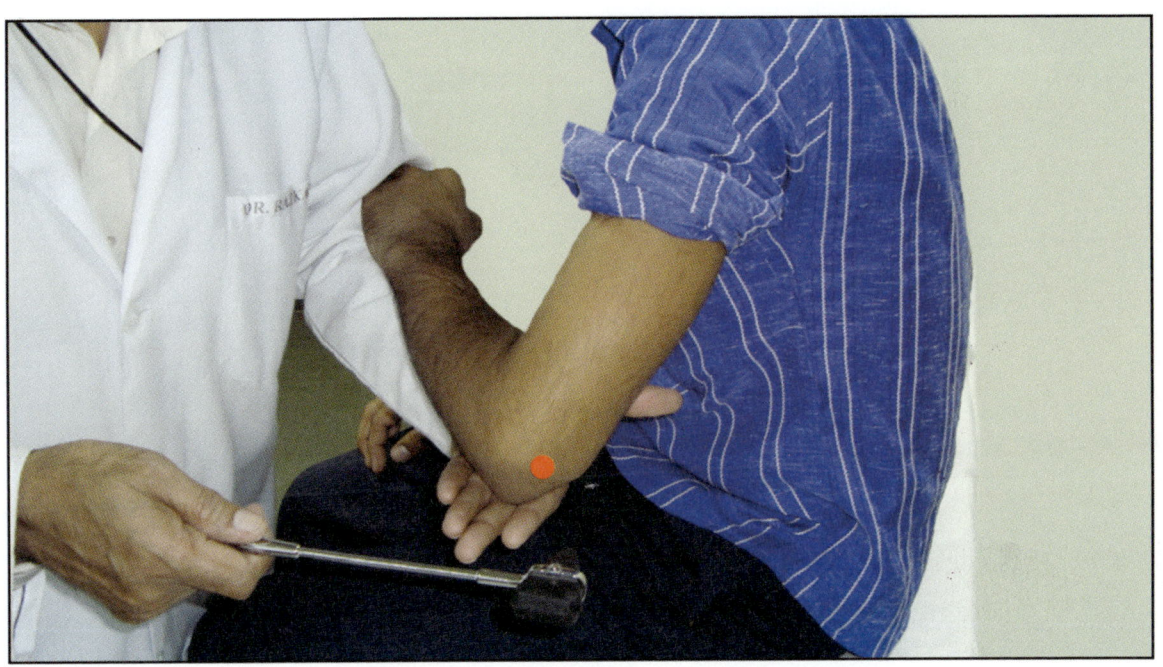

(b) Left

Fig. 3.28.6: To elicit triceps reflex in sitting position.

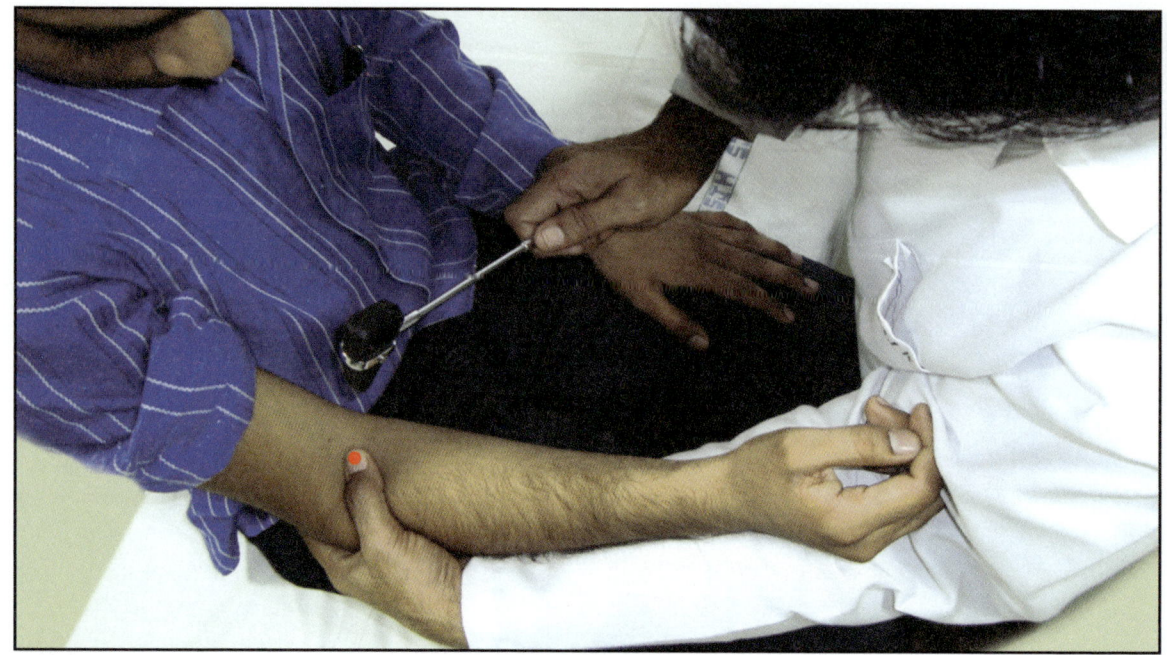

(a) Right

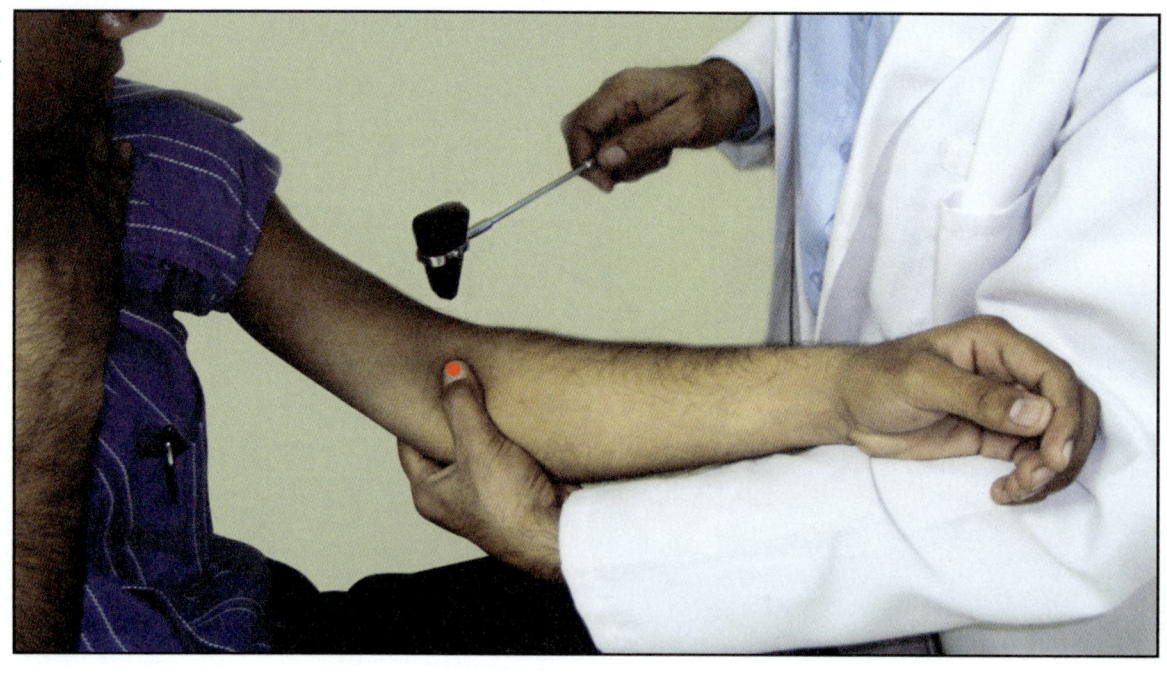

(b) Left

Fig. 3.28.7: To elicit biceps reflex in sitting position.

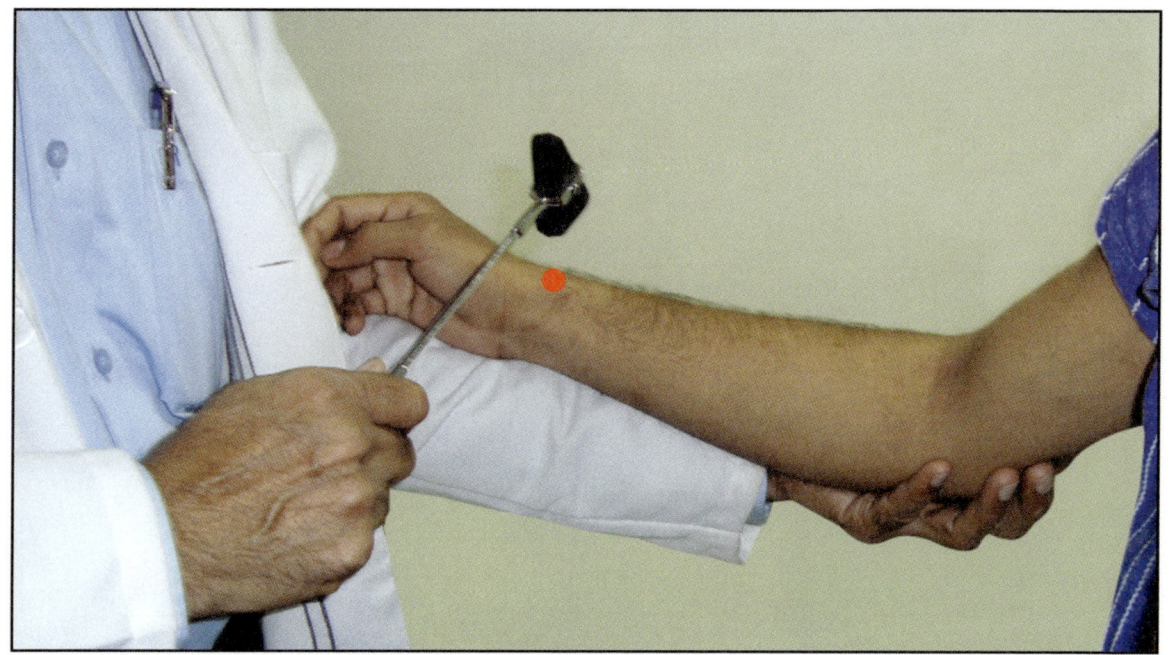

(a) Right

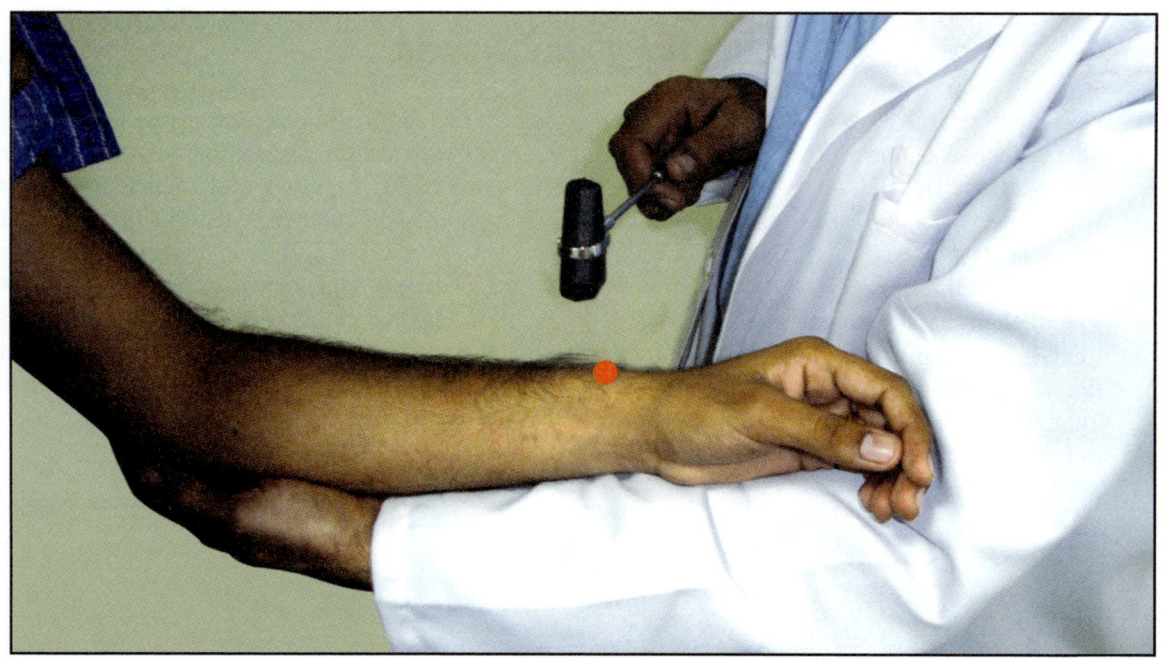

(b) Left

Fig. 3.28.8: To elicit supinator reflex in sitting position.

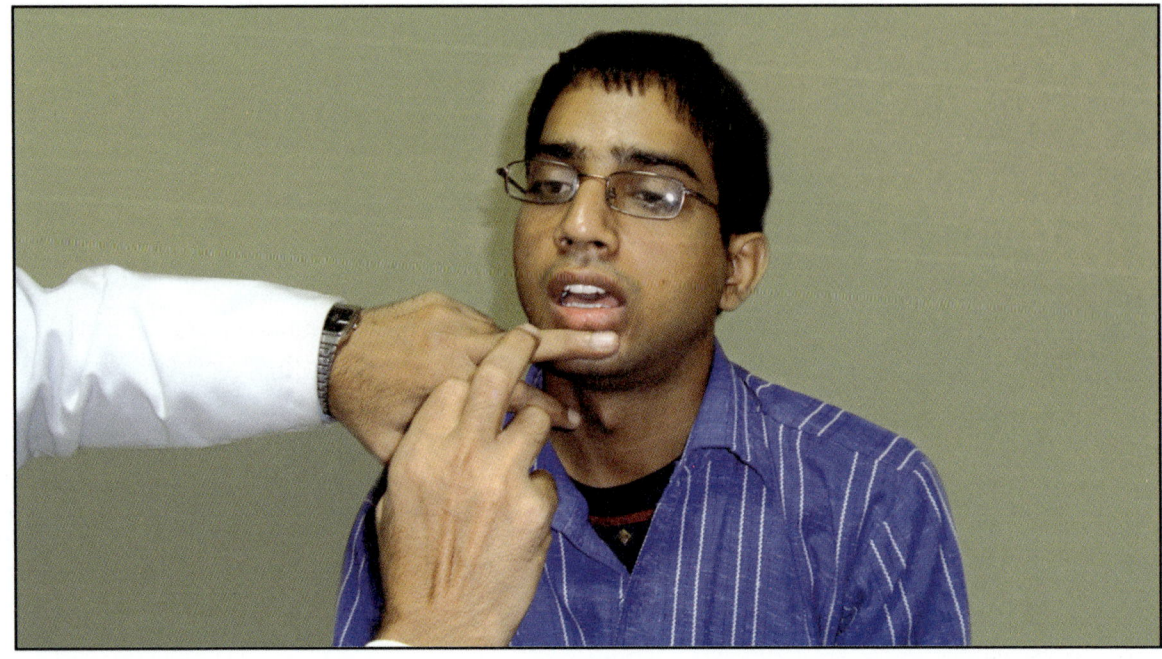

Fig. 3.28.9: To elicit jaw jerk.

QUESTIONS AND ANSWER

1. What is reflex arc?
2. What happen to tendon reflexes in upper motor neuron lesion?
3. What happen to tendon reflexes in lower motor neuron lesion?
4. What is stretch reflex?
5. How to elicit the various reflexes?
6. What is the Babinski's sign? What is the clinical significance of it?
7. What is reinforcement (Jendrassik's mano-euvre) and how it works?

Ans. If there is no response during eliciting the deep reflexes ask the subject to hook the fingers of two hands together and then to pull them against one another as hard as possible or to make a clench fist with ipsilateral hand (Jendrassik's manoeuvre or reinforcement). By doing this manoeuvre there is increase in α motor neuron discharge which increases the sensitivity of muscle spindle (responsible for stretch reflex).

8. How to grade reflexes?

These nerves have their cell bodies in brain. There are twelve pairs of the cranial nerves. Some are afferent (sensory), some are efferent (motor) and some contain both the fibres are called mixes nerves.

First (Olfactory) Nerve

It is a sensory nerve. The central processes from olfactory epithelium passes to olfactory area of cerebral cortex (the uncus of the parahippocampal gyrus).

For testing the sense of smell, have three small bottles, one containing some oil of clove, second oil of peppermint and the third some tincture of asafoetida. Common bedside substances such as soap, fruit or garlic may also be used. Irrigating substances like ammonia should not be used to test smell sensation. Each nostril should be tested separately. In anosmia the sense should of smell is abolished. Hyposmia is reduction of sense of smell. Perversion of sense of smell is called parosmia.

Second (Optic) Nerve

It is a sensory nerve. Sensory fibres originate from photoreceptors and finally go to visual cortex. For testing optic nerve visual acuity, visual fields and colour vision are examined.

Third (Oculomotor) Nerve, Fourth (Trochlear) Nerve and Sixth (Abducent) Nerve

They control ocular movements so considered together. They are mixed nerves. They bring sensations from proprioceptors in the eye muscles.

Fibres of these nerves take origin from a series of nuclei which begin in the floor of sylvian aqueduct and extending up to the fourth ventricle. Abducent nerve innervates the lateral (external) rectus muscle and trochlear innervates the superior oblique muscle. All other extraocular muscles, the sphincter pupillae,

muscles of accommodation, and the levator palpebrae superioris are supplied by oculomotor nerve.

Different types of movements of eyeball are shown in Fig. 3.29.1.

Role of extraocular muscle in movement of eye ball is shown below (Fig 3.29.2).

How to Test?

1. Look for *ptosis* (drooping of upper eyelid); *squint* (abnormality of ocular movement in which the visual axes do not meet at the point of fixation); and *nystagmus* (involuntary rhythmic to and fro movements of eyeball).

2. **Test for ocular movements:** Ask the subject to follow the movement of examiners finger with his eyes in superior, medial, inferior lateral and oblique directions.

3. Examination of pupil:
   (i) Size and shape of the pupil in both the eyes.
   (ii) Pupillary reflexes
       (a) Light reflex
       (b) Accommodation reflex

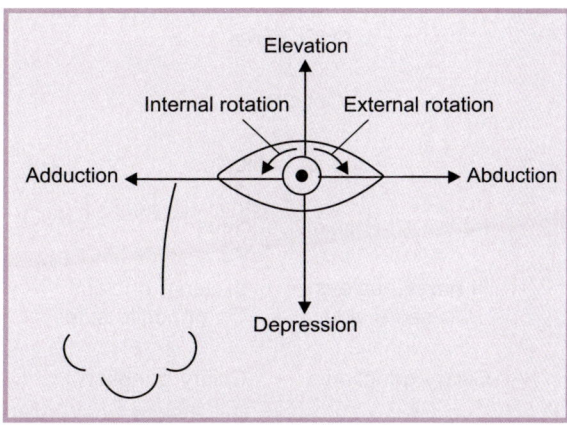

Fig. 3.29.1: Various types of movements of eyeball produced by extraocular muscles.

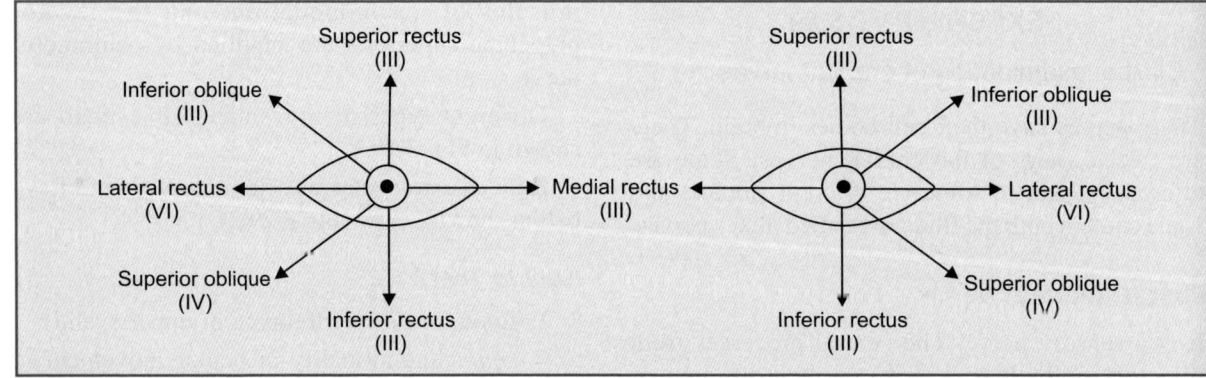

Fig. 3.29.2: Direction of movements produced by different extraocular muscles and their nerve supply.

(a) Light Reflex

Direct light reflex: It is done with the help of a torch in dim light room. Each eye is examined separately. Ask the subject to see at a distant object. Through a bright light with the help of torch by bring it from later side of the eye. Immediately observe the size of the pupil. Normally it should constrict.

Indirect (consensual) reflex: Project the light in one eye only and observe the response in other eye. In this reflex other eye also shows constriction of pupil. To prevent entry of light in other eye, the other hand is placed at the nose in between the eyes.

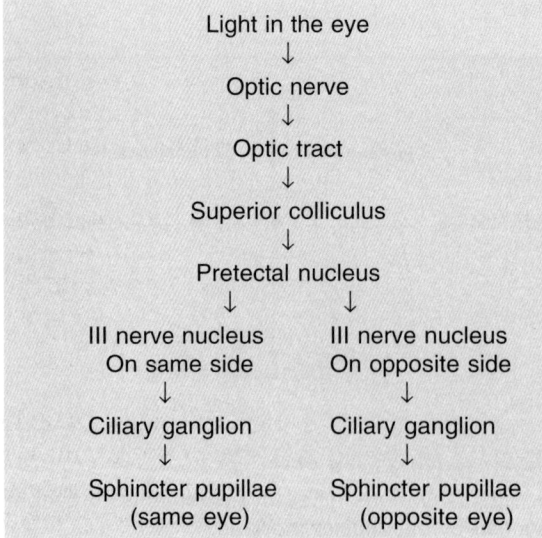

Pathway for light reflex.

(b) Accommodation Reflex

When a person asked to see a near object from distant object certain changes are taking place to see the near object clearly. These are

1. Increase in the power of the lens by contraction of ciliary muscles.

2. Constriction of pupil which cause to decrease spherical and chromatic aberrations, intensity of light entering into the eye and to increase the depth of focus.

3. Convergence of visual axis due to contraction of medial rectus muscle.

How to Do?

Ask the subject to look at distant object and then he is asked to see at the tip of pen or pencil held in front of the subject. Increase in the power of the lens (change on anterior surface of lens) can only be seen by changes in Purkinje–Sanson image.

Construction of pupil and convergence (adduction) can be observed.

Fifth (Trigeminal) Nerve

It is a mixed nerve. Sensory roots take origin from gasserian ganglion (trigeminal ganglion) in pons and motor nucleus is located in floor of fourth ventricle. Nerve divides in three divisions, ophthalmic division, maxillary division and mandibular division (Fig. 3.29.3).

Pathway of Accommodation Reflex

Blurring of image $\longrightarrow$ optic nerve $\longrightarrow$ optic chiasma $\longrightarrow$ optic tract $\longrightarrow$ superior colliculus

$\downarrow$

- Ciliary muscles,
- Sphincter pupillae, $\longleftarrow$ III nerve muscles $\longleftarrow$ Visual cortex $\longleftarrow$ Optic radiations
- Medial rectus

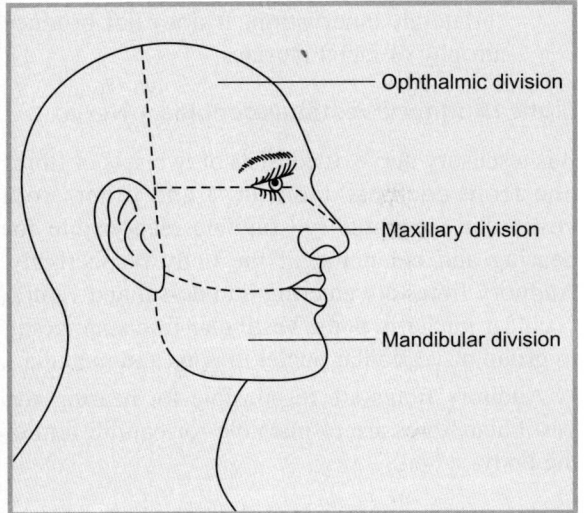

Fig. 3.29.3: Areas of face supplied by various divisions of trigeminal nerve.

1. *Ophthalmic division*: It supplies the conjunctival surface of the upper lid only and skin of medial part of nose as far as its tip, upper eye lids, the forehead and scalp up to vertex.
2. *Maxillary divisions*: It supplies the check, the front of the temple, the lower eyelid, sides of the nose, upper lid, upper teeth, the mucous membrane of nose, upper part of pharynx, roof of the mouth, parts of soft palate tonsils and cornea.
3. *Mandibular division*: It supplies lower part of the face, lower lip, the ear, tongue, lower teeth and salivary glands. Its motor root supplies all the muscles of mastication except buccinator which is supplied by facial nerve.

How to Test?

A. Sensory Part

1. Test for various sensations (touch, pain, pressure and temperature) over the skin and mucous membrane supplied by this nerve.
2. Testing corneal reflex: Ask the subject to look at some distant object, then lightly touch the lateral edge of the cornea with the help of a light wisp of cotton. It leads to blinking of the subject. Compare the reflex on opposite side also.
3. Testing of the taste: Taste sensation is rarely carried by trigeminal nerve. Taste sensation from anterior two-thirds from the tongue is carried by chorda tympani to facial nerve and from the posterior one-third it carried by glassopharyngeal nerve.

B. Motor Part

Ask the subject to clench his teeth, the temporalis and masseter muscle should be stand out with equal prominence on each side which can be confirmed by palpation.

Ask the subject to open his mouth, in case of paralysis the jaw will deviate towards the paralysed side because of push by healthy external pterygoid muscle on the opposite side.

Seventh (Facial) Nerve

It is a mixed nerve. The facial nerve muscles is situated in the pons, lateral to that of the abducent nerve. It receives the taste fibres from anterior two-thirds of tongue through (lingual) chorda tympani nerve.

A. Motor Part

All the muscles of face and scalp are supplied by facial nerve except levator palpebral superioris which is supplied by occulomotor nerve. It also supply to buccinaton, stapedius and styloid muscles.

Look for facial expression, furrows over forehead, nasolabial fold, angle of the mouth and width of the palpebral fissure. In case of paralysis expressions are lost on affected side, nasolabial fold is less pronounced, eye is more widely open. Saliva and any fluid he drinks, may escape from the affected angle of the mouth.

Tests

1. Ask the subject to shut his eyes as tightly as he can. Note that affected eye is either not closed at all. Try also to open the eyes while the subject attempts to keep them closed.

2. Ask the subject to whistle. Affected person is not able to do.

3. Ask him to smile or show his upper teeth. The mouth is then drawn to the healthy side.

4. Ask him to inflate his mouth with his air and blow out his cheeks. Tap with the finger in turn on each inflated cheek. Air can be made to escape from the mouth more easily on the weak side.

B. Sensory Part

From anterior two-thirds of tongue lingual nerve carries the sensation and through the chorda tympani going to the facial nerve. To test the sense of taste use strong solution of sugar (for sweet) and common salt (for salt); and weak solutions of citric acid (for sour) and quinine (for bitter). These are applied with the help of glass rod to the surface of the protruded tongue and if the test is recognised indicate or write about the taste. The quinine solution should be tested in the last as its effect is more lasting than that of others. After each taste mouth must be rinsed. Both the anterior and posterior part of the right and the left halves of the tongue should be tested separately. Difference between infranuclear lesion (LMN) and supranuclear lesion (UMN).

(i) *Infranuclear lesion* (lesion distal to the nucleus of facial nerve): This results in paralysis of both upper and lower part of the face, with atrophy of the facial muscles. It also causes loss of taste in anterior two-thirds portion of tongue.

(ii) *Supranuclear lesions* (lesions above the nucleus of facial nerve): This mainly results in paralysis of lower half of face because muscles of upper part of face has double (bilateral) innervation. It does not produce atrophy of facial muscles.

Eight (Auditory/Vestibulocochlear) Nerve

It is a sensory nerve. It consists of two sets of fibres one from cochlear (auditory) and other from vestibular apparatus (vestibular) responsible for hearing and balancing of the body respectively. Auditory fibres are entering into dorsal and ventral cochlear nuclei in pons. Vestibular fibres are going to group of vestibular nuclei in pons and medulla.

Auditory fibres are responsible for hearing and vestibular fibres are responsible for equilibrium of the body.

A. Tests for Auditory (Cochlear) Fibres

Various hearing tests are done which are helpful in finding out hearing loss.

They are as follows:

1. Watch test
2. Tuning fork tests
3. Audiometery

1. Watch Test

It is a simple and rough test only applicable when loss of hearing is not much. After closing the eyes of the subject find out the distance at which he is able to hear tickling sound of a watch. Repeat on opposite side also.

2. Tuning Fork Tests

These tests are used to find out the type of deafness. These tests are done by using tuning forks vibrate at

256 or 512 Hz (cps), since the apex of the cochlea contains the units which respond to the lower OCTACAVES (16–32–64–128–256–512–1024).

(i) Rinne Test

Give proper instruction to the subject about the test. Strike the prongs of the tuning fork on wooden table or on rubber pad from the side of the prong after holding it from the base.

Place the base of the vibrating tuning fork on the mastoid process behind the ear. Ask the patient when he stop hearing the vibrations (Fig. 3.29.4a).

Now bring the prong of tuning fork close to the auditory meatus and ask whether he is able to hear it or not (Fig. 3.29.4b).

Normally the subject is able to hear the vibration when it is brought in front of the ear from the mastoid process (air conduction is better than the bone conduction). This is referred as Rinne test positive.

In conduction deafness, subject is not able to hear when tuning fork is brought near auditory meatus from mastoid process. Here bone conduction becomes better than air conduction. The test is repeated on other side also.

(ii) Weber Test

Give the proper instruction to the subject regarding the test.

Vibrate the tuning fork as in Rinne test and place the base of this on the centre of forehead (Fig. 3.29.5) or vertex.

Ask the subject whether sound heard in both the ears equal or it is better in the one ear.

In normal individual sound heard in both the ears is equal.

If the sound heard better in the defective ears, it is because of absence of masking effect of environmental noise (shows conduction deafness in defective ear). If the sound heard better in the normal ear it shows that there is nerve deafness in the defective ear.

(iii) Schwabach Test

In this test bone conduction of the subject is compared with that of normal subject (examiner).

Place a vibrating tuning fork over the subject's forehead. When he is not able to hear any more transfer it to your forehead.

If you are able to hear it, this shows there is hearing loss in the subject because of nerve deafness.

In case of conduction deafness in the subject he is able to hear longer than you (examiner).

3. Audiometery

Loss of hearing can be measured accurately with the help of audiometer. It is discussed in detail in the separate practical.

Ninth (Glossopharyngeal) Nerve

It is a mixed nerve. The glossopharyngeal, vagus and accessory nerves arise, from above downward, in an elongated nucleus in the floor of fourth ventricle.

It contains taste fibres from posterior third of the tongue (bitter taste).

Motor fibres supply to stylopharyngeus muscle (help in swallowing).

Secreto-motor fibres supply the parotid gland.

How to test?

Test for taste sensation (for bitter) in positive one-third of the tongue.

Tickle at the back of pharynx, either with finger or with a swab stick and note its reflex contraction (Palatal reflex).

Tenth (Vagus) Nerve

It is a mixed nerve. Motor fibres supply to involuntary muscles of heart, respiration and gastrointestinal tract; voluntary muscles of pharynx, larynx and soft palate. Sensory fibres are distributed to mucous membrane of larynx, pharynx and soft palate.

Paralysis of this nerve leads to regurgitation of fluids through the nose during swallowing due to defective elevation of the soft palate, because of incomplete closure of nasopharynx nasal tone present in voice (egg as eng) and voice becomes hoarse and deep.

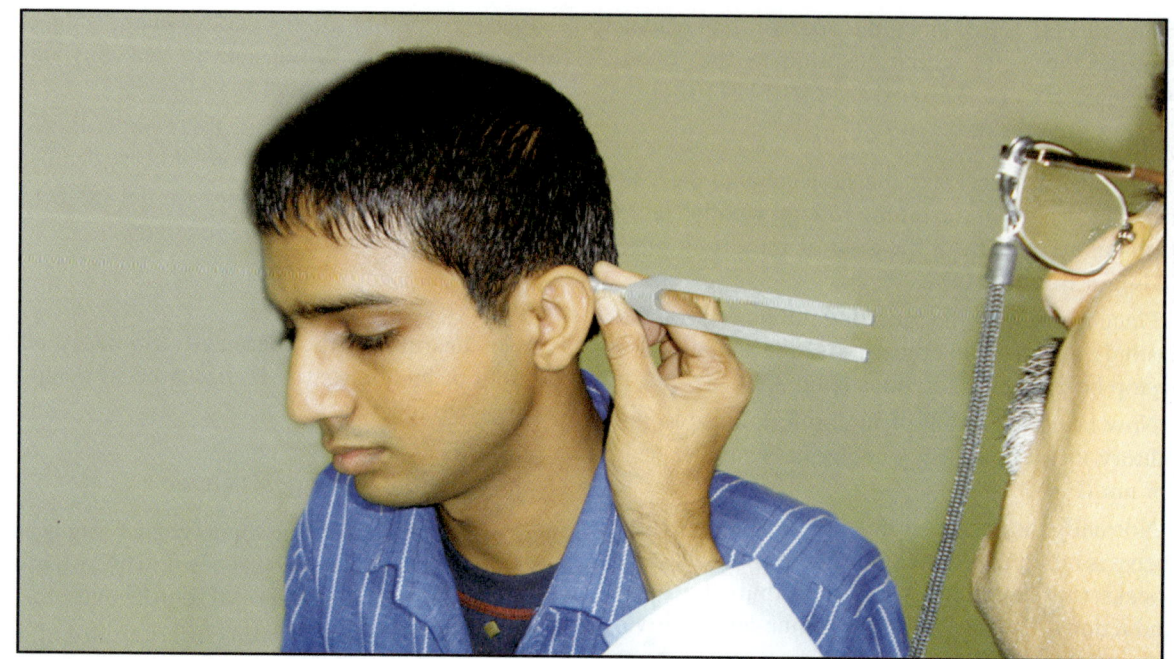

(a)

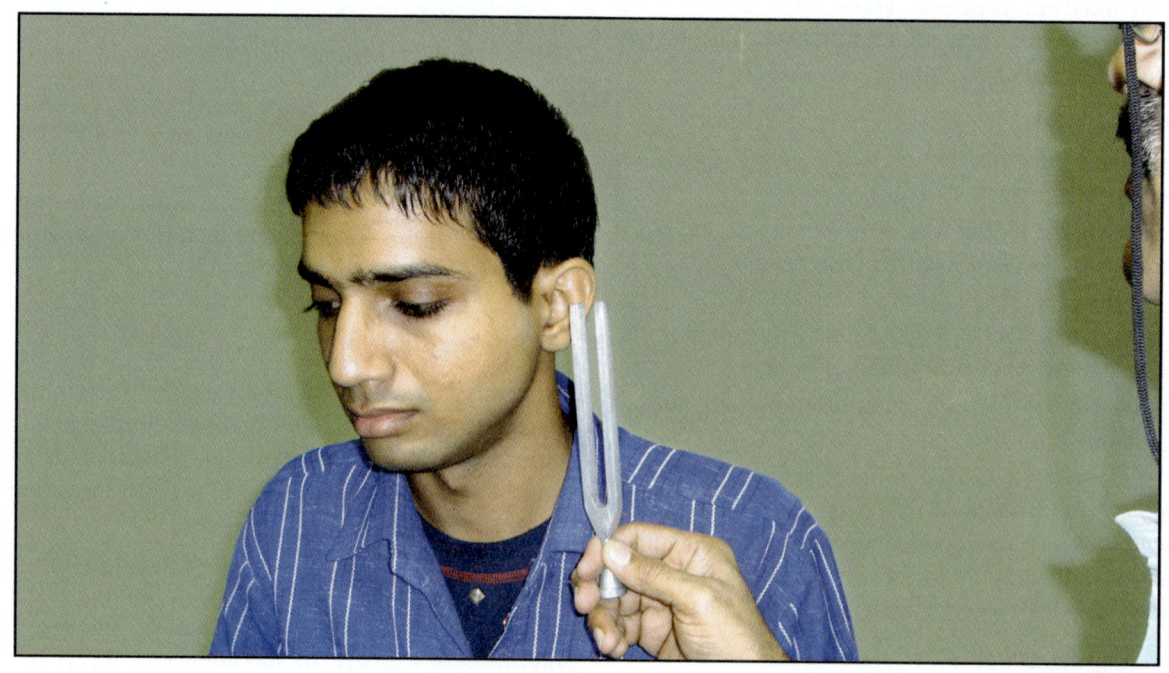

(b)

Fig. 3.29.4: To perform Rinne test

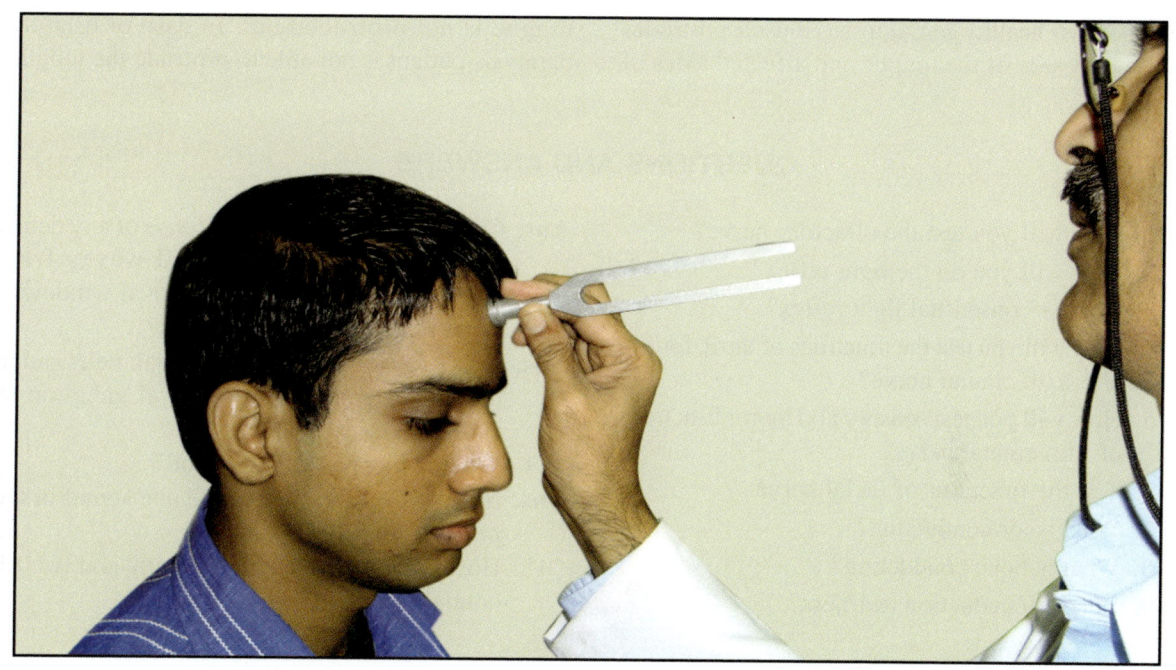

Fig. 3.29.5: To perform Weber test.

How to Test?

1. Palatal reflex
2. Ask the subject to say 'Ah' and observe the movements of both sides of palatal arch.

   Normal: Both the palatal arch shows equal movement and uvula remains in the midline.

   If one side paralysed, arch of this side remains flat and uvula moves towards healthy side.

   In both side paralysis soft palate remains motionless.
3. Laryngoscopy is done to see the movements of vocal cords.

Eleventh (Spinal Accessory) Nerve

It is a motor nerve. Cranial part arises from medulla oblongata spinal part arises from spinal nucleus of lateral part of anterior gray column of the spinal cord extending up to fifth cervical segment.

How to Test?

1. *Power of sternocleidomastoid muscle*

   (i) Chin is rotated to one side and apply the resistance to oppose the movement to the other side. It done in both the sides.

   (ii) Ask the subject to flex the head against passive resistance of the examiner's hand.

2. *Power of trapezius muscle*

   (i) Look for drooping of should be on the affected side.

   (ii) Ask the subject to shrug his shoulders while the examiner apply the passive resistance on them from above.

Twelfth (Hypoglossal) Nerve

The hypoglossal nerve arises from a nucleus in the lower part of the floor of the fourth ventricle. It is a purely motor nerve supplying to the muscles of tongue.

How to test?

Ask the subject to protrude his tongue. In case of unilateral paralysis tongue deviates towards the affected side, because healthy genioglossus muscle protrudes the healthy side of the tongue and affected sides of tongue is not protruded out. In case of bilateral paralysis patient is not able to protrude the tongue.

QUESTIONS AND ANSWERS

1. How will you test the olfactory nerve?
2. How will you do the light reflex?
3. What is consensual light reflex?
4. How will you test the functions of third, fourth, and sixth cranial nerve?
5. How will you test sensory and motor functions of fifth cranial nerve?
6. Test the functions of facial nerve.
7. What is air conduction?
8. What is bone conduction?
9. What is conduction deafness?

Ans. Conductions deafness is because of any defect in the conduction of sound waves from external auditory canal to the oval window.

10. What is nerve/central deafness?

Ans. It is because of damage in the hair cells and in the neural pathway from spiral ganglion to auditory cortex.

11. What is the masking of sound?

Ans. It is the inability to hear the one sound in the presence of other sound.

12. How will you test tenth, eleventh, and twelfth cranial nerves?

EXPERIMENT 3.30A

Recording of Electroencephalogram (EEG)

APPARATUS

EEG machine or multichannel polyrite or physiograph for bipolar recording, electrodes and jelly (paste).

PRINCIPLE

Electrical activity of cerebral cortex is recorded by placing the electrodes on the scalp. If the electrical activity is directly recorded by placing the electrodes on the surface of the cerebral cortex, it is called as **Electrocorticogram** (ECG).

EEG is probably because of current flow in fluctuating dipoles on the dendrites of cortical cells and cell bodies.

PROCEDURE

EEG can be recorded by two methods: Using bipolar leads (on EEG machine or multichannel polyrite) and unipolar leads (on student physiograph).

Bipolar lead method: 8 pairs (16) of electrodes are used to record EEG.

Unipolar lead method: There are to electrodes, one is acting as an active or exploring electrodes and other is indifferent electrode. Indifferent electrode is placed on the ear lobule. Active electrode is place in the specific area on the scalp from where we want to record EEG. Potential is recorded between these two points. Body is also earthed by applying the other electrode on the other ear lobule.

Subject is asked lie comfortable on the bed in a dark room. Active electrode is applied at the centre of the forehead or at vertex after cleaning the scalp with spirit swab. Similarly indifferent electrode is applied on the one ear lobule. On the other ear lobule third electrode is applied to earth the body.

Sensitivity of the physiograph is adjusted at 100 µV on 200 µV and base line is brought in the centre of the recording paper.

Now record is taken after asking the subject to close his eyes. Effect of various factors is recorded as follows:

1. *Normal*: Record with closed eyes.
2. *Clapping*: Take the record after clapping.
3. Ask him to open the eyes (a block is recorded).
4. *Thinking*: He is asked to do a calculation without speaking with closed eyes.
5. *Light*: Effect of light can be recorded with closed eye also.
6. *Tactile stimuli*: Touch the body part of the subject is different areas and take the record of the subject with his eyes closed.

Normal EEG

Following electrical waves are seen in EEG (Table 3.30a.1)

Normal record of EEG, shown in Fig. 3.30a.1.

Factors affecting EEG.

A. Physiological factors

B. Pathological factors

C. Others

A. Physiological Factors

1. Any type of sensory stimulus leads to change a wave pattern and there is production of high frequency low voltage waves. It is called as desynchronisation or a block.
2. *Sleep*: In non-REM sleep, pattern of EEG changes from high frequency, low amplitude to low frequency and high amplitude (D waves). But in stage II there are bursts of a like waves in-between sleep spindles. In REM sleep EEG having low voltage high frequency graph.

Table 3.30a.1: Features of various ECG waves.

S.No.	Waves	Frequency	Voltage mV
1.	α	8–12/sec	50
2.	β	18–30/sec	5–10
3.	θ	4–7/sec	10
4.	δ	<1/sec	20–200

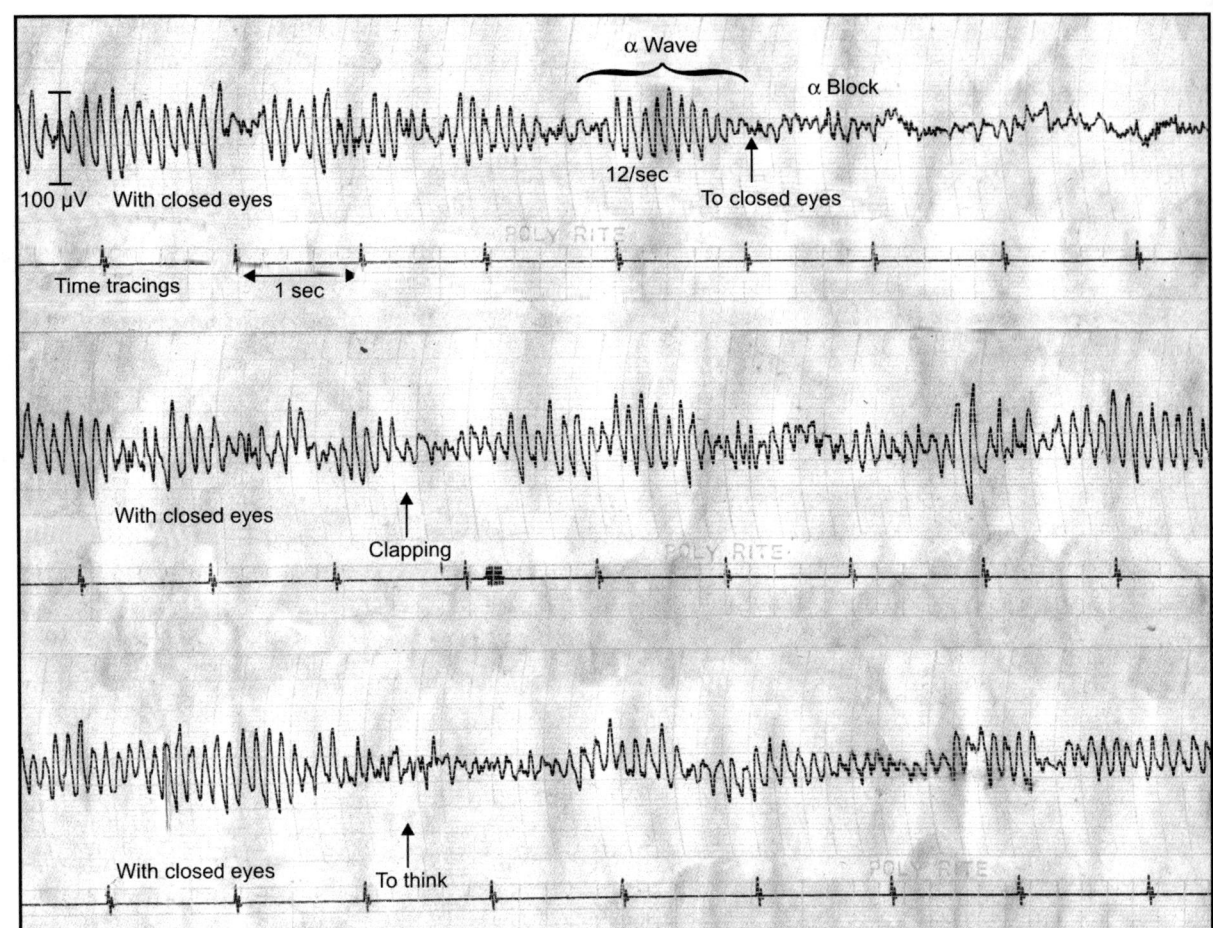

Fig. 3.30a.1: Electroencephalogram recorded on polyrite using bipolar lead.

B. Pathological Factors

1. Grand mal epileptic seizures: Fast activity during tonic phase, slow wave preceded by spike at the time of each clonic jerk. After completion of attack slow waves are present.

2. Petit mal epilepsy: Typical rounded wave preceded by spike and there are about three such doubles per second. In between attack there is no abnormality.

3. Brain tumour, abscess and subdural hematoma: There are slow waves (D wave) in localised area.

4. Comma due to any cause leads to D waves.

C. Others

Anaesthesia: There is slowing of wave pattern with increase in voltage but voltage goes on decreasing with increase in dose.

QUESTIONS

1. What is EEG?
2. What is the physiological base of EEG?
3. What are the various waves present in EEG?
4. What is α-block or desynchronisation?
5. What is the clinical application of EEG?

EXPERIMENT 3.30B

Recording of auditory and visual reaction time

APPARATUS

Audiovisual reaction time instrument (RTM-608, Medicaid, Chandigarh).

This instrument is made up of two parts separated by a black sheet placed vertically in the centre. One part has lights of different colours (red, green, and yellow) and the switches to put them off.

A small speaker is also present in this part to give sound signal. An additional switch is also present to put the sound signal off. There are two small sockets to connect the foot switch and head-phone.

On the second part of the instrument there are various switches to give the different signals to the subject. This part is fitted with a quarts clock which displays time in 1/10 of millisecond (0.0001 sec). This instrument works at domestic (220 volt AC) electricity supply.

THEORY

Reaction time is the time interval between the application of a stimulus and appropriate voluntary response by a subject. The response is primarily governed by the ability of an individual to concentrate and to establish a muscular attitude of readiness. The reaction time indicates the time lost between application of a stimulus and appearance of its end effects.

For visual reaction time light stimulus of different colours is given and subject is asked to put the light off.

For auditory reaction time sound stimulus is given and subject is asked to switch off the sound.

Reaction time is facilitated by alertness, training and concentration. It is inhibited by distraction, advancing age and muscular weakness.

PROCEDURE

Switch on the instrument. Ask the subject to sit on a stool comfortably in a quite room. Explain to the subject about the test. For visual reaction time subject is asked to concentrate on the specific light and as soon as he sees this he is supposed to put the light off. Note down the time from the display of the clock. Before taking the next reading clock is reset by pressing the small switch. Measure the reaction time for light of different colours. For auditory reaction time he is asked to concentrate on the sound and he is supposed to put the sound off. Take at least three readings and least is considered the final reading. Measure the reaction time with right hand and left hand of the subject. With the help of foot switch we can measure the reaction time of right foot and left foot. Enter the various readings in the Table 3.30 b.1.

OBSERVATIONS AND RESULTS

Table 3.30b.1: Audiovisual reaction time.					
Limb involved	Reaction time	Reading - 1	Reading - 2	Reading - 3	Least reading
Right hand	Visual - red Auditory				
Left hand	Visual – red Auditory				
Right foot	Visual – red Auditory				
Left foot	Visual - red Auditory				

Factors effecting reaction time: (1) Limb involved in switching off the stimulus. (2) Colour of the light stimulus.

EXPERIMENT 3.31

Audiometry

With the help of audiometer we can find out the loss of hearing at specific frequency (auditory acuity). With this instrument we can record threshold of sound perceived by the individual at different frequencies through air conduction as well as bone conduction. The procedure is called as audiometry.

Audiogram is a record show hearing status by air conduction as well bone conduction. Audiometer is a device having electronic oscillator, which produce sounds of different frequencies (150 to 8000 Hz) and intensities (–10 to 100 dB). Frequency and amplitude of sound can be adjusted with the knob provided. Headphones are therefore air conduction and a knob is therefore bone conduction.

PROCEDURE

The test is conducted in the sound proof room. Each ear is tested separately for air conduction as well as for bone conduction.

Proper instructions are given to the subject regarding the test.

He is asked to wear the headphone and a hand switch is given to him.

He is asked to press the switch whenever he hears the sound. Threshold intensity is found out for various frequencies of sound ranging from 250 to 8000 Hz for both the ears. Apply the knob behind the ear on mastoid process and find out the threshold intensity for all the frequencies as done above.

A graph is plotted with all the threshold values on audiometer paper.

SIGNIFICANCE

Test is used to assess the degree of deafness, the type of deafness (conduction deafness, nerve deafness) and to assess the frequency range, in which deafness is most affected. Thus hearing aid can be designed to overcome some of the hearing problems of the individual patient (Fig.3.31.1).

QUESTIONS AND ANSWERS

1. What is nerve deafness?
2. What is conduction deafness?
3. What is ossicular conduction?

Ans. Conduction of sound waves through the ear ossicles is known as ossicular conduction. Practically it is called as air conduction.

4. What is bone conduction?

Ans. Conduction of sound waves through bone (skull) is called as bone conduction.

5. What is air conduction?

Ans. Theoretically the conduction of sound waves from the tympanic membrane to the round window through the air present in middle ear is called as air conduction (not playing much role in hearing) but practically air conduction means the conduction of sound waves through the ear ossicles.

6. What are the common causes for conduction deafness?

Ans. Wax and foreign body in the external auditory canal, destruction of auditory ossicles and thickening of eardrum are the most common causes of conduction deafness.

7. What are the causes of nerve deafness?

Ans. Causes of nerve deafness are:
   (i) Use of certain antibiotics e.g. strepto-mycin and gentamicin.
   (ii) Prolonged exposure to noise.
   (iii) Tumours of vestibulocochlear nerve.
   (iv) Vascular damage in the medulla.

8. What are the frequencies of voice of normal man and woman?

Ans. Frequency of voice of a normal man is 120 Hz and a woman is 250 Hz.

9. What is the range of frequency of sound, audible to human ear?

Ans. Human ears are able to hear the frequencies of the sound range from 20 to 20000 Hz.

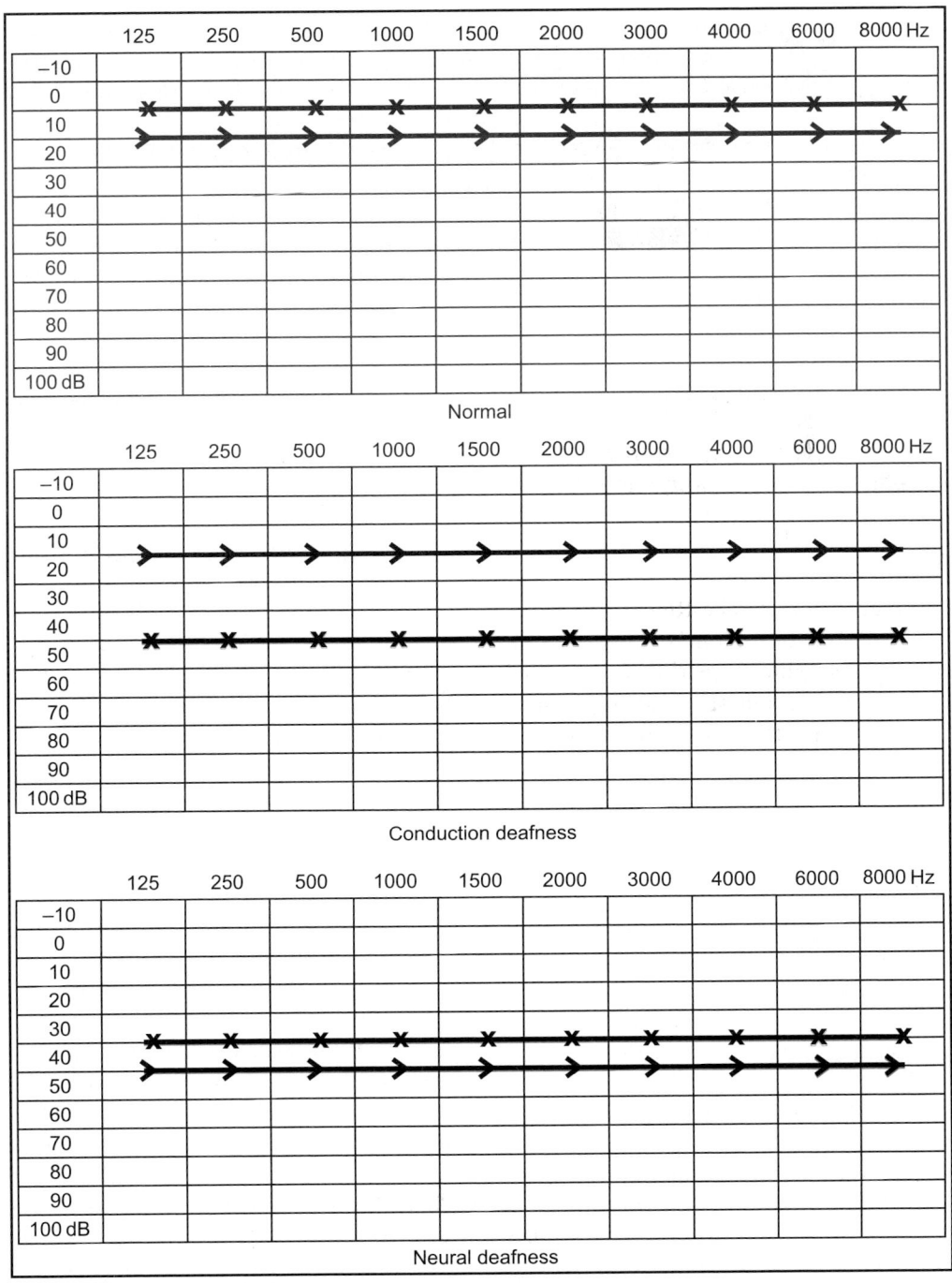

Fig. 3.31.1: Audiograms.

Mammalian Experiments
(For Postgraduate Students)

To perfuse the isolated heart of rabbit and study the effect of various drugs and ions

APPARATUS

Langendroff's apparatus, Locke-Ringer's solution, thermometer, Polyrite/Student's physiograph/ kymograph, oxygen cylinder, petri dish, nembutal (pentobarbitone) or chloralose, dissecting instruments and solution of various drugs and ions.

PRINCIPLE

Isolated rabbit's heart is perfused with Locke-Ringer's solution in a suitable environment, and effects of various drugs are studied. Mechanical changes are converted into electrical signals with the help of force transducer and recorded on Student's physiograph/ polyrite/kymograph (without transducer).

Langendroff's Apparatus

It consists of a rectangular Perspex container having a spiral tube of glass which is connected at its upper end to the Mariotte bottle through a Y-shaped glass tube and at lower end to the cannula through a rubber tube. Container is filled with water. It contains heating coil which maintains the temperature of water to 37 °C with the help of thermostat mechanism. On the base of the apparatus there are two pulleys which is used to connect the apex of

the heart to the transducer with the help of a thread. There is a three-way glass cannula, which is connected to the heart, the thermometer and the mercury manometer (Fig.4.1.1).

Composition of Locke-Ringer's Solution

NaCl : 0.92 gm (maintains isotonicity)
KCl : 0.042 gm (excitation & contraction)
$CaCl_2$: 0.024 gm (excitation & contraction)
$NaHCO_3$: 0.015 gm (maintain pH)
Dextrose : 0.1 gm (provide nutrition)

Distilled water to make it 100 ml (pH of Locke's solution is 7.1 to 7.6)

PROCEDURE

Fill the Mariotte bottles with the Locke-Ringer's solution and maintained the oxygenation of the solution. The apparatus is put on to warm the water of the container.

Rabbit is anaesthetised by giving pentobarbitone (nembutal 30 mg/ kg i.v.) or phenobarbitone (barbitone sodium 80 mg/kg i.v.) or chloralose (100 mg/kg i.v. or i.p.) or urethane (0.5–1.5 g/kg aq.solution i.v. or i.p.) or ketamine (2 mg/kg i.v.). An incision is given in mid-line starting from xiphisternum to the base of the neck. Now xiphisternum is lifted with forceps and various cartilages are cut on both sides of the sternum and heart is exposed. Identify the aorta and other vessels, and cut the aorta leaving one centimeter at its origin.

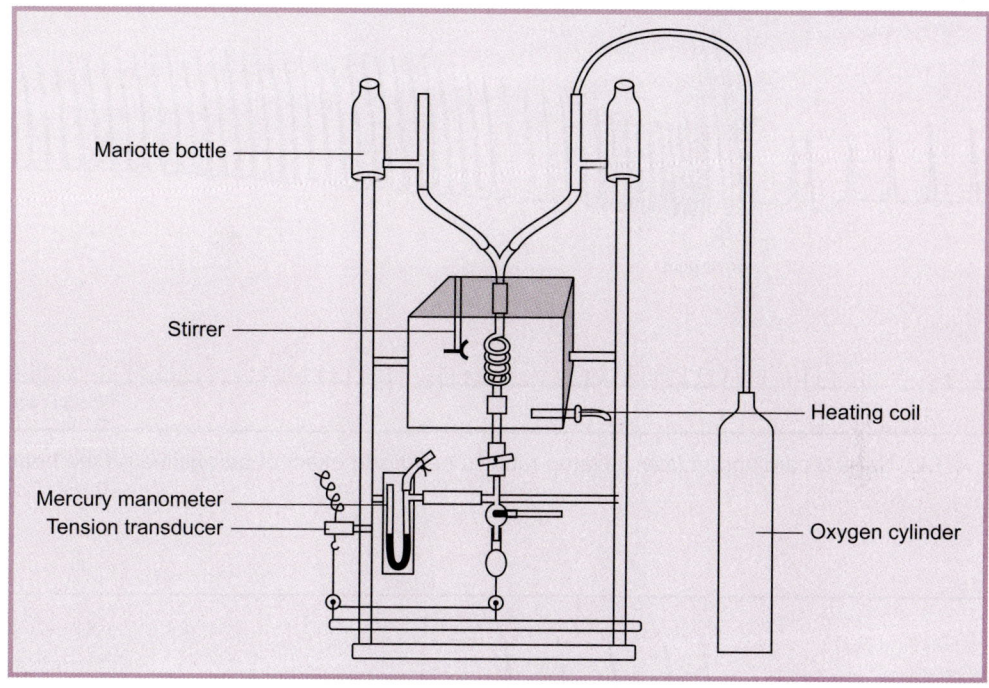

Fig. 4.1.1: Langendroff's apparatus.

Now all the vessels are cut and heart is transferred to well oxygenated ice cold Locke-Ringer's solution in a petri dish. It is repeatedly pressed with the help of fingers in the Locke's solution to push out blood from the heart, which might clot in coronary vessels.

Now cut the pericardium properly and transfer the heart to the Langendroff's apparatus. Aorta is tied over cannula and perfusion pressure is maintained about 50 to 70 mm of Hg. It is done with the help of the clamp present over the rubber tube between cannula and spiral glass tube. Locke's solution is oxygenated in Mariotte bottle. Maintain the temperature of the Locke's solution strictly at 37 °C. A hooked alpine is passed through the apex of the heart, taking care that it should not puncture the ventricle; and with the help of a thread it is connected to the transducer through the pulleys. The base line and sensitivity of the physiogaph is adjusted according to the requirement.

Normal cardiogram is recorded on Student's physiograph at the 2.5 mm/sec speed of the paper.

Now inject 0.5 ml of adrenaline solution (1:10,000) in the rubber tube just above the cannula and take the record (Fig.4.1.2).

Flush the heart with Locke's solution and get it normalised. Inject 0.5 ml of 1 % solution of calcium chloride and take the record (Fig.4.1.3)

Now inject 0.5 ml, of 1:1,00,000 solution of acetylcholine and take the record. After this inject 1.0 ml ,1 % solution of atropine and again study the effect of acetylcholine (Fig. 4.1.4).

Now inject 0.5 ml of 1 to 2 % solution of sodium chloride and take the record (Fig. 4.1.3).

In the end study the effect of 1% solution of potassium chloride (Fig. 4.1.3).

Effect of change in perfusion pressure can also be studied by regulating the flow of Locke's solution.

Effects of Various Drugs

Adrenaline: Responsible for increase in heart rate (positive chronotropic effect) and increase in

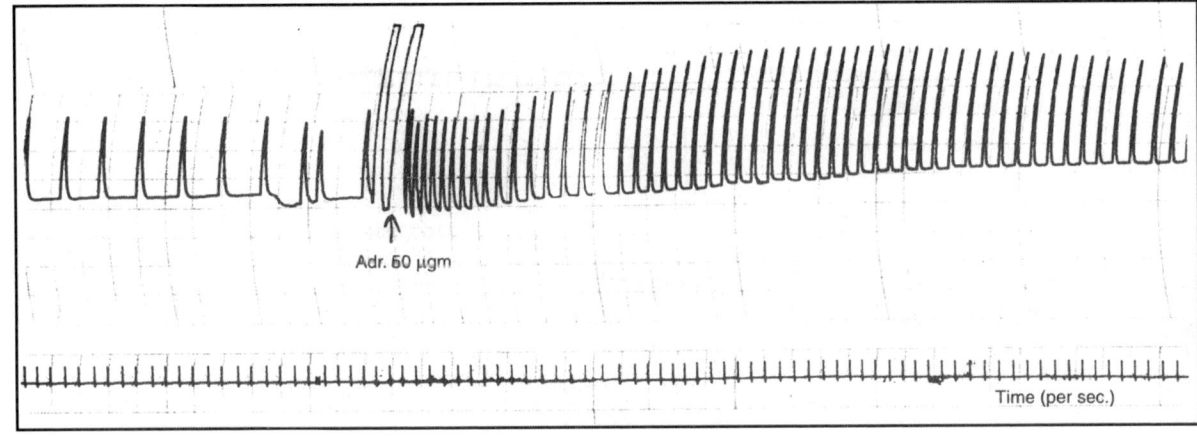

Adr. 50 μgm

Time (per sec.)

Fig. 4.1.2: Normal cardiogram from isolated rabbit's heart and effect of adrenaline on the heart.

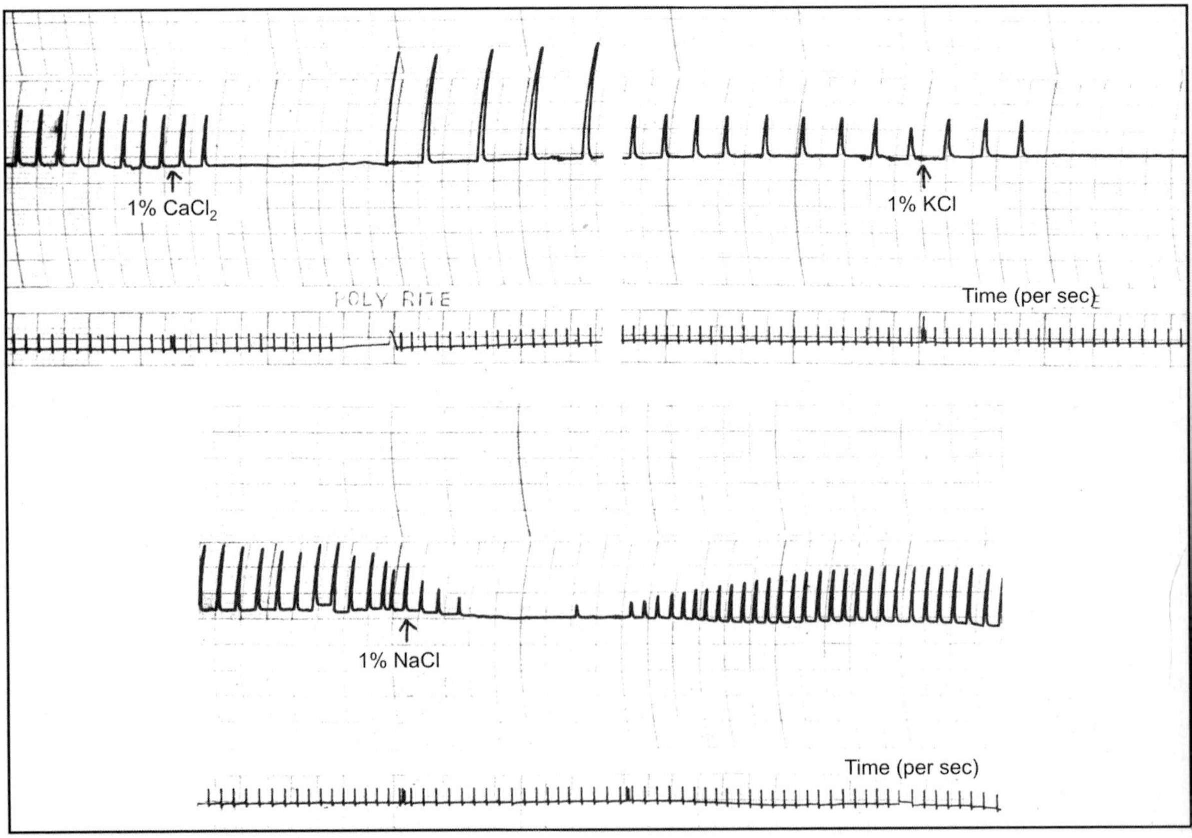

1% CaCl$_2$

HOLY RITE

1% KCl

Time (per sec.)

1% NaCl

Time (per sec)

Time (per sec)

Fig. 4.1.3: Effect of calcium chloride, potassium chloride and sodium chloride on rabbit heart.

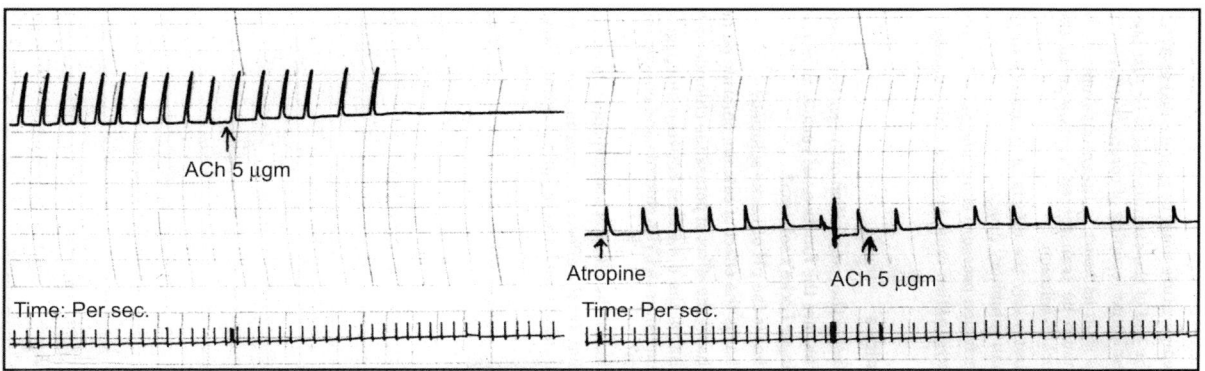

Fig. 4.1.4: Effect of acetylcholine on rabbit's heart (cardiogram).

amplitude of contraction (positive inotropic effect). It acts through beta-1 receptors, causes increase in permeability of Na^+ so facilitates the depolarization and increase the heart rate. It also increases Ca^{++} entry in to the cell and responsible for increase in amplitude of contraction.

Acetylcholine: It causes decrease in heart rate (negative chronotropic effect) and decrease in amplitude of contraction (negative inotropic effect). It is acting through cholinergic (muscarinic) receptors. It increases potassium permeability leading to efflux of K^+ in the nodal tissue and causes decrease in heart rate. It causes decrease in Ca^{++} influx leading to decrease in force of contraction. Atropine blocks muscarinic receptors, this is why acetylcholine fails to produce its effects after atropine.

Calcium chloride: Calcium ions are required during contraction in actin and myosin coupling leading to increase in amplitude of contraction. It further responsible for sustained contraction and heart stops in systole.

Sodium chloride: Because of competitive inhibition of calcium ions there is inhibition of heart which causes decrease in heart rate and force of contraction.

Potassium chloride: It prevents out flow of K^+ during depolarization causing delay in depolarization, ultimately heart stops in diastole.

Precautions

1. Temperature must be maintained at 37 °C.
2. The end of the cannula should lie just above the semilunar (opening of coronary arteries) valve.
3. As soon as heart is taken out from the body it should be transferred quickly into the cold Locke's solution.
4. First study the effects of excitatory drugs and than inhibitory drugs.
5. Perfusion pressure should be 50 to 70 mm Hg.
6. Oxygenation must be done continuously.

QUESTIONS

1. What is the composition of Locke-Ringer's solution?
2. What are the functions of various ingredients of Locke-Ringer's solution?
3. What is the pH of Locke's solution?
4. What is the effect of calcium chloride on heart?
5. What is the effect of potassium chloride on heart?
6. What is the difference between stoppage of the heart after calcium chloride and potassium chloride?
7. What is the effect of sodium chloride on heart?
8. What are the effects and mechanism of action of adrenaline and acetylcholine on the heart?

EXPERIMENT 4.2

To study the movements of small intestine of rabbit and study the effects of various drugs and ions

APPARATUS

Dale's organ bath, kymograph, time marker, tyrode solution, oxygen cylinder, dissection instruments, nembutal (pentobarbitone) or chloralose, thermometer, frontal writing lever, thread, needle, petri dish, pasticin and solution of acetylcholine, atropine, adrenaline, histamine, calcium chloride and barium chloride.

Principle

When isolated piece of rabbit's intestine is placed into the similar environment as that of extracellular fluid, it shows the property of autorythmicity and the effects of various drugs can be studied on it.

Dale's Organ Bath

It consists of a Perspex rectangular chamber which contains a glass tube (vessel) of 50 ml capacity fixed in the centre of the bath, a bent glass tube open at both the ends used to supply oxygen to tyrode solution and to tie one end of the piece of intestine, a heating coil with thermostat mechanism, a stirrer, and two metallic side rods to fix the bent glass tube and frontal writing lever (Fig.4.2.1).

Composition of Tyrode Solution

pH of Tyrode solution is 7.4 to 7.6. Its constituents are as follows

NaCl   – 0.8 gm (maintain isotonicity and electrical activity)
KCl   – 0.02 gm (electrical activity of muscle)
CaCl   – 0.02 gm (excitation and contraction)
$MgCl_2$ – 0.01 gm (excitation and contraction)
$NaHCO_3$ – 0.1 gm (maintains pH)

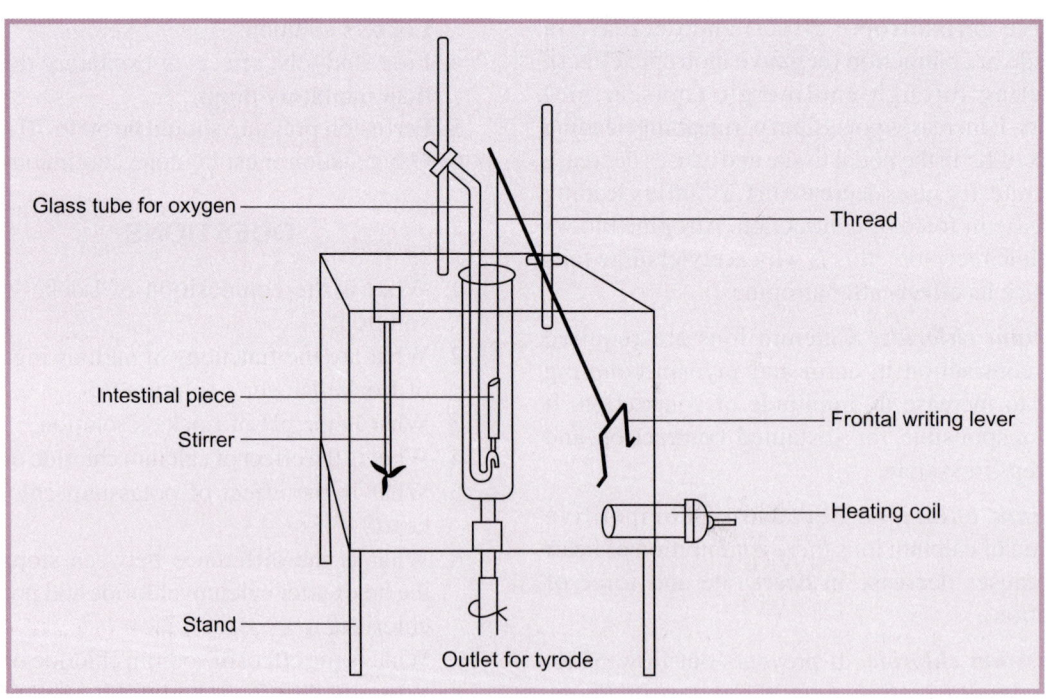

Fig. 4.2.1: Dale's organ bath.

NaH_2PO_4 – 0.005 gm (maintains pH)

Glucose   – 0.1 gm (provide nutrition)

Distilled water to make it 100 ml

PROCEDURE

Fill the Dale's organ bath with water and put it on.

Rabbit is anaesthetised by giving nembutal or chloralose. Open the abdomen by giving the incision in the upper part at midline. Dissect out about 3 to 4 cm long pieces of duodenal or jejunal part of small intestine (this area is acting as pacemaker for intestinal movements and having maximum frequency of movements). Transfer the pieces to the tyrode solution maintained at 37°C in petri dish. Wash the pieces with the warm tyrode solution with the help of a syringe and transfer them in clean tyrode solution.

Now make a loop of thread at one end of the piece with the help of a needle and tie a piece of thread at other end, diagonal to the loop at first end. Loop of the thread is put over hooked end of bent glass tube

and by holding the free end of thread it is transferred to inner vessel of the bath which is filled with tyrode solution. Tie the free end of the tread to the one arm of (balanced) frontal writing lever. About one gram of pasticin is put towards writing side of the lever from the fulcrum so that there will be slight stretch on the piece of intestine. Temperature of the bath should be maintained at 37 °C.

Record the normal intestinal movements on kymograph drum at 2.5 mm per second speed.

Now add 0.5 ml of acetylcholine solution of strength 1:1,00,000 and take the record (Fig. 4.2.2).

Drain the tyrode solution from the vessel through the outlet present at the base of the vessel and fill it with fresh tyrode solution after rinsing it 2–3 times.

Add 1 ml 1% solution of atropine in the vessel with the help of a syringe and wait for two minutes. Now again add 0.5 ml acetylcholine solution and take the record (Fig. 4.2.2).

Now again rinse the vessel properly and study the effect of 1 % solution of barium chloride, 1%

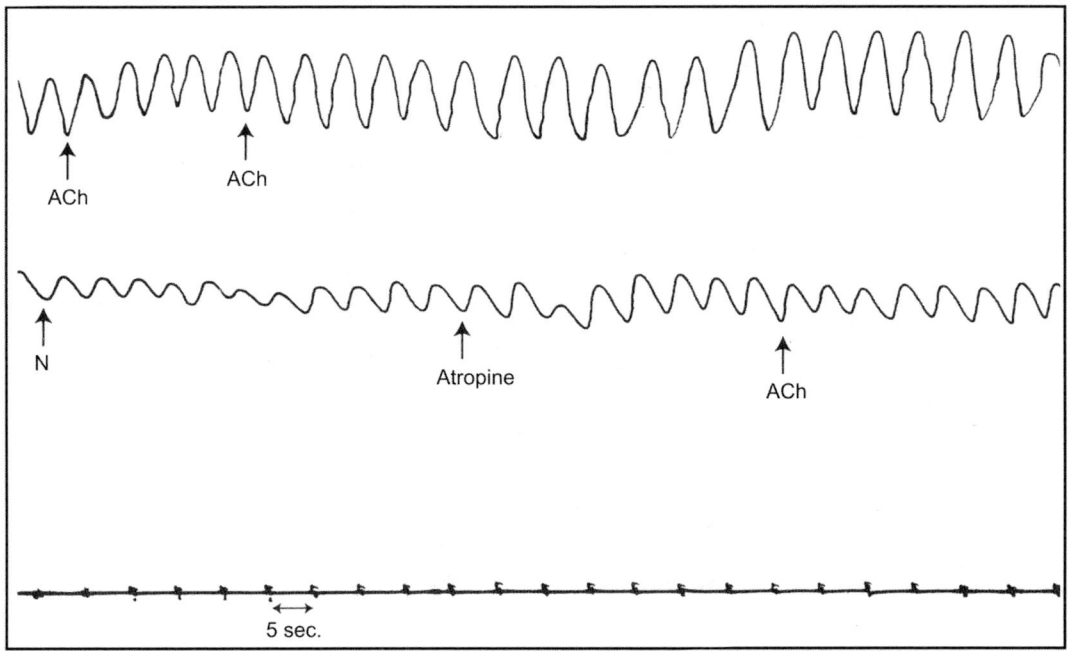

Fig. 4.2.2: Effect of acetylcholine on intestinal movement of isolated rabbit's intestine.

solution of calcium chloride (Fig. 4.2.3), 0.01% solution of histamine and 0.01% solution of adrenaline, i.e. 1:10,000 (Fig. 4.2.4).

Effect of Various Drugs

Acetylcholine: It is responsible for increase in frequency and amplitude (tone) of contraction. It is because of increase in permeability of Na^+ and Ca^{++} leading to influx of these ions. It acts through the cholinergic (muscarinic) receptors that can be blocked by atropine.

Barium chloride: It is responsible for increase in amplitude of contraction (tone). This is not through the receptors rather it is having the direct effect on smooth muscles. This effect cannot be blocked by atropine.

Calcium chloride: It increases the amplitude of contraction.

Histamine: It increases the frequency of contractions. It is having direct stimulatory effect on smooth muscles. It also facilitates the action of acetylcholine.

Adrenaline: It decreases the frequency of contractions and tone of the smooth muscles. It causes hyperpolarization of the membrane and decreases the frequency of spike potential. Through

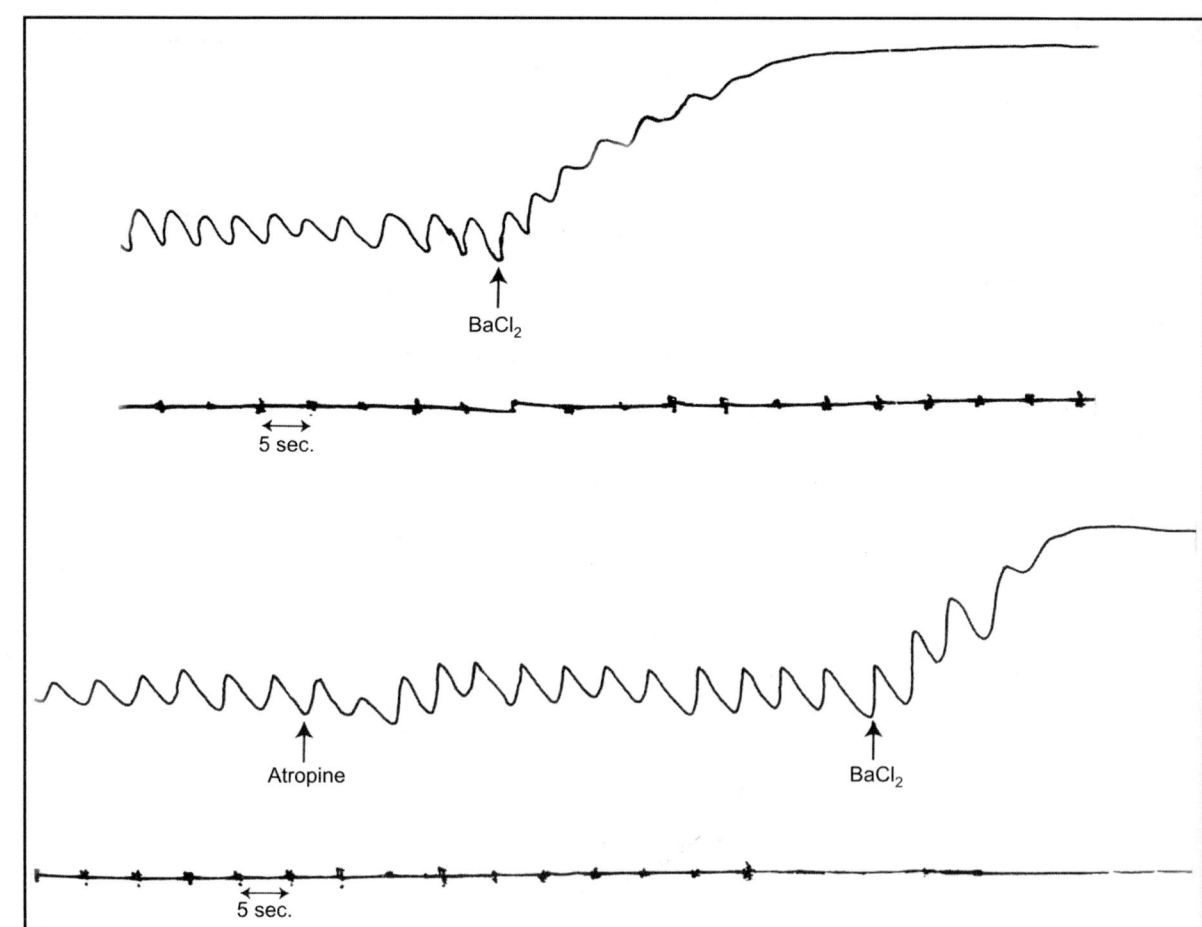

Fig. 4.2.3: Effect of barium chloride on intestinal movements of isolated rabbit's intestine.

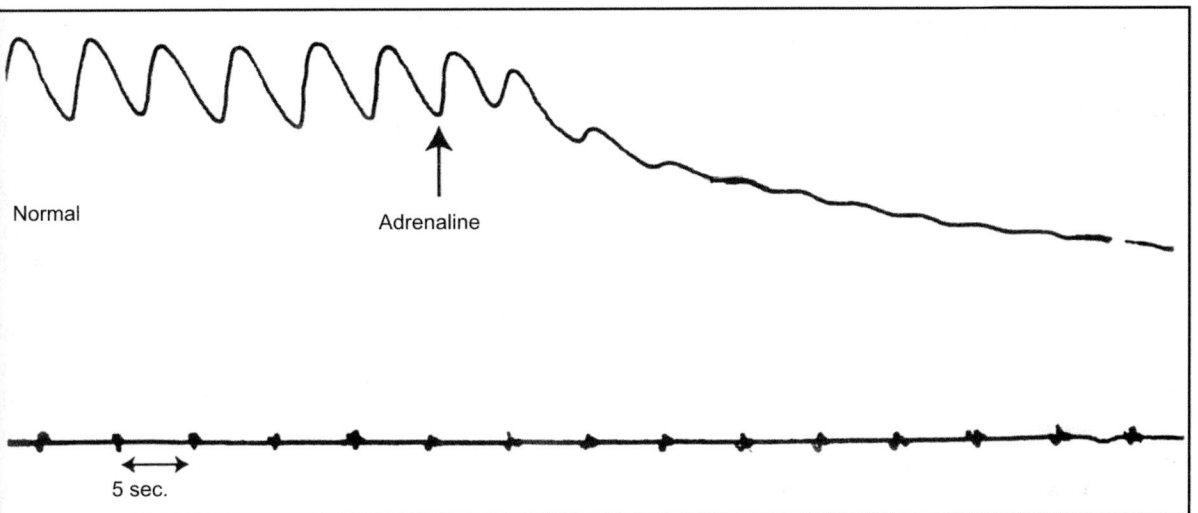

Normal

Adrenaline

5 sec.

Fig. 4.2.4: Effect of adrenaline on intestinal movements of isolated rabbit's intestine.

alpha receptors it leads to calcium efflux and decreases the force of contraction.

PRECAUTIONS

1. Temperature should be maintained at 37 °C.
2. Effect of excitatory drugs should be studied first.
3. After studying the effect of one drug, piece of intestine should be washed properly by rinsing the vessel.
4. Oxygenation of tyrode solution should done continuously.

QUESTIONS

1. What is the composition of tyrode solution?
2. What are the functions of various ingredients of tyrode solution?

3. What are the differences between the actions of acetylcholine and barium chloride?
4. What are the effects of adrenaline on intestinal movements?
5. What is the effect of histamine on intestinal movements and what is its mechanism action?
6. What is the effect of calcium chloride on intestinal movements?
7. What is the effect of barium chloride on intestinal movements?
8. What is the capacity of central glass tube (vessel)?
9. Why we add the extra plasticin towards writing side of frontal writing lever?
10. What are the various different types of intestinal movements?
11. Why the thread is tied at other end of the piece of intestine diagonal to the first one?

EXPERIMENT 4.3

To measure the blood volume of a rabbit by dye dilution method

APPARATUS

Evans blue dye, photocalorimeter, heparin, Wintrobe's tube, intravenous catheters, hypodermic syringe and needles (gauze number 26), test tubes, tracheostomy tube, and nembutal.

Principle

The plasma volume is estimated by dye dilution method and with the help of haematocrit (PCV) total blood volume is calculated.

The known quantity of Evans blue (T-1824) dye is injected, which combines with albumin in the plasma, after ten minutes a blood sample is taken and concentration of dye in the plasma is measured.

Plasma volume is calculated as follows.

$$\text{Plasma volume} = \frac{\text{Total dye injected}}{\text{Concentration of dye in plasma after ten minutes}}$$

$$\text{Blood volume} = \text{Plasma volume} \times \frac{100}{100 - \text{PCV}}$$

Photocalorimeter

It consists of a photocell connected to a galvanometer and a light source (Fig.4.3.1).

Light is passed through solution and it falls on the photocell through the filter. The type of filter used depends on the colour of the solution. For red coloured solution blue filter and for blue coloured solution red filter is used. As light falls on the photocell it leads to deflection in the galvanometer and it gives the optical density of the solution.

Concentration of the dye can be calculated with the help of optical density of the plasma containing dye (ODT), concentration of dye in standard solution (Conc.S) and optical density of standard solution (ODS) as follows.

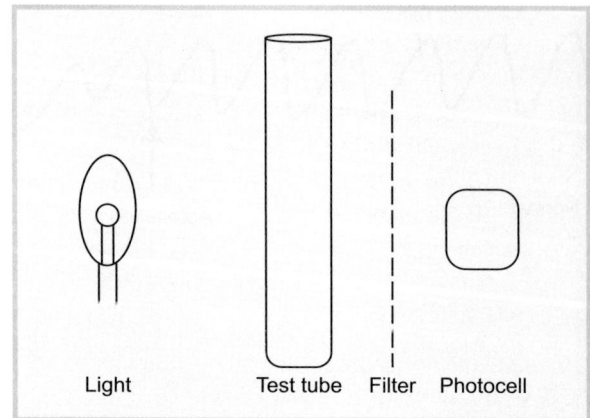

Light   Test tube   Filter   Photocell

Fig. 4.3.1: Basic diagram of photocalorimeter.

Concentration of dye in test solution (plasma)

$$= \frac{\text{ODS}}{\text{ODS}} \times \text{Conc. S}$$

Evans Blue (T–1824) Dye

It is nontoxic dye and dose not attach to any cell of the blood. It combines with albumin in the blood, very slowly leaks in extracellular fluid and slowly excreted by the kidneys.

PROCEDURE

Give nembutal (phenobarbitone) intravenously (40 mg per kg body weight) through the pinna vein with gauze 26 hypodermic needle or chloralose intraperitonialy (30 mg per kg body weight). Make sure that corneal reflex is absent. After anaesthetizing the animal, do the tracheostomy.

Introduce two catheters, one on each side of both the femoral veins after proper surgery. Take about 4 to 5 ml of blood in heparinised syringe. Fill the Wintrobe's tube with the blood and rest of the blood is transferred into the test tube. Both the blood samples are centrifuged at 3000 rmp for 30 minutes. Note down the PCV from the Wintrobe's tube. Separate out the plasma from the test tube and utilise it for two purposes, one to calibrate the photocalorimeter (blank solution) and other to prepare standard solution of the dye.

Inject 1.2 mg of dye (in 1 ml DW) through the femoral vein of one side and collect about four ml of blood sample after ten minutes of injection of the dye from the opposite vein. Centrifuge the blood and separate out the plasma (test solution).

Measure the optical density of standard solution (ODS) and of test solution (ODT) on photo-calorimeter.

CALCULATIONS

Calculate the concentration of the dye in the plasma (test solution) with the help of the formula given above.

Calculate the plasma volume as follows.

Plasma volume of the rabbit

$$= \frac{\text{Amount of the dye injected}}{\text{Concentration of the dye in plasma}}$$

Blood volume of the rabbit

$$= \text{Plasma volume of rabbit} \times \frac{100}{100 - \text{PCV}}$$

PRECAUTIONS

1. Overdose of anaesthesia must be avoided.
2. Standard solution should be made very accurately.

Factors Affecting Blood Volume

Normal blood volume in a rabbit is about 80 ml/kg body weight.

1. Dehydration.
2. Haemorrhage.
3. Burns.
4. Vomiting and diarrhoea.

QUESTIONS

1. How much is the blood volume in rabbit?
2. What are the various factors effecting the blood volume?
3. Why Evans blue dye is used to measure the blood volume?

EXPERIMENT 4.4

Recording of blood pressure and respiration in dog / rabbit and study the effect of various drugs on it

APPARATUS

Multichannel polyrite or student's physiograph with pressure transducer, thermistor (temperature transducer), sphygmomanometer with water sealed bottle for calibration of polyrite, surgical instruments, tracheostomy tube, artificial respirator, nembutal (pentobarbitone) solution, heparin, thread, arterial and venous catheter, three-way cannula, hypodermic syringes and solution of adrenaline, noradrenaline, acetylcholine, atropine.

PROCEDURE

A. Anaesthesia

There are so many anaesthetic agents, which can be given to the animal. These are barbiturates (pentobarbitone, phenobarbitone, barbitone), chloralose, urethane and paraldehyde. Prepare about 20 ml solution of nembutal of strength 30 mg/ml by dissolving it in distilled water.

Weigh the dog and give a dose of pentobarbitone 6% aqueous solution (nembutal 30 mg/kg body weight) intravenously slowly (ideally nembutal is dissolved in 10 % alcohol).

Phenobarbitone (80 mg/kg 10% aqueous solution i.v.) or barbitone sodium or chloralose (0.5–1.5 g/kg i.v. 25% aqueous solution or 37% aq. solution i.p.) can be given to rabbit. Ketamine 2 mg/kg i.v. can also be used (human dose) as an anaesthetic in rabbit.

There are four stages of anaesthesia.

I. *Stage of analgesia*: Pain dulled but consciousness retained.

II. *Stage of excitement*: Consciousness lost, abolition of controlling centres which leads to subconscious manifestations.

III. *Stage of surgical anaesthesia*: There are four planes in this stage but we are concerned with light and deep surgical anaesthesia. In light surgical anaesthesia respiration is thoracic and regular, pupil fixed and central and not dilated, eyelash reflex absent but corneal reflex is intact. In deep surgical anaesthesia respiration is regular but abdominal, undilated fixed central pupil and corneal reflex is absent. If anaesthesia becomes light animal starts to react with surgeon's manipulation and corneal reflex appears.

IV. *Stage of impending overdose*: Pupil becomes dilated and fixed.

B. Dissection

Hold the tongue with the help of artery forceps to avoid back fall of tongue. Tie the legs of the animal on the experimental table with the help of strings.

Tracheostomy is done by giving an incision in midline about one cm above the suprasternal notch. After cutting the skin and subcutaneous tissue, all the muscles are separated to reach up to trachea. Tracheostomy tube is put in to the trachea after 'T' shaped incision in trachea. Here you have to more careful to avoid the passage of blood in to trachea during giving incision.

After tracheostomy femoral artery and vein are catheterised to record the blood pressure and inject the drug respectively.

Steps for Arterial and Venous Catheterization

Fill the arterial or venous catheter with heparinised saline. Feel the pulsations of femoral artery in the ventromedial aspect of the thigh (area of femoral triangle). Clean this area with normal saline or with 1% antiseptic solution (Savlon). With the help of the thumb push the skin overlying the femoral artery on one side and give a cut parallel to the vessels on the skin to the length of about one and a half inches to two inches. Separate out the connective tissue overlying the vessels and pass two pieces of thread below each vessel separately. Apply the clamps on the femoral vein proximally as well as distally and give a 'V' shaped nick in the vein between two clamps. Apply a knot to the thread already passed below the vein towards distal clamp. Push the tip of the catheter in to the vein through the cut. Push the catheter in the vein for about two to three inches. Apply the knot to the thread placed near the proximal clamp to fix the catheter properly. Now remove the clamps from the vein. Same procedure is repeated for catheterizing the femoral artery. One has to be more careful because blood pressure in the artery is very high as compared to vein.

Arterial catheter must be flushed time and again with heparinised saline to avoid blockage of the catheter because of coagulation of blood.

C. Calibration of Polyrite/Physiograph

After putting the polyrite on, adjust the sensitivity and connect the pressure transducer to a BP apparatus (which is further connected to water sealed bottle) through the three-way cannula. Now the pressure is increased with the help of bulb of the BP apparatus and markings of calibration are taken on polyrite with increase in pressure of 20 mm of Hg each time, till it reaches to 200 mm of Hg. After this the transducer is closed and disconnected from the manometer. This is connected with arterial catheter and knob is turned on to record the blood pressure.

D. Recording of Blood Pressure

Record the normal blood pressure. With the help of the thermal transducer record the respiration (In case of Student's physiograph, blood pressure and respiration are recorded on two different physiographs). Time tracing should also be recorded simultaneously. Speed of the polyrite paper should be 2.5 mm per second.

Inject the different doses (10 mg, 50 mg) of adrenaline and take the record (Fig.4.4.1). Dose in relation to quantity and volume is shown in Table 4.4.1.

Inject the different doses (100 mg, 500 mg) of acetylcholine and take the record (Fig.4.4.2).

Now inject 0.6 mg of atropine and then inject acetylcholine and take the record (Fig.4.4.2).

Effects of Various Drugs

Adrenaline

It increases the systolic as well as diastolic blood pressure. It is because of its positive inotropic and chronotropic action. Rise in the diastolic pressure is less, leading to increase in pulse pressure. It is not a good vasoconstrictor so rise in diastolic pressure is less. The higher doses of adrenaline cause inhibition of respiration, which is called as adrenaline apnoea.

Noradrenaline

It also increases systolic as well as diastolic blood pressure. It is again because of its positive inotropic and chronotropic action through beta 1 receptors. It is a powerful vasoconstrictor as compared to adrenaline, so the rise is more in diastolic blood pressure and there is no increase in pulse pressure.

Table 4.4.1: Relationship of the quantity of drug with its strength.					
gm / 100 ml	mg / 100 ml	mg / 10 ml	μg / 10 ml	μg/ml	Strength
1	1000	100	1,00,000	10,000	1:100
0.1	100	10	10,000	1000	1:1000
0.01	10	1	1000	100	1:10,000
0.001	1	0.1	100	10	1:1,00,000
0.0001	0.1	0.001	10	1	1:10,00,000

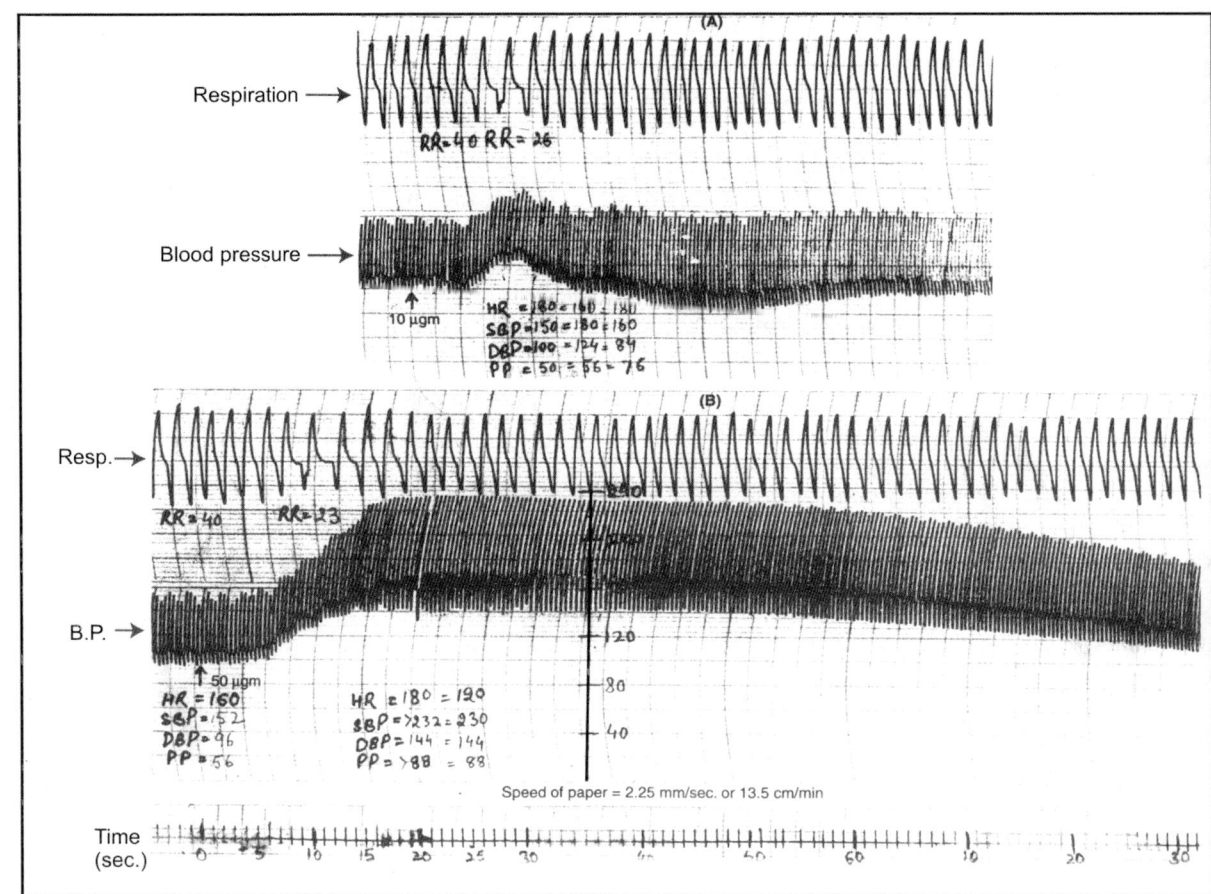

Fig. 4.4.1: Effect of adrenaline on blood pressure and respiration in dog (A: low dose; B: high dose).

Acetylcholine

It leads to decrease in both systolic and diastolic blood pressure. It is because of its negative inotropic and chronotopic action. It also causes vasodilatation and decreases peripheral resistance. Effect of acetylcholine can be abolished by injecting atropine, which is a muscarinic receptor blocking agent.

There is reflex increase in respiratory rate because of marked decrease in blood pressure.

PRECAUTIONS

1. Anaesthesia should be given carefully and must avoid over doses.

2. Flush the arterial and venous catheters with heparinised saline off and on to avoid blocking of the cannula because of blood clot.

3. Do not disturb the sensitivity of polyrite or physiograph once it is calibrated.

4. Keep the respirator ready to tackle the arrest of respiration in emergency.

QUESTIONS

1. What is the effect of adrenaline on blood pressure?

2. Why there is increase in pulse pressure after injection of adrenaline in the animal?

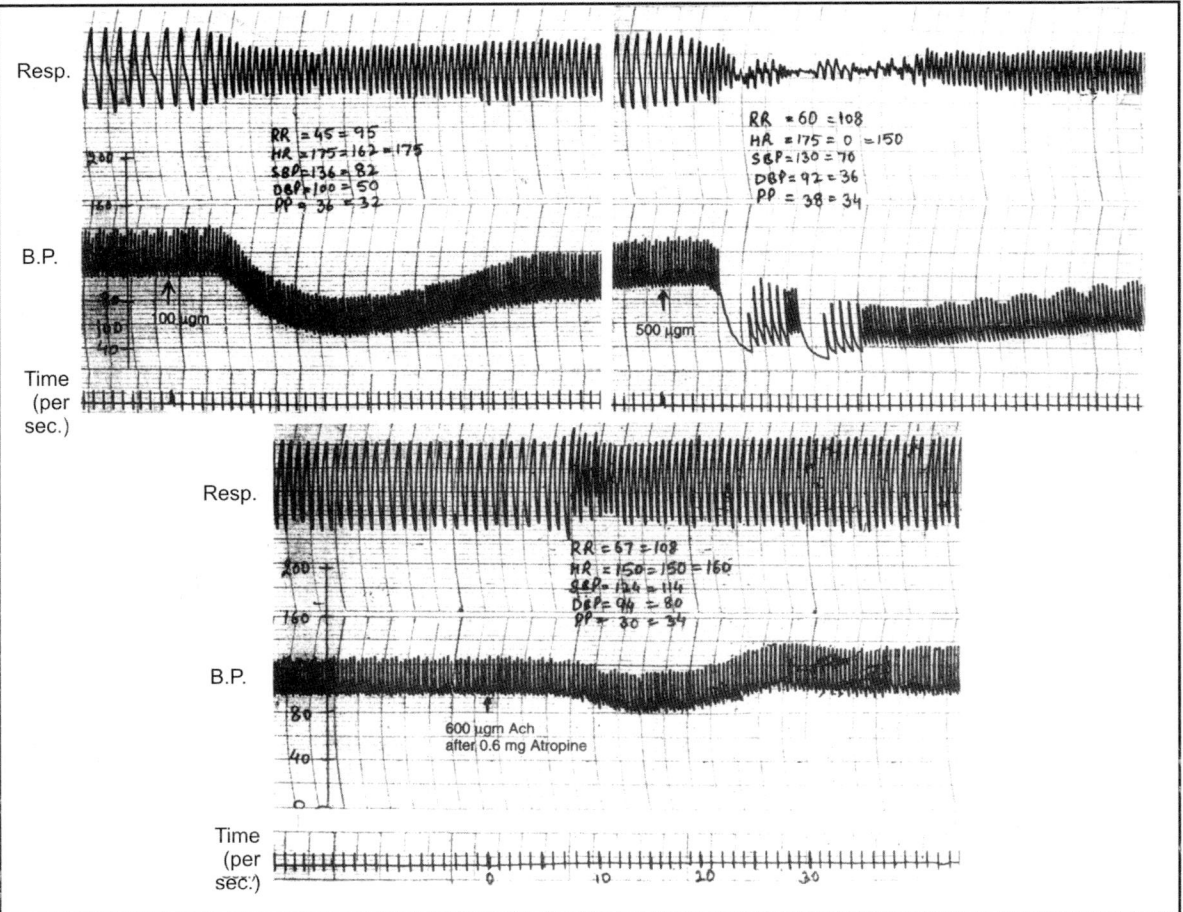

Fig. 4.4.2: Effect of acetylcholine on blood pressure and respiration in dog.

3. What is the difference between adrenaline and noradrenaline as far as blood pressure is concerned?

4. What are the effects of acetylcholine on blood pressure and respiration?

5. Which drug is used to block the effect of acetylcholine and what is its mechanism of action?

6. What is the effect of higher dose of adrenaline on respiration?

EXPERIMENT 4.5

Recording of blood pressure and respiration in dog / rabbit and study the effect of vagus nerve and carotid sinus stimulation

APPARATUS

Multichannel polyrite or student's physiograph with pressure transducer, thermistor, student's stimulator, blood pressure apparatus with water sealed bottle for calibration of physiograph, surgical instruments, tracheostomy tube, three-way cannula, nembutal solution, heparin, thread, arterial and venous catheter, hypodermic syringes.

PROCEDURE

Anaesthetise the dog by giving nembutal intravenously as described in Exp. 4.4.

Insert arterial and venous catheter in femoral artery and vein respectively after performing the tracheostomy.

Identify carotid sheath lying on either side of trachea, feel for carotid pulsations dissect bluntly and expose carotid artery and vagus nerve on both the sides. Pass separate thread around carotid artery and vagus nerve.

Clean the common carotid artery up to its bifurcation and identify carotid sinus at the origin of internal carotid artery taking care that sinus nerve should not get damaged during the dissection.

Put the polyrite or physiographs on and calibrate them at specific sensitivity as described in previous chapter.

Record the normal blood pressure and respiration at 2.5 mm/sec speed (Fig. 4.5.1). Respiration is recorded by putting the thermistor at the one opening of tracheostomy tube.

Now stimulate right and left vagus one by one with stimuli of different frequencies (10 & 20 per sec) and different strengths (10 & 20 volt) (Fig 4.5.1).

Cut the right vagus and stimulate its central and peripheral ends and take the record (Fig 4.5.2).

Stimulate the carotid sinuses mechanically by rolling them between thumb and index finger and take the record (Fig 4.5.3). The sinus may also be stimulated by inflation of venous balloon in the sinus (Fig 4.5.4).

Stimulate the sinuses electrically and take the tracings (Fig 4.5.5).

Study the effect of occlusion of common carotid artery (Fig 4.5.6).

At the end of the practical animal may be sacrificed by giving overdose of anaesthesia.

Effect of Stimulation of Intact Vagus

It causes inhibition of respiration and decrease in blood pressure. With higher frequency and strength of stimulus there will be complete inhibition of heart and respiration. After stoppage of vagal stimulation there is reflex increase in ventilation and increase in blood pressure.

Effect of Stimulation of Central End of Cut Vagus

There will be complete inhibition of respiration and increase in blood pressure. Rise in BP is because of apnoea.

Effect of Stimulation of Peripheral End of Cut Vagus

Because of inhibition of heart it is responsible for decrease in the blood pressure. There may be stimulation of respiration as result of fall in the blood pressure.

Effect of Mechanical Stimulation of Carotid Sinus

It responsible for decrease in the heart rate and blood pressure. There may be stimulation of respiration. Similar effects will be there with electrical stimulation of sinus but the effect are more pronounced.

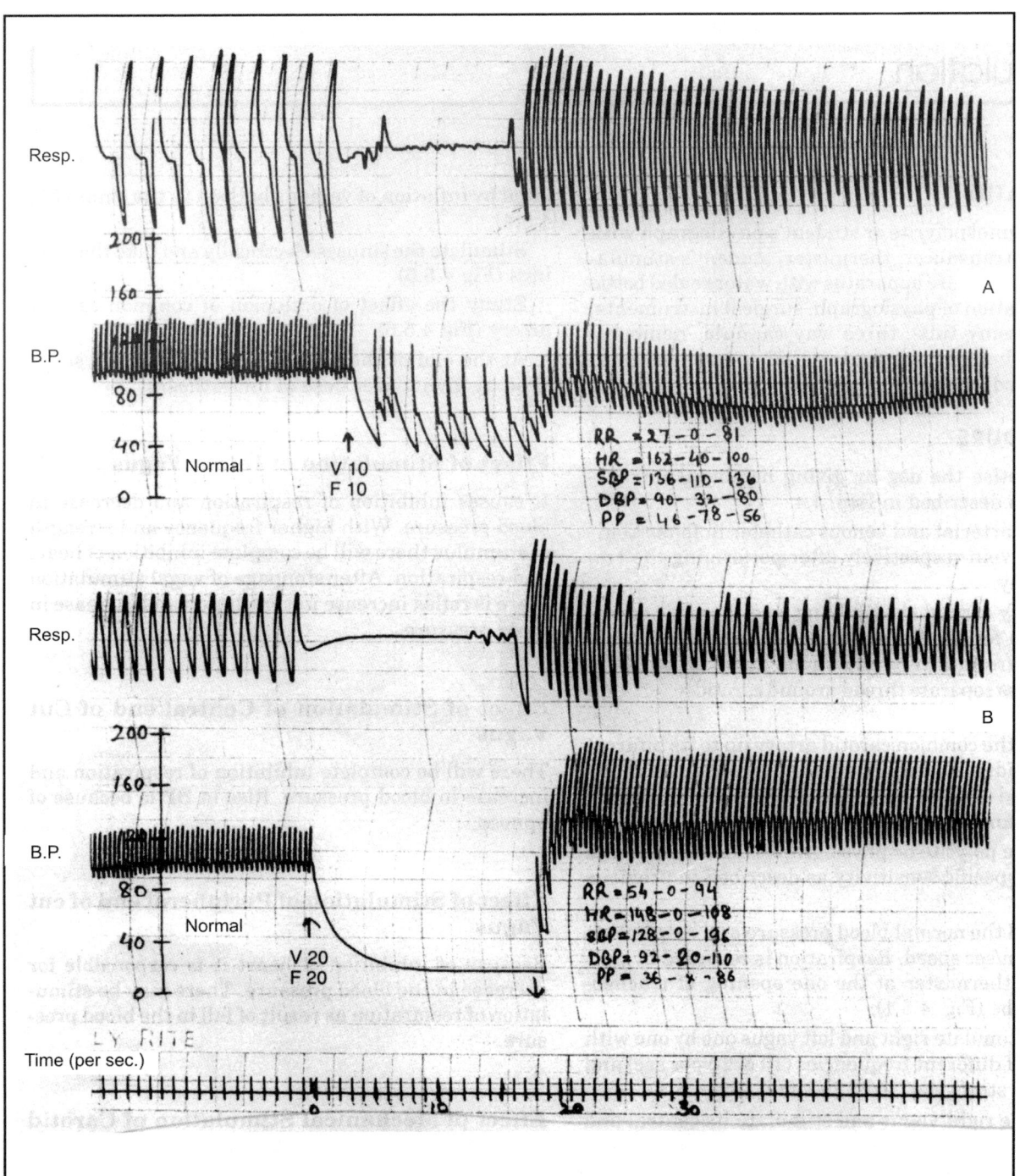

Fig. 4.5.1: Effect of vagus (intact) stimulation on BP and respiration in dog with different strength of stimuli (A 10 volt, 10 cyc/sec, B 20 volt, 20 cycles/sec).

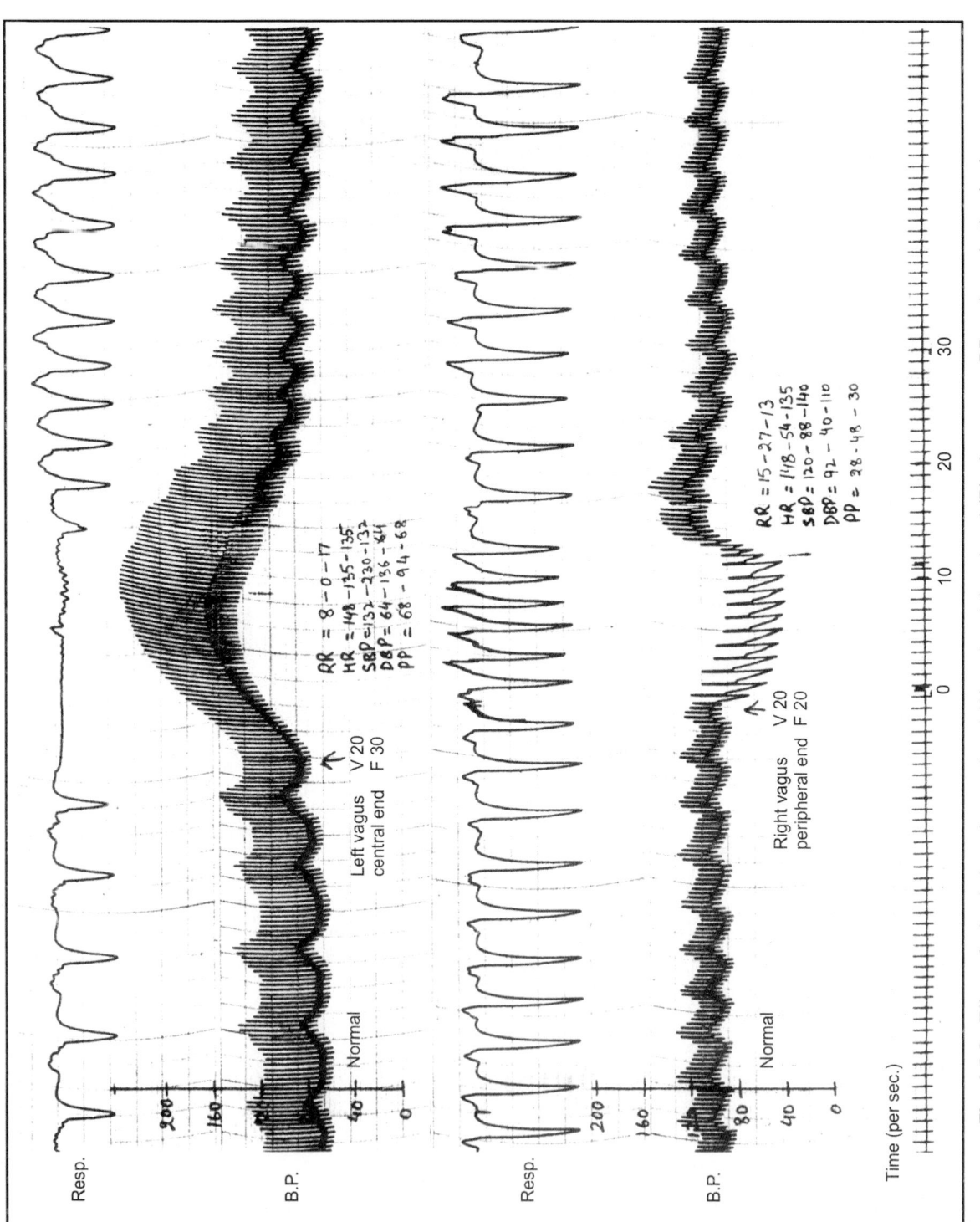

Fig. 4.5.2: Effect of stimulation of central end (A) and peripheral end (B) of vagus on BP and respiration in dog.

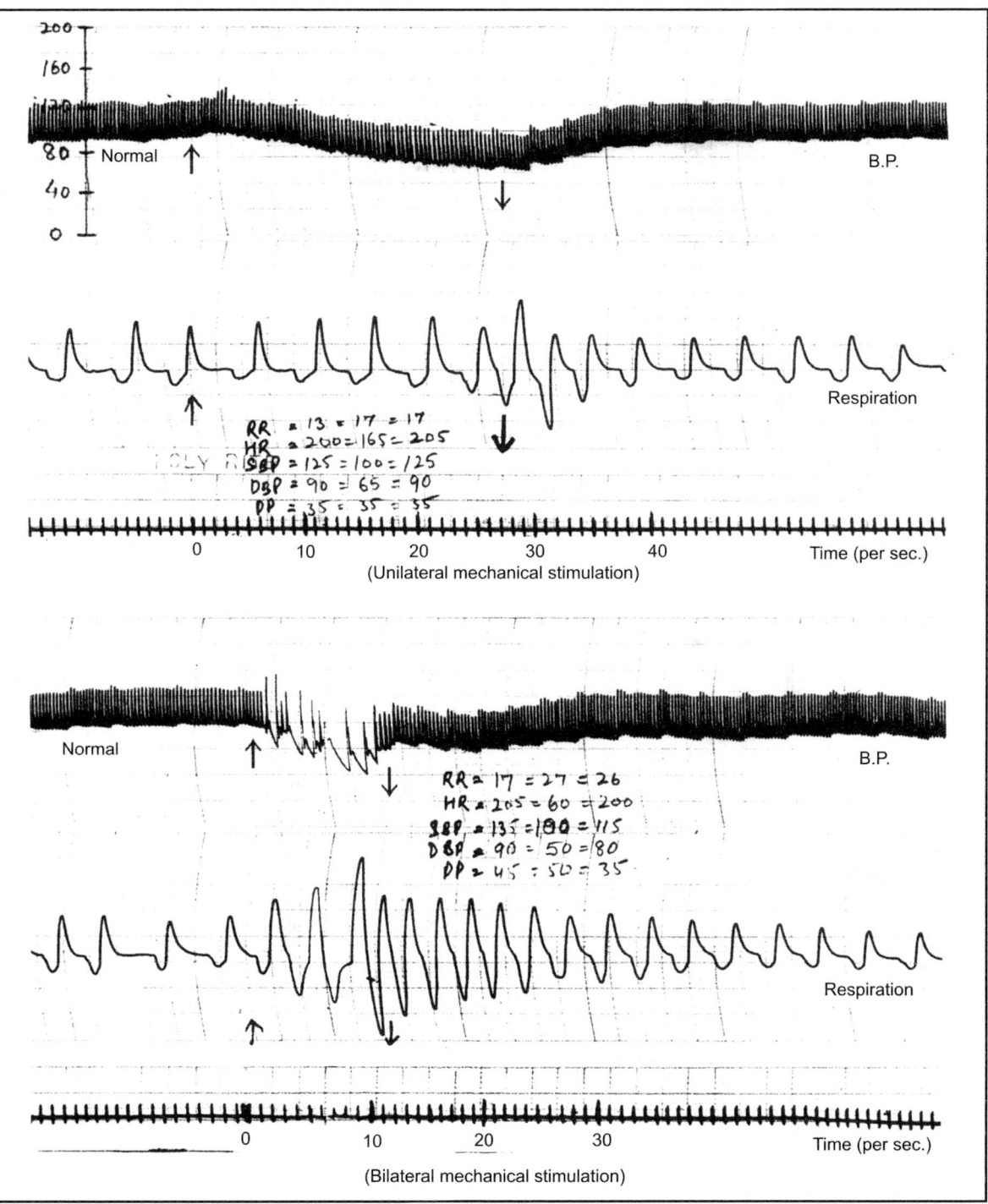

Fig. 4.5.3: Effect of mechanical stimulation (pinching) of carotid sinus on BP and respiration in dog.

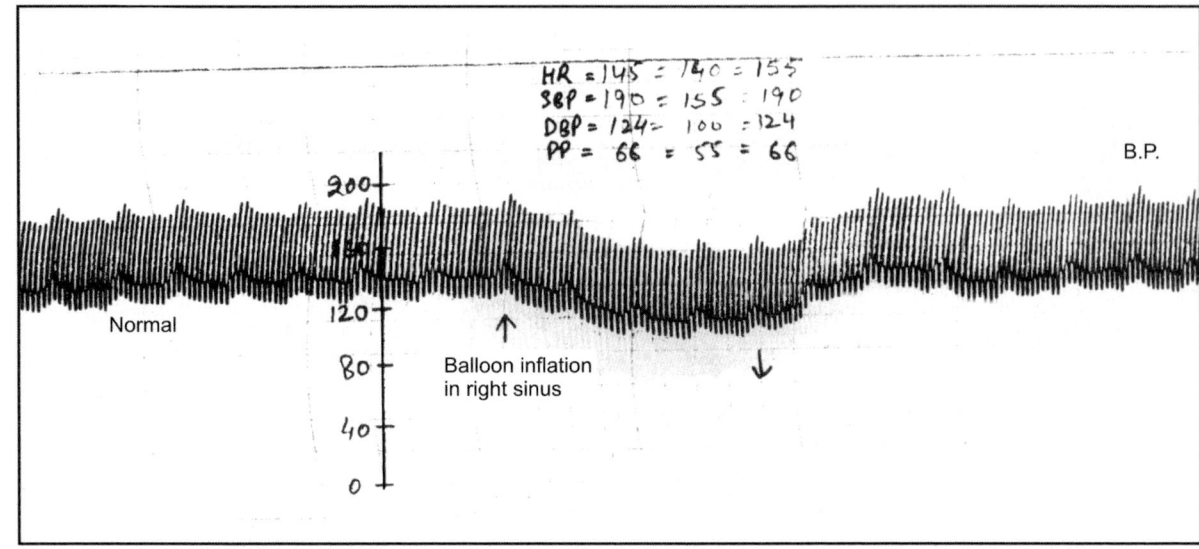

Fig. 4.5.4: Effect of stimulation of sinus by inflation of balloon in the sinus on blood pressure in dog.

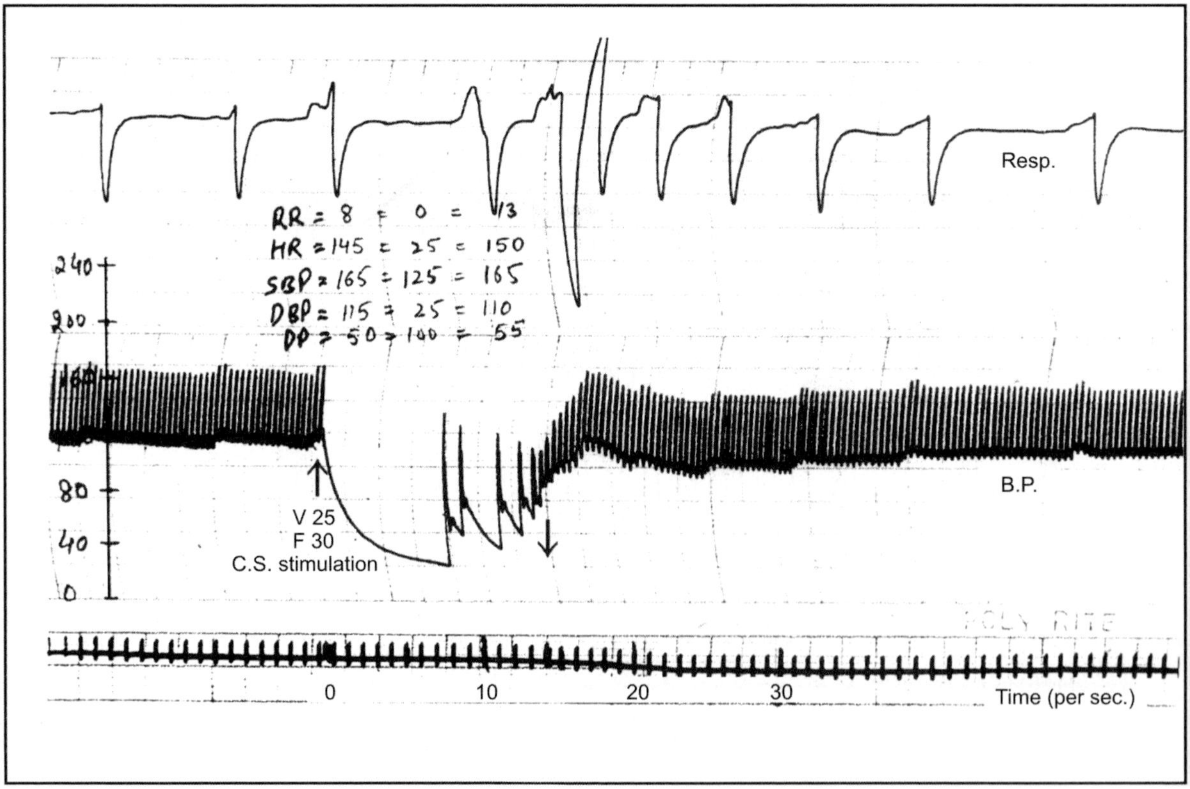

Fig. 4.5.5: Effect of electrical stimulation of carotid sinus on BP and respiration in dog.

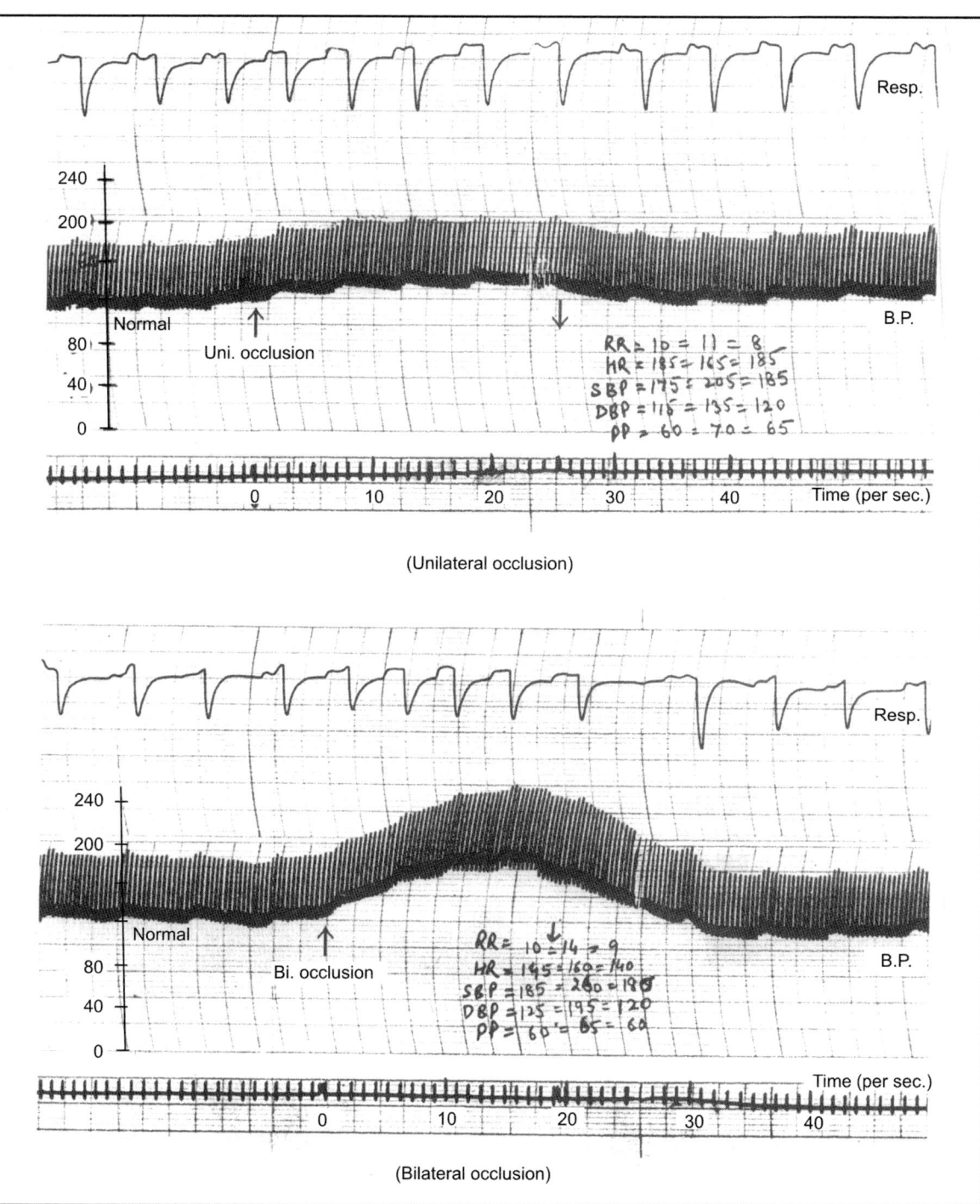

Fig. 4.5.6: Effect of carotid artery occlusion on BP and respiration in dog.

Effects of Occlusion of Common Carotid Arteries

Bilateral occlusion of common carotid arteries is responsible for increase in blood pressure. It is because of decreased discharge from the baroreceptors. There may be slight stimulation of respiration.

PRECAUTIONS

1. Flush the arterial catheter off and on with heparinised saline to avoid blocking of catheter because of blood clot.
2. Should not disturb the sensitivity of physiograph once it is calibrated.
3. Take care that you should not damage the sinus nerve during dissection of carotid sinus.

4. Do not occlude both the carotid arteries for long time. It may lead to death of the animal.
5. Keep the respirator ready to tackle arrest of respiration in emergency.

QUESTIONS

1. What is the effect of stimulation of intact vagus on BP and respiration?
2. What are the differences between stimulation of central and peripheral cut ends of vagus?
3. What are the effects of stimulation of carotid sinus on BP and respiration?
4. What are the effect of occlusion of common carotid arteries on BP and respiration?

EXPERIMENT 4.6

To study the effect of splanchnic nerve stimulation and haemorrhage on blood pressure, respiration and urine formation in dog.

APPARATUS

Four channel polyrite with pressure transducer, thermistor (temperature transducer), sphygmo-manometer with water sealed bottle for calibration of polyrite, surgical instruments, tracheostomy tube, ureteric cannulae, intravenous set, artificial respi-rator, Nembutal (Pentobarbitone) solution, heparin, thread, arterial and venous catheter, three-way cannula, hypodermic syringes and intravenous fluids.

PROCEDURE

A. Anaesthesia

There are so many anaesthetic agents, which can be given to the animal. These are barbiturates (Pentobarbitone, Phenobarbitone, Barbitone), chloralose, urethane and paraldehyde. Prepare about 20 ml solution of Nembutal of strength 30 mg / ml by dissolving it in distilled water.

Weigh the dog and give a dose of Pentobarbitone 6% aqueous solution (Nembutal 30 mg / kg body weight) intravenously slowly (Ideally Nembutal is dissolved in 10 % alcohol).

B. General Dissection

Hold the tongue with the help of artery forceps to avoid the back fall of the tongue. Tie the legs of the animal on the experimental table with the help of strings.

Tracheostomy is done by giving an incision in midline about one cm above the suprasternal notch. After cutting the skin and subcutaneous tissue, all the muscles are separated to reach up to trachea. Tracheostomy tube is put in to the trachea after 'T' shaped incision in trachea. Here you have to more

careful to avoid the passage of blood in to trachea during giving incision. After tracheostomy femoral artery and vein are catheterised to record the blood pressure and inject the drug respectively.

Arterial catheter must be flushed time and again with heparinised saline to avoid blockage of the catheter because of coagulation of blood.

C. Calibration of Polyrite

After putting the polyrite on, adjust the sensitivity and connect the pressure transducer to a BP apparatus (which is further connected to water sealed bottle) through the three-way cannula. Now the pressure is increased with the help of bulb of the BP apparatus and markings of calibration are taken on polyrite with increase in pressure of 20 mm of Hg each time, till it reaches to 200 mm of Hg. After this the transducer is closed and disconnected from the manometer. This is connected with arterial catheter and knob is turned on to record the blood pressure.

D. Dissection for Splanchnic Nerve Exposure

An incision is given in parallel to the right costal margin and various muscles are separated. Right adrenal is exposed then suprarenal vein is confirmed. Now confirm the splanchnic nerve crossing this vein. Clear the nerve carefully and pass a thread around it. It can be further confirmed by stretching the nerve that leads to reflex inhibition of respiration.

E. Dissection for Ureters Catheterisation

Midline incision is given in suprapubic area and muscles are separated out to reach in the abdominal cavity. Identify both the ureters and after giving a nick introduce the catheters in them and tie them properly so that there will not be any leakage of urine.

F. Recording of Various Parameters

Record the normal blood pressure with the help of pressure transducer. With the help of the thermal transducer record the respiration (In case of Students physiograph blood pressure and respiration are recorded on two different physiographs). Time tracing should also be recorded simultaneously. Speed of the polyrite paper should be 2.5 mm per second. Urinary output is recorded with the help of photocell drop by drop. Slow intravenous saline is given with the help of i.v. set and normal saline bottle.

G. Stimulation of Splanchnic Nerve

Stimulate the nerve with threshold strength of stimulus with the help student stimulator and record the effects (Fig. 4.6.1).

H. To Induce Haemorrhage

About 350 ml of blood was drained from the femoral artery into empty i.v. bottle in three stages of 100 ml,100 ml and 150 ml and effects were recorded. To record the Mayer's waves speed of the polyrite was further slowed down. The blood which was

drained, re-infused to see weather the haemorrhagic shock induced was reversible or irreversible.

OBSERVATIONS AND RESULTS

Effect of splanchnic nerve stimulation: This nerve is a sympathetic nerve containing it is because of release of catecholamine from adrenal medulla. There will be complete inhibition preganglionic sympathetic fibres coming from T 5 to T 12 spinal segment. The fibres going to the adrenal medulla are preganglionic because they don't relay in sympathetic ganglion. Two peaks were observed as a rise in blood pressure (Fig 4.6.1). First rise in BP is a direct neural effect because of contraction of splanchnic vessels. Second effect is because of release of catecholamine from the adrenal medulla. Increase in pulse pressure during second peak also indicates the release of adrenaline from adrenal medulla. There is inhibition of respiration during

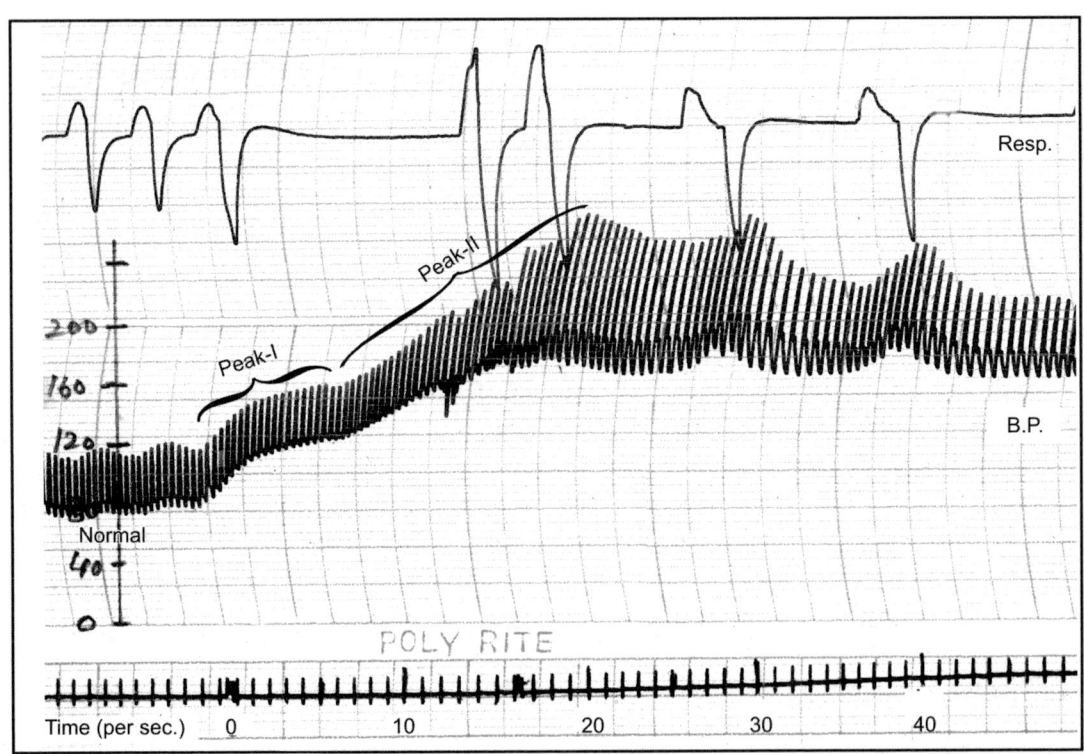

Fig. 4.6.1: Effect of splanchnic nerve stimulation on BP and respiration in anaesthetized dog.

neural response. As this inhibition of respiration is not seen during second phase of increase in BP which shows that it is not adrenergic apnoea.

Effect of haemorrhage: About 350 ml of blood was drained. SBP, DBP and pulse pressure went on decreasing with increase in the loss of blood. Respiratory rate also went on increasing and urinary output was decreased (Fig 4.6.2). *Traube Hering waves* are observed as a normal fluctuation in BP as a result of respiration they are seen even before inducing the haemorrhage.

Mayer waves are observed when there is sufficient fall in BP (Fig 4.6.2). These waves are because of stimulation of chemoreceptors. When BP falls below 90 mmHg baroreceptors loose their function and blood pressure falls further which leads to stimulation of chemoreceptors. Chemoreceptors increase BP as

it approach 80–90 mmHg it causes fall in the BP again and this cycle goes on. The frequency of Mayer wave is about two to three per minute. After recording the effect of haemorrhage the blood is infused back through the vein. In case of reversible shock BP come to its previous level. In case of irreversible shock BP does not rise and animal dies.

QUESTIONS

1. What is shock?
2. What are reversible and irreversible shocks?
3. What are Mayer waves and what is the cause of their production?
4. What happens to BP, respiration and urinary output during haemorrhage?

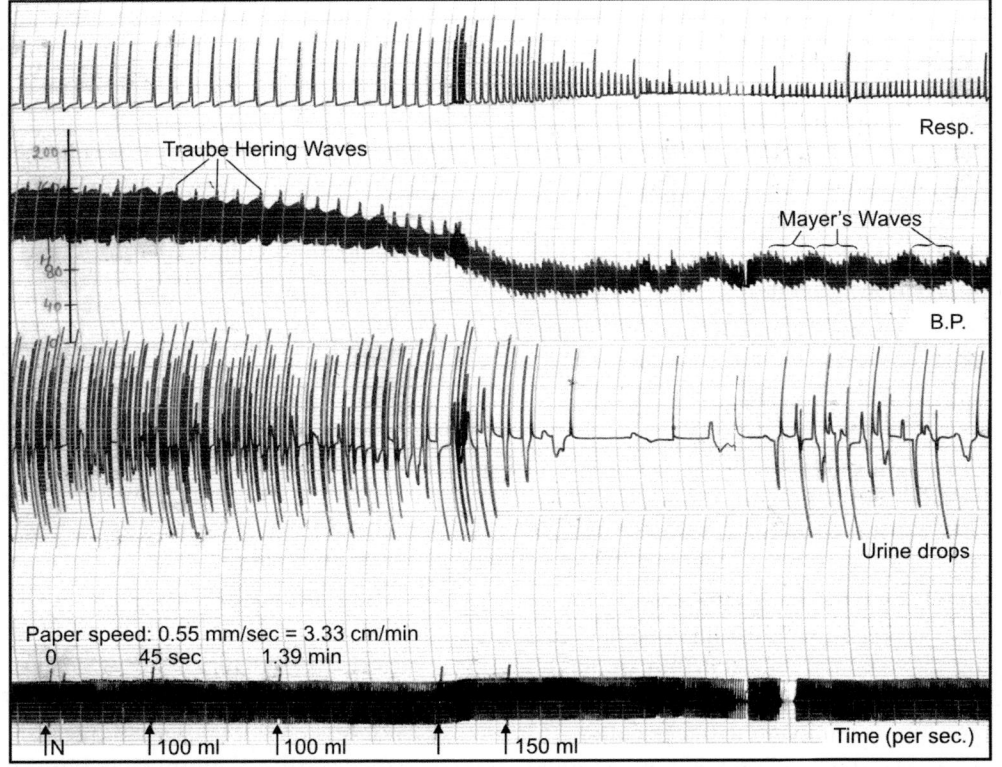

Fig. 4.6.2: Effect of haemorrhage on BP, respiration and urinary output in anaesthetized dog.

EXPERIMENT 4.7

Effect of various chemicals on urine formation in dog.

APPARATUS

Three channel polyrite with pressure transducer, thermistor (temperature transducer), sphygmo-manometer with water sealed bottle for calibration of polyrite, surgical instruments, tracheostomy tube, ureteric cannulae, intravenous set, nembutal (pentobarbitone) solution, heparin, thread, arterial and venous catheter, three way cannula, normal saline, 5% dextrose, 20% dextrose, 20% mannitol, 10% sodium chloride, adrenaline and hypodermic syringes.

PROCEDURE

A. Anaesthesia

There are so many anaesthetic agents, which can be given to the animal. These are barbiturates (pentobarbitone, phenobarbitone, barbitone), chloralose, urethane and paraldehyde. Prepare about 20 ml solution of nembutal of strength 30 mg/ml by dissolving it in distilled water.

Weigh the dog and give a dose of Pentobarbitone 6% aqueous solution (Nembutal 30 mg/kg body weight) intravenously slowly (Ideally nembutal is dissolved in 10 % alcohol).

B. General Dissection

Hold the tongue with the help of artery forceps to avoid the back fall of the tongue. Tie the legs of the animal on the experimental table with the help of strings.

Tracheostomy is done by giving an incision in midline about one cm above the suprasternal notch. After cutting the skin and subcutaneous tissue, all the muscles are separated to reach up to trachea. Tracheostomy tube is put in to the trachea after "T" shaped incision in trachea. Here you have to more careful to avoid the passage of blood in to trachea

during giving incision. After tracheostomy femoral artery and vein are catheterised to record the blood pressure and inject the drug respectively.

Arterial catheter must be flushed time and again with heparinised saline to avoid blockage of the catheter because of coagulation of blood.

C. Dissection for Ureters Catheterization

Midline incision is given in suprapubic area and muscles are separated out to reach in the abdominal cavity. Identify both the ureters and after giving a nick introduce the catheters in them and tie them properly so that there will not be any leakage of urine.

D. Calibration of Polyrite

After putting the polyrite on, adjust the sensitivity and connect the pressure transducer to a BP apparatus (which is further connected to water sealed bottle) through the three-way cannula. Now the pressure is increased with the help of bulb of the BP apparatus and markings of calibration are taken on polyrite with increase in pressure of 20 mm of Hg each time, till it reaches to 200 mm of Hg. After this the transducer is closed and disconnected from the manometer. This is connected with arterial catheter and knob is turned on to record the blood pressure.

E. Recording of the Effects of Various Chemicals

1. **Normal saline:** Normal record is taken of BP and urinary output at slow speed of the polyrite (2 mm per second). Now 100 ml of normal saline is infused within a minute and the effect is recorded (Fig 4.7.1).

2. **Effect of 5% Dextrose:** 100 ml of 5% dextrose is infused with in a minute and the effect is recorded. Dextrose acts as a diuretic in two ways: one as an osmotic diuretic and second as a forced diuretic (Fig 4.7.2).

3. **Effect of 10% Sodium chloride:** 5 ml of 10% Sodium chloride solution injected through the

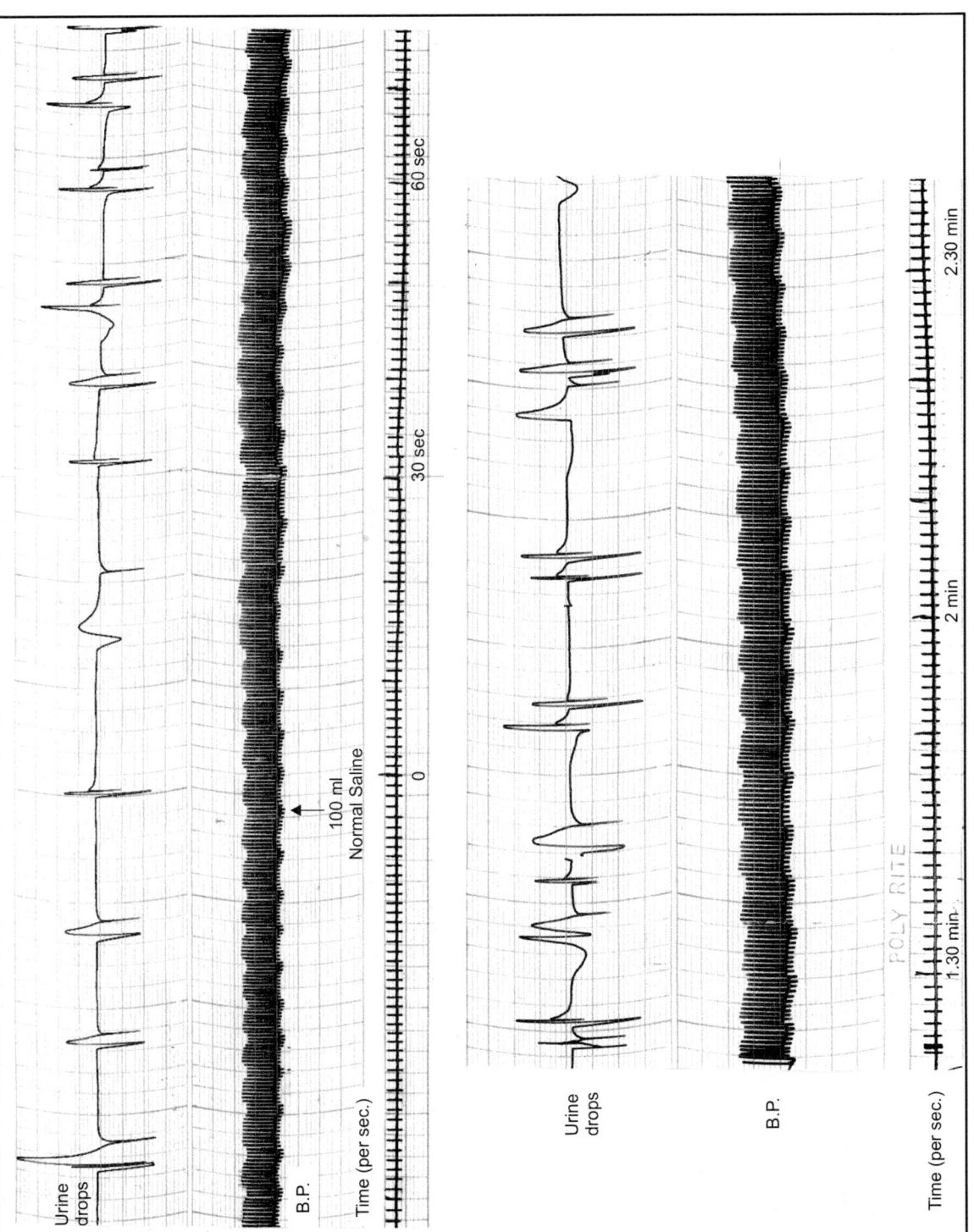

Fig. 4.7.1: Effect infusion of 100 ml normal saline on urinary output in anaesthetized dog.

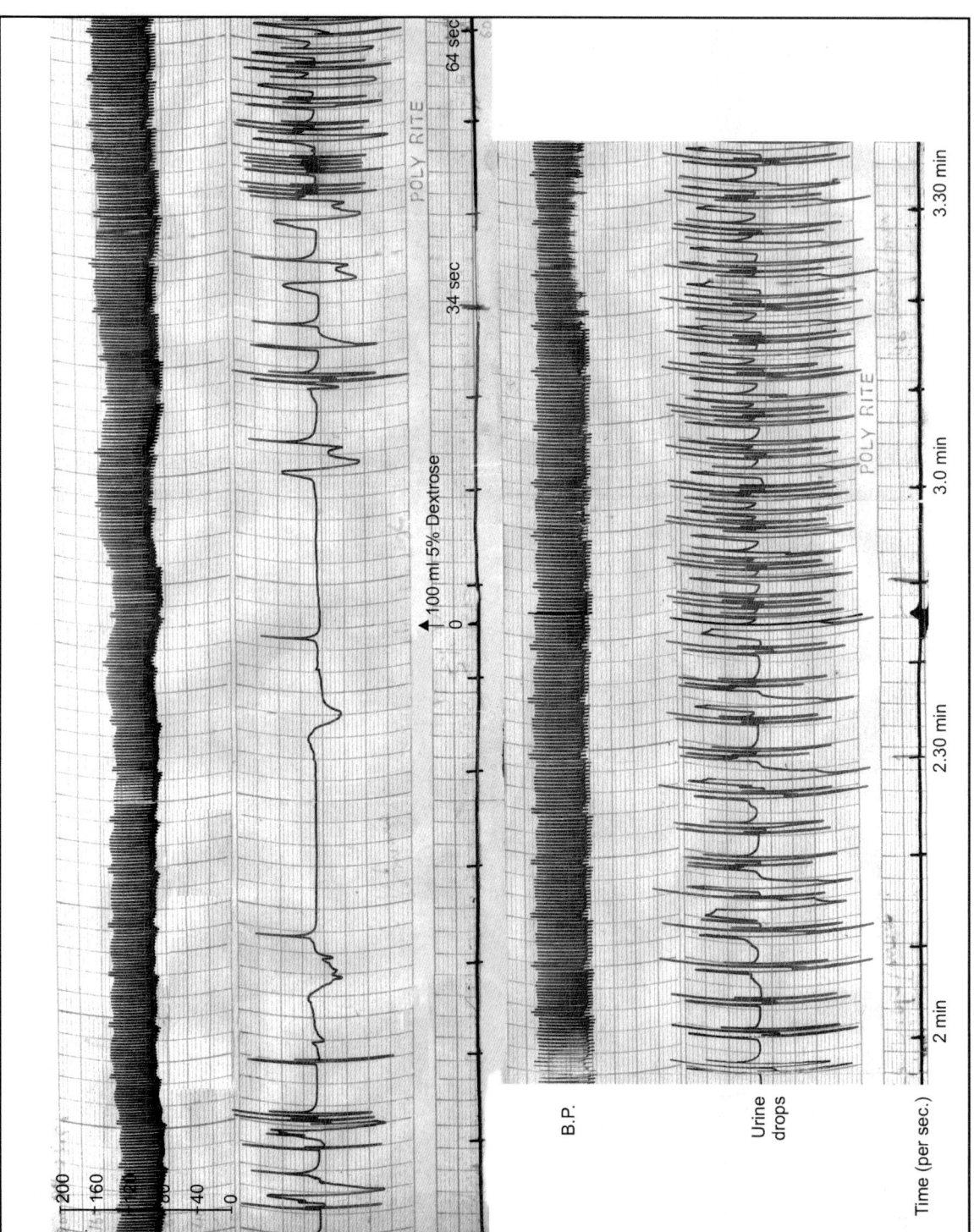

Fig. 4.7.2: Effect of 100 ml 5% Dextrose infusion on urinary output and BP in anaesthetized dog.

venous catheter and its effect is recorded. It acts as an osmotic diuretic. Fall in the BP is because of local vasodilator effect on smooth muscle fibres of blood vessels (Fig 4.7.3).

4. **Effect of 10% Sodium sulphate:** 5 ml 10% solution of sodium sulphate is given through venous catheter and the effects are recorded. It acts as an osmotic diuretic and causes increase urinary output (Fig 4.7.4).

5. **Effect of 20% Dextrose:** 5 ml of 20% dextrose solution is injected through the venous catheter and effects are recorded. It acts as an osmotic diuretic and causes increase in urinary output (Fig 4.7.5).

6. **Effect of 20% Mannitol:** 5 ml of 20% mannitol solution is injected through the venous catheter and effects are recorded. It is a potent osmotic diuretic and causes increase in urinary output.

7. **Effect of adrenaline:** Inject 1 ml 1:10000 adrenaline solution through venous cannula and record its effect. It causes decrease in urine formation in spite of marked increase in blood pressure (Fig 4.7.6). Catecholamines have vasoconstrictor effect on inter lobular arteries and afferent arterioles so the blood flow to the kidneys is markedly decreased. Norepinephrine has more potent effect as compared to epinephrine. Angiotensin II causes mainly constriction of efferent arteriole and leads to increase in renal blood flow.

F. Effect of Vagus Nerve Stimulation

Stimulate the vagus nerve and record the effects. It will lead to decrease in urinary output as a result of decrease in blood flow to the kidneys (Fig 4.7.7).

G. Effect of Splanchnic Nerve Stimulation

Stimulate the splanchnic nerve and record the effects. Stimulation of splanchnic nerve causes renal vasoconstriction leading to marked reduction in urinary output (Fig 4.7.8).

REFERENCE BOOKS

1. Experimental Physiology for medical students by DT Harris, HP Gilding, and WAM Smart. 6th Edition, 1963. London J & A Churchill Ltd.

2. Fundamental of Experimental Pharmacology by MN Ghosh, 1971.

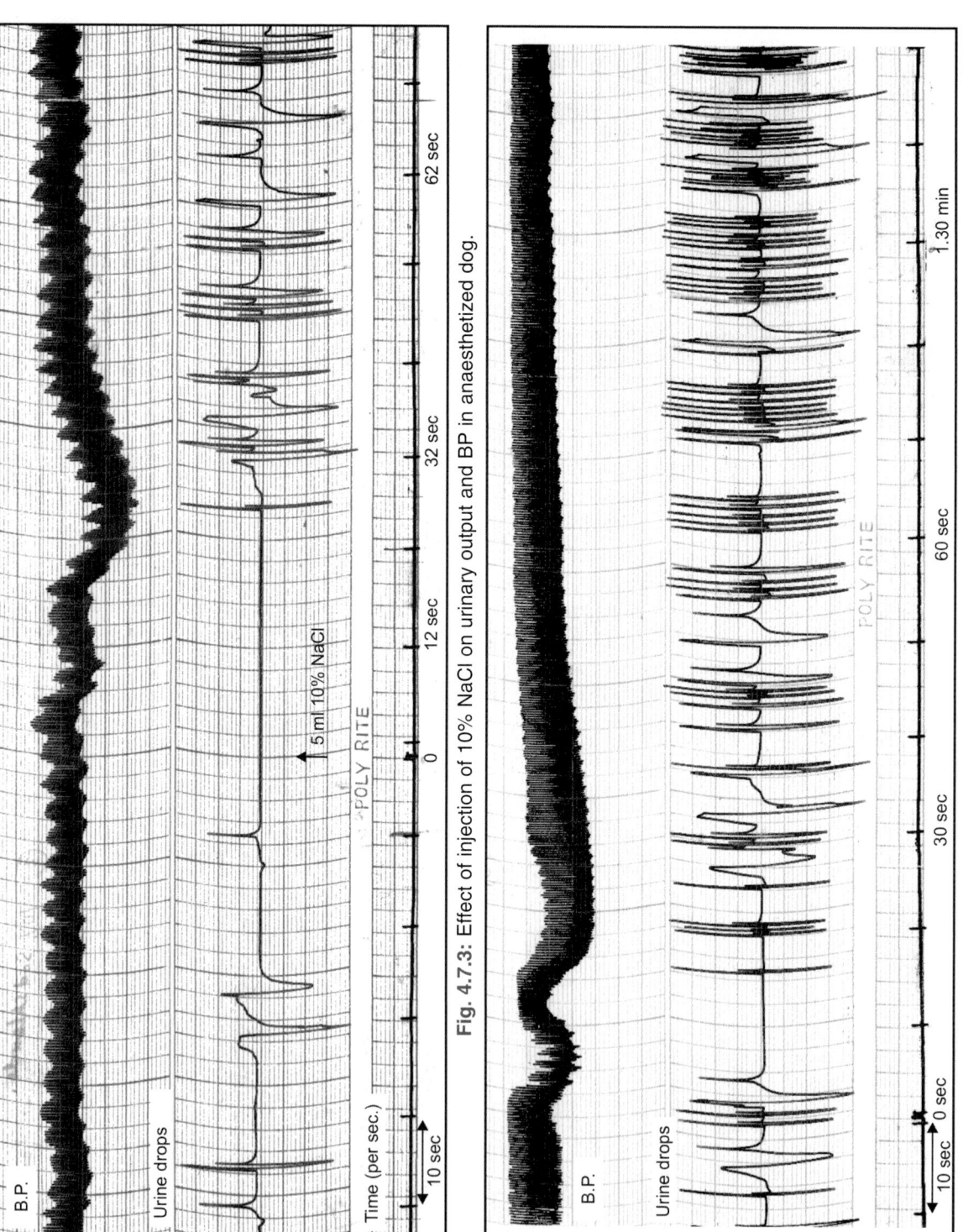

Fig. 4.7.3: Effect of injection of 10% NaCl on urinary output and BP in anaesthetized dog.

Fig. 4.7.4: Effect infusion of 5 ml 10% Na_2SO_4 on urinary output and BP in anaesthetized dog.

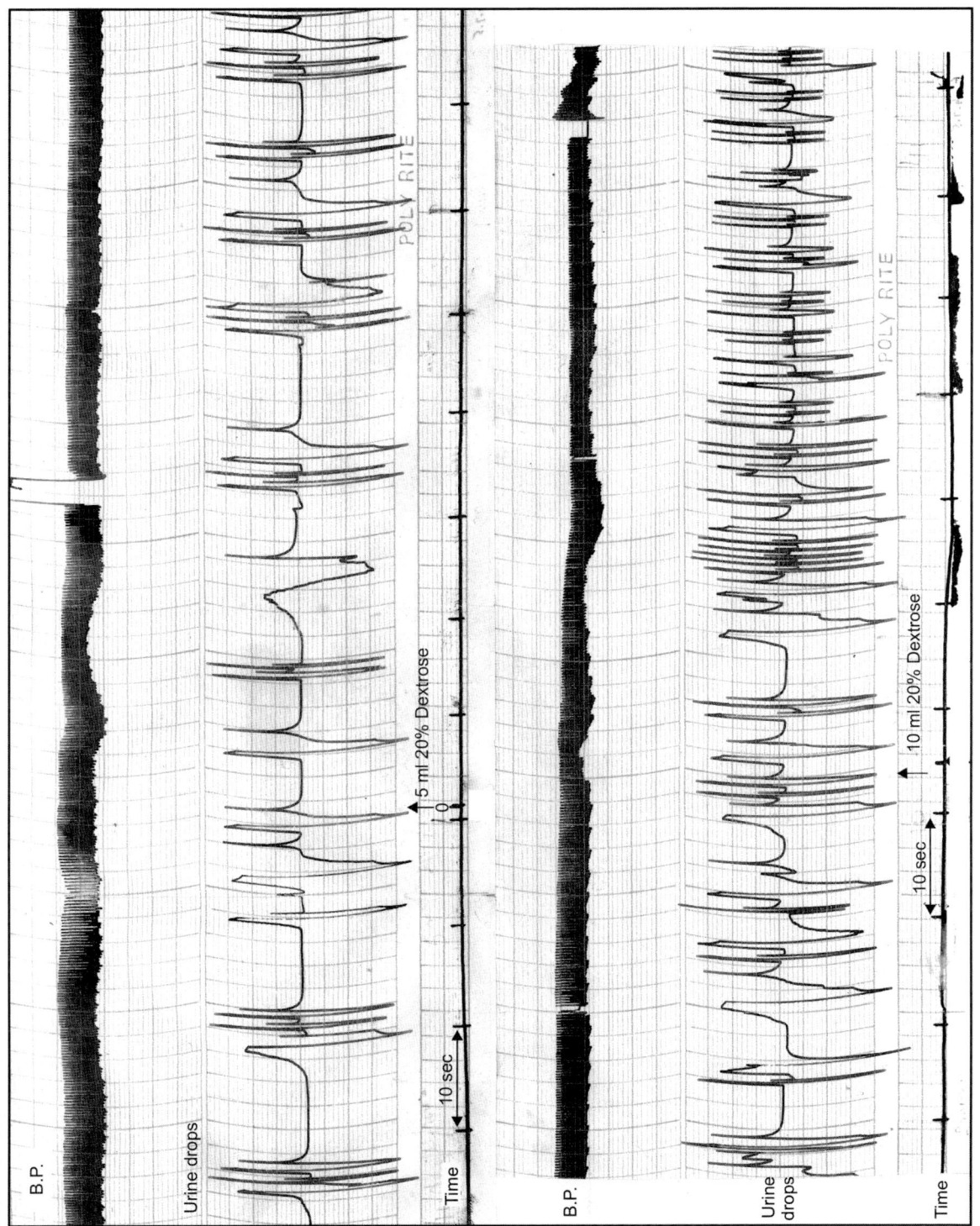

Fig. 4.7.5: Effect of 5 ml and 10 ml 20% Dextrose on injection urinary output and BP in anaesthetized dog.

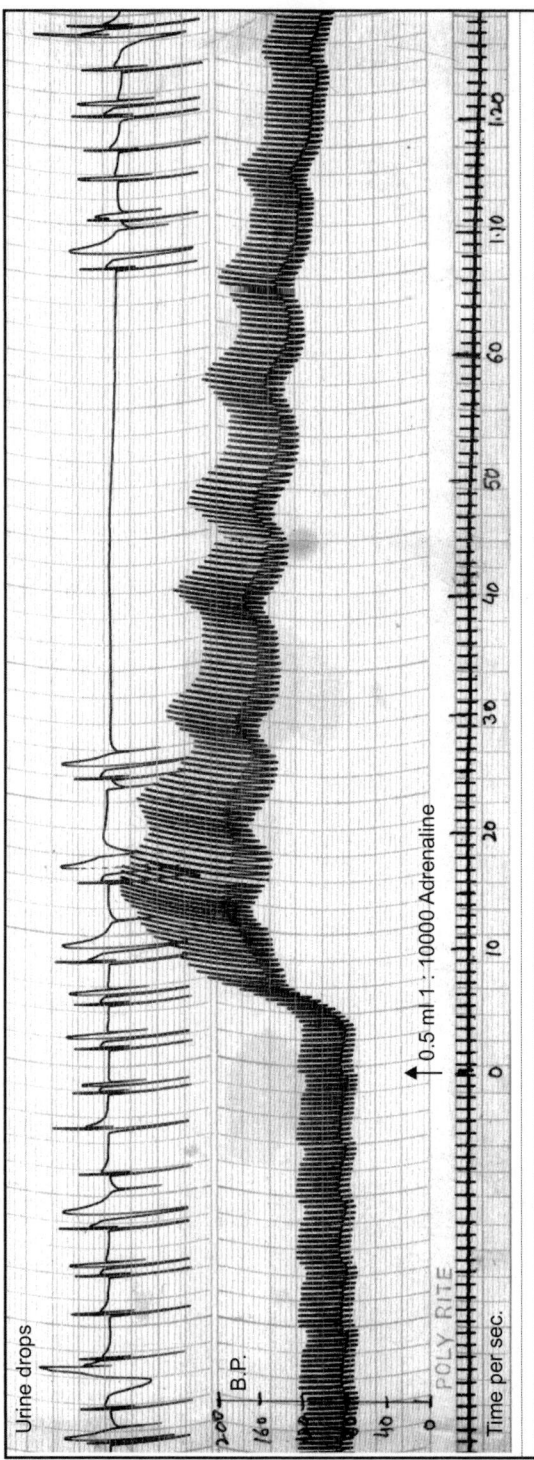

Urine drops

B.P.

0.5 ml 1 : 10000 Adrenaline

Time per sec.

POLY RITE

Fig. 4.7.6: Effect of Adrenaline on BP and urine output in anaesthetized dog.

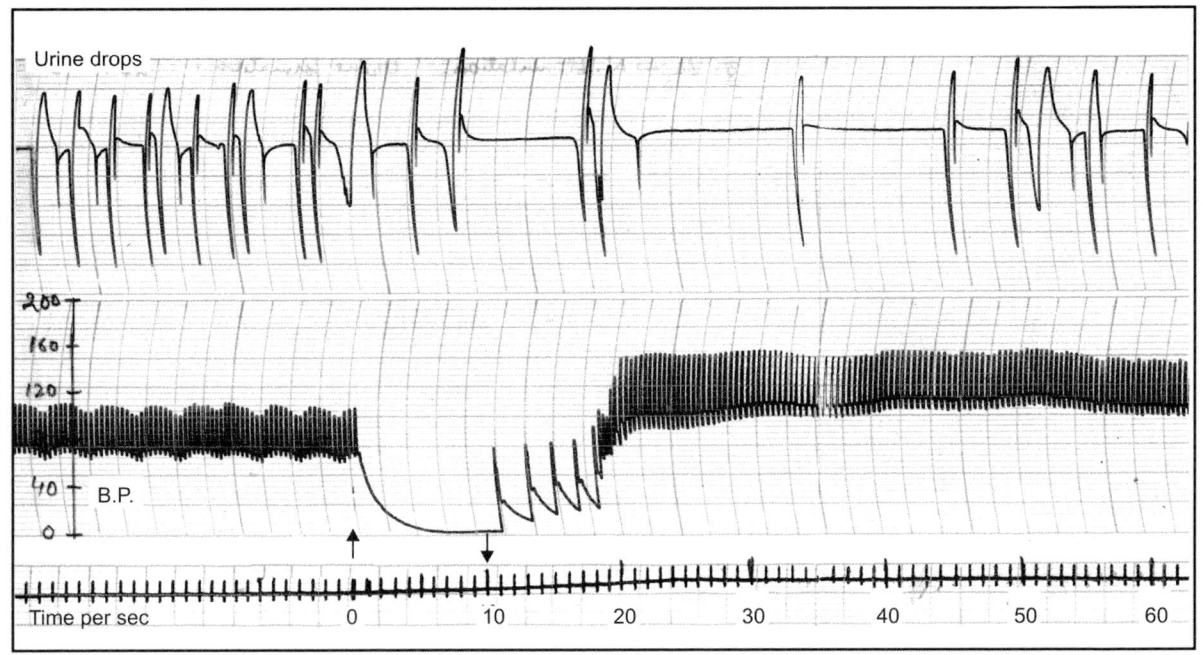

Fig. 4.7.7: Effect of vagus stimulation on BP and urine output in anaesthetized dog.

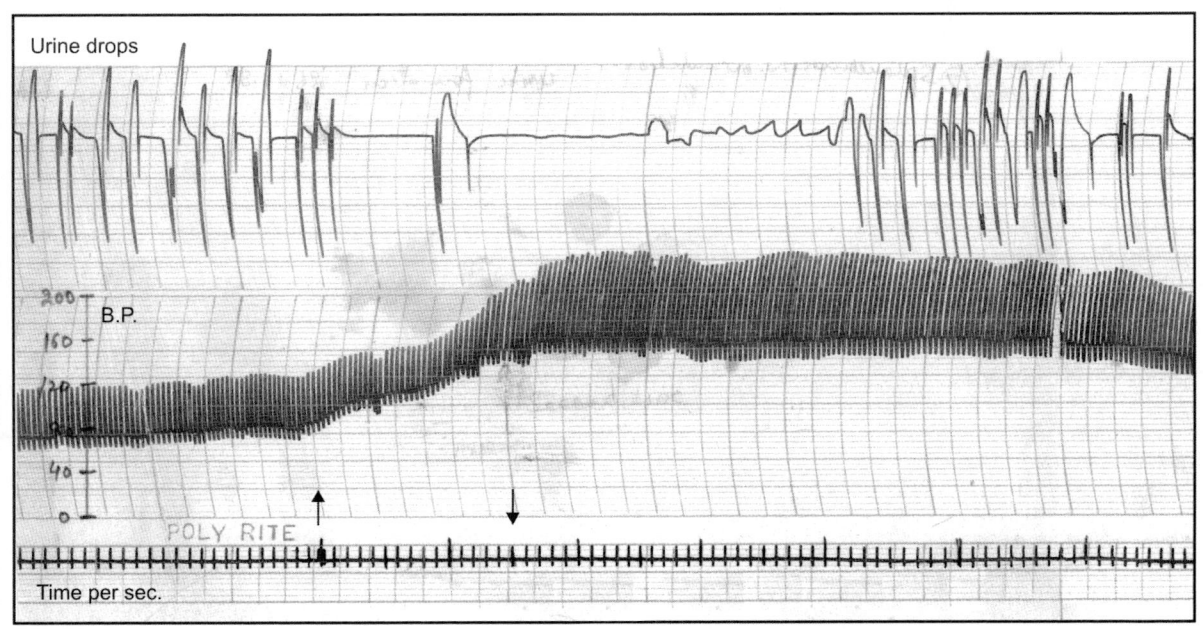

Fig. 4.7.8: Effect of splanchnic nerve stimulation on BP and urinary output in anaesthelized dog.

Index